101 REASONS WHY I'M A VEGETARIAN

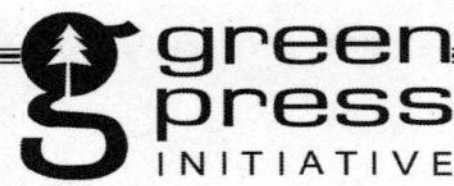

Lantern Books has elected to print this title on Rolland Enviro Natural a 100% post-consumer recycled paper, processed chlorine-free. As a result, we have saved the following resources:

15 Trees (40' tall and 6-8" diameter)
6,147 Gallons of Wastewater
2,472 Kilowatt Hours of Electricity
678 Pounds of Solid Waste
1,331 Pounds of Greenhouse Gases

As part of Lantern Books' commitment to the environment we have joined the Green Press Initiative, a nonprofit organization supporting publishers in using fiber that is not sourced from ancient or endangered forests. We hope that you, the reader, will support Lantern and the Green Press Initiative in our endeavor to preserve the ancient forests and the natural systems on which all life depends. One way is to buy books that cost a little more but make a positive commitment to the environment not only in their words, but in the paper that they were written on.

For more information, visit www.greenpressinitiative.org

101 REASONS WHY I'M A VEGETARIAN

Pamela Rice

Lantern Books · New York
A Division of Booklight Inc.

2005
Lantern Books
One Union Square West, Suite 201
New York, NY 10003

Cover design by Josh Hooten

Printed in the United States of America

Library of Congress Cataloging-in-Publication Data

Rice, Pamela, 1955-
101 reasons why I'm a vegetarian / Pamela Rice.
p. cm.
Includes bibliographical references and index.
ISBN 1-59056-075-2 (alk. paper)
1. Vegetarianism. I. Title. II. Title: One hundred and one reasons why I'm a vegetarian. III. Title: One hundred one reasons why I'm a vegetarian.
RM236.R495 2005
613.2'62—dc22

2005006069

Table of Contents

Acknowledgments

First, and foremost, I want to express a deep-felt gratitude to my husband, Alan Rice. He fully shares my interest in this subject and has supported my work in every way and on many levels, including several readings of the manuscript. His insight can be found on every page. Furthermore, he has brought reams of valuable reference material to the project. This book could not have been written without him.

Next, I want to thank Martin Rowe for believing in my work and bringing me on board as an author with Lantern Books. He also has read this book in manuscript form, offering numerous valuable suggestions, including, "Let the facts speak for themselves, Pam." And thank you, Sarah Gallogly, managing editor of Lantern Books, for a superb editing job.

I also want to thank several people who read selections from the manuscript. I am grateful to Michael Greger, M.D., T. Colin Campbell, Ph.D., and David Wolfson, Esq., for their input. Laura Heifetz was able to read most chapters, maintaining a high level of enthusiasm for the tedium of fact checking. Steve Ruder provided fresh, discerning eyes in one of the latter stages of production. And thank you, "master wordsmith" Jesse Legue, for making numerous headline suggestions, several dozen of which became part of the book.

My career as a writer has, since 1992, been intertwined with the activities of the VivaVegie Society, an educational organization that I founded in 1991 and later incorporated as a nonprofit in 1997. The group has regularly engaged in publishing projects, vegetarian street outreach, and the establishment of the first Vegetarian Center in the United States in 1999. Literally thousands of people have lent their support to this group either as volunteers or financial supporters, in great ways and in small. Extensive archives at the Center have been indispensable to me in this endeavor.

I am exceedingly thankful to everyone who volunteered their time or made a donation to, or a purchase from, the society. Special people in this category include Norbert Banholzer, David Sielaff, NALITH, Martin Rowe, Alex Press, Joy Pierson and Bart Potenza, William and Terri Choi, Bernie G., Glen Boisseau Becker, Mia MacDonald, Jessie Legue, Judea Johnson, Elena Romanova, Janet Bloor, Marian Cole, Nadine Miral, Craig Filipacchi, Tom Thompson, and my sister Julia Fauci. I apologize to any supporters or contributors whom I have inadvertently omitted.

Special thanks must be extended to Alex Press and Glen Boisseau Becker, both top-notch copy editors, who through the years labored heroically on *The VivaVine: The Vegetarian-Issues Magazine*, which was published by the VivaVegie Society. In doing so, they not only made that publication great but also taught me countless writing skills at the same time. I am forever grateful.

I wish to express a deep appreciation to my parents, Ted and Lucille Teisler, for the love and encouragement they have always given me. They taught me that to do the right thing often means feeling a responsibility to the world—both present and future. Dinner-table conversation has always tended to migrate to issues of political and moral ideals, and I thank them for this. Furthermore, I'd like to thank my parents-in-law, Howard and Jean Rice, for the love and support they also have given me. In addition, thank you, Kim Rosenthal, for being a vegetarian and showing me that your lifestyle was an option for me, too.

I would also like to acknowledge two history instructors, Leon Stein, Ph.D., and Alex DeGrand, Ph.D., who made my already excellent experience at Roosevelt University (Chicago) particularly rewarding. They inspired me to forever be a student of history, whether in or outside of an academic setting.

Each of the chapters, or "reasons," contained herein has been distilled from volumes of material written by people who have dedicated their lives to subjects I may only allude to with a single sentence. Many are on the cutting edge in their respective fields and frequently, in the profoundest of ways, have served to inspire me and my work. My hope is that by mentioning them as necessary in the text and in the references I have done something, however small, to honor them. In this regard, I would like to mention John Robbins by name. His book, *Diet for a New America*—in addition to a weekend conference at the annual Summerfest of the North American Vegetarian Society—was the impetus for my own vegetarian epiphany.

Finally, this is a book overflowing with facts. Every endeavor has been made to interpret and communicate them correctly. I take full responsibility for the content. Comments, complaints, criticisms, and compliments may be sent to 101reasons@vivavegie.org. The "101 Reasons" Web site is located at http://www.vivavegie.org/101book/.

Introduction

We humans are an opportunistic species—not the least when it comes to the foods we eat. I still remember my seventh-grade science teacher in LaGrange Park, Illinois, confidently explaining that humans are omnivores. Our diet consists of both plants and animals, she said. Indeed, with an open-mindedness about foods, our species has been able not only to survive but to succeed.

I have since observed that, beyond survival, humans have preferences. Our kind tends, in fact, to choose meat whenever it can. Until recently, this was a choice few people even had the opportunity to make. So historically, most of the world has existed on vegetarian or near-vegetarian diets.

Today we have deviated far away from this historical norm. Not only are societies with primarily plant-based diets eating increasingly more meat, but the meat-eating cultures such as our own have taken gluttony to extremes. Today, European and American cultures in particular have come to consume aberrant quantities of extremely fatty meat, milk, eggs, chicken, and fish. We can, it seems, so we do.

Throughout the ages, cultures have tended to engage in ceremony and ritual sacrifice when slaughtering animals. We've gone beyond this, too. We've now "advanced" to a place where, I can only suppose, we feel we have the luxury of relegating the consumption of meat to a mundane activity. These days, people effortlessly purchase plastic-wrapped cuts of meat, slaughtered by others, without a thought or a prayer. Most see this activity, and attendant attitude, as their right—witness the uproar when Reagan-administration budget crunchers attempted to make tofu into a meat substitute for the school lunch program.

Physiologically there is of course another story. Humans resemble the herbivores far more closely than the mammalian carnivores. Our jaws allow lateral movement for grinding fibrous plant material. Carnivore jaws, perfectly designed for tearing flesh, only move hinge-like up and down. The human digestive tract, like those of herbivores, is particularly long—again, good for processing plant foods. Carnivore digestive tracts are relatively short so that meat, which becomes toxic inside the body, is quickly expelled before poisons can accumulate. Moreover, meat in the human diet is found to cause arterial walls to harden with plaque—a phenomenon that never occurs in carnivores, only herbivores. The most obvious aspect of true carnivores is their menacing, elongated canine teeth, large mouths, and claws. They will, in fact, swallow their food whole. Humans possess short canines, small mouths, and no claws. We were able to eat only scavenged meat before weapons were developed. Ultimately, humans not only survive on all-plant diets, they thrive. An all-meat diet will, on the other hand, shorten a person's life greatly.

As for those well-worn meat-eater mantras—our species has *always* eaten meat; we are meat eaters because that is our place on the food chain; meat tastes good, etc.—I'm not going to dispute these statements, except to say that they sound more like excuses than reasons to eat meat.

My goal for this book is not to argue with people's beliefs (a futile endeavor in any case) but to appeal to our capacity for reason. Collectively, we humans may have an innate desire to eat meat, but our physical make-up also includes a very large brain, which has been used to overcome countless barriers that were also considered insurmountable. To hope that humanity will choose to transcend its nature and adopt vegetarianism is indeed to aim high. Still, our brain has allowed us to achieve some pretty amazing things. Surely it can secure our ultimate survival on earth by anticipating looming dangers, not the least of which are the ones we inflict upon ourselves with our collective meat habit.

Look at all the lives that are saved by modern weather reporting. Consider this book as just another forecast—similar, perhaps, to one that warns of an advancing hurricane. It endeavors to provide hope and even solace in knowledge. At the same time it should instill a healthy fear about the consequences of current trends. It even offers a solution—a simple and, once explored, delicious one at that.

In the end, we can choose to undermine our bodies' exquisite mechanisms that keep us healthy. We can continue to foster a grievous alienation from the natural world with efficient but cruel systems of livestock production. We can perish by our own hands on a planet ruined by the environmental ravages of our carnivorous desires. Or we can embrace life by creating a vegetarian world.

Frequently asked questions

Why isn't your book arranged in categories?

This book has a long history in pamphlet form. For nearly a decade and a half it has existed in various updated editions as a quick-read list—about an eighth the length of this book. Vegetarians could use it as a pass-along item for those who asked them about their diet. It has always jumped from subject to subject. Indeed, any person wanting to read just the *health* or the *environmental* or the *animal* or the *social* or the *economic* reasons was always hard-pressed to do so. By design, I have taken away that which might otherwise have offered a user-friendly function in order to present the big picture. As far as I am concerned, there is only one category here: vegetarianism. And I aim to communicate to each reader—despite his or her special interests—the full breadth of that topic. If I have done my job, this book will unfold into a rich amalgam of disparate subjects—one that connects the dots for those who may have heard just one or a few aspects of the vegetarian argument. For those who still take issue with this approach, I offer the "reasons by category" page (p. xvii). A comprehensive index is also provided.

Why so many references?

I hope that everyone who reads this book takes some time to read through or at least consult the references. Naturally, these sources serve to verify the words that are in the text. But their titles also impart knowledge, often in telling and even amusing ways. Moreover, by listing so many articles I wish to show the extent of mainstream reportage that essentially supports vegetarianism, albeit not usually with that intent.

During a stint when I published a vegetarian journal, I always made sure to include a section entitled "Vegetarian News"—mainstream news reconstituted to a vegetarian mindset. If this notion seems alien for now, it shouldn't after a read-through of this book.

Is there a spiritual element to this book?

No, not in the traditional sense. There is a spirited element, however. I seem to have limitless energy to root out information that either supports the vegetarian lifestyle or indicts conventional eating habits and their production techniques. I have made every effort to avoid sentimentality and dogma, trusting that my readers can reach a proper conclusion after learning the facts. Beliefs (my own and others') come into play, but not without hypothesis, observation, and the weight of evidence. There is but one quote from the Bible, and except for this isolated case, there are no references from religious sources. Again, I cannot argue with faith.

Where do we go from here?

Though this book is an attempt to investigate every good reason to adopt the vegetarian lifestyle—however remote—it is worlds away from being exhaustive. My best hope is that it will in time inspire a flood of other investigations. Surely, every "reason" could be a volume on its own. At this writing, unfortunately, vegetarianism does not even have its own section in bookstores, so there is plenty left to explore! We have, no less, a culture to build.

Beyond this, I'm always of the hope that the type of information I uncover inspires a political response. I long for vegetarians to become a constituent force—one that has coalesced to the point of having a voice in policy decisions. So far, vegetarianism is largely viewed as little more than a peculiar dietary lifestyle that some people choose for...who knows why. This book, I hope, explains the serious consequences of the choice to eat meat. Though I'm not sure we vegetarians are ready to call meat eaters our adversaries in the usual sense, I do think that it is high time that those who choose meat pay the true cost of their predilection (see reason #44). At the minimum, meat eaters should have to pay for the environmental damages associated with their lifestyle. I'm afraid that no less than an avalanche of grassroots organizing will be required to transform this idea into public policies that take away all subsidies to meat.

Why is your book so negative?

Admittedly, this book could have just as easily been entitled *101 Reasons Why I Don't Eat Meat.* Without question, I do not spare the reader when I describe the downside of our collective meat-centered diet. It soon becomes apparent that there is more than a little unpleasantness in the information I impart. This was unavoidable; the subject lends itself to this kind of treatment. There is nothing pretty about the meat industry.

On the other hand, I view vegetarianism as the norm. I believe that if humans the world over suddenly adopted vegetarianism, it would not necessarily be good or bad, just the way life was meant to be. And given this, there is no need to defend it. On the other hand, the moment humanity deviates from this neutral position, there is much to be said.

Acronyms used in this book

ACS	American Cancer Society
AICR	American Institute for Cancer Research
AMR	advanced meat recovery
AP	Associated Press
AQMD	South Coast Air Quality Management District (CA)
ARS/USDA	Agriculture Research Service/U.S. Department of Agriculture
BBC	British Broadcasting Service
BSE	bovine spongiform encephalopathy
CAFO	Confined Animal Feeding Operation
CAST	Council for Agricultural Science and Technology
CBC	Canadian Broadcasting Corporation
CIWF	Compassion in World Farming, UK (an animal protection organization)
CMAB	California Milk Advisory Board
CRP	Conservation Reserve Program
CSPI	Center for Science in the Public Interest
CSU	Colorado State University
CVM	Center for Veterinary Medicine
CWD	chronic wasting disease
DDT	dichlorodiphenyltrichloroethane (an organochlorine insecticide)
DEIP	Dairy Export Incentive Program
DHA	docosahexaenoic acid (an essential nutrient)
DNS	Division of Nutritional Sciences, Cornell University
ENN	Environmental News Network
EPA	Environmental Protection Agency
EPA	eicosapentaenoic acid (an essential nutrient)
EQIP	Environmental Quality Incentives Program
ERS/USDA	Economic Research Service/U.S. Department of Agriculture
EU	European Union
FAO/UN	Food and Agriculture Organization of the U.N.
FDA	Food and Drug Administration
FDA/CVM	Food and Drug Administration/Center for Veterinary Medicine
FMD	foot and mouth disease
FSIS	Food Safety and Inspection Service
FTC	Federal Trade Commission
GERD	gastroesophageal reflux disease
GM	genetically modified
HAB	harmful algal bloom

HACCP	Hazard Analysis and Critical Control Point
HCAs	heterocyclic amines
HFA	Human Farming Association (an animal rights organization)
IBP	formerly Iowa Beef Packers, now just IBP
IFPRI	International Food Policy Research Institute
KFC	formerly Kentucky Fried Chicken, now just KFC
MAP	Market Access Program
MAP	mycobacterium paratuberculosis (dairy cow disease)
NALITH	Nature, Life, Truth, and Health (a charity)
NAMP	North American Meat Processors
NASD	National Association of Securities Dealers
NCEP	National Cholesterol Education Program
NHLBI	National Heart, Lung, and Blood Institute
NIH	National Institutes of Health
NOAA	National Oceanic and Atmospheric Administration
NPR	National Public Radio
NRDC	National Resources Defense Council
PAHs	polycyclic aromatic hydrocarbons
PBS	Public Broadcasting Service
PCB	polychlorinated biphenyls
PCRM	Physicians Committee for Responsible Medicine
PETA	People for the Ethical Treatment of Animals
PMS	premenstrual syndrome
RMRS	Rocky Mountain Research Station
RSPCA	Royal Society for the Prevention of Cruelty to Animals (UK)
S.T.O.P.	Safe Tables Our Priority (a food-safety citizens group)
SARS	Severe Acute Respiratory Syndrome
SIV	simian immunodeficiency viruses
SHBG	sex hormone binding globulin
TSEs	transmissible spongiform encephalopathies
UK	United Kingdom
UN	United Nations
UNEP	United Nations Environment Program
UPC	United Poultry Concerns (an animal rights organization)
UPI	United Press International
USDA	United States Department of Agriculture
USGS	U.S. Geological Survey
vCJD	new variant Creutzfeldt-Jakob disease
WHO	World Health Organization
WTO	World Trade Organization
WWF	World Wide Fund for Nature

Reasons by category

General animal issues: 5, 12, 14, 36, 41, 50, 55, 59, 63, 78, 87

Cruelty to specific species: 6, 30, 53, 58, 82, 94, 99

Contamination and sanitation: 6, 25, 31, 35, 54, 70, 72, 79, 91, 93, 95

Dead animals and where they go: 15, 40, 46, 76, 80

Animal drugs, disease: 17, 18, 28, 32, 65, 83

Environmental issues: 8, 20, 27, 34, 42, 52, 61, 62, 66, 69, 84, 89, 101

Hazards for fish: 4, 21, 39, 45, 47, 64, 68, 71, 92, 98

Human health: 2, 16, 23, 24, 33, 81, 85, 88

Human nutrition: 9, 19, 26, 37, 43, 48, 49, 67, 74, 77, 90, 96, 100

The nitrogen cycle, manure: 3, 13, 29, 38, 56, 60, 73,

Social and economic issues: 1, 10, 11, 22, 44, 51, 57, 75, 86, 97

1 Gratifying consumers

PACKAGES OF WOE

"Increasingly, our consumers insist on defining what is produced. . . . The food system now is clearly consumer-driven."—former USDA secretary Ann Veneman[1]

It all starts, or perhaps ends, with those tidy packages of meat in the supermarket display case—glistening, beckoning, and, from the looks of things, completely harmless. But to keep what's in those packages up to precise market spec requires a vast production machine of unprecedented proportions—one with a reach so phenomenal that a popular cable-television series would document it as one of the world's "modern marvels."[2] Today's consumer blithely eats animal-based foods that are consistent in taste and quality, precise in desirable fat content, inexpensively priced, and available without exception in every grocery store in America, no matter how remote. And in order to keep those packages jumping off the shelves, our fickle supermarket-ambling shopper must be spared any notion of the real costs or realities behind the scenes.

Read any speech by any recent USDA secretary and you'll probably find the words "consumer-driven" somewhere in the text. Consumer fancy is the given, and from this all seems to be justified, no matter that industrially produced meat has fostered systems that destroy ecosystems, threaten public health, inflict suffering on animals, exploit workers, and unravel the richness of the rural social fabric.

Bodies by science

Though there are exceptions, most meat dollars today go to those farmers who gave in to USDA pressure, the message heard since the 1950s: "Get big or get out." Aided over the last half-century by a confluence of technological innovations and cheap inputs, producers of chickens, hogs, and cows, primarily, have been able to place their livestock indoors and under rigid systems of control, often in unfathomable numbers.

On the surface, the advances may appear positive. Genetic manipulation has made the animals better able to withstand the intensive conditions and to mature faster. Drugs have been developed to speed growth on less feed. And trait tinkering has brought forth a uniformity in breeds, designed in fact to custom-fit automated machinery. With indoor confinement, geneticists now concentrate their efforts on breeding animals with flesh that is consistent in taste and texture. No longer is a breed favored because of its special ability to stand up to conditions defined by climates or local diseases and pests.

The hidden costs

An assembly-line model may be suitable for plastic cups or electronic goods, but not for meat. This now-immense industry that produces all this precision and efficiency has ushered in industrial methods that pose unique risks. For one, the mass grinding and pooling of carcasses regularly leads to food-poisoning outbreaks that affect victims over geographic expanses without limit.

Other dangers stem from the derivation of feed from animal-protein by-product; the misuse of antibiotics; the titanic hoarding of land, energy and water; and the profuse generation of manure.

Furthermore, while such advances gave those farmers and processors who adopted them the economic edge, they also worked to shake out the smaller concerns that didn't. By the end of the twentieth century we had headlines like the following from *Business Week*: "Will agribusiness plow under the family farm?" The article recounted what it described as "rampant consolidation" in the nation's farm sector. Alas, the trend has left us with two million nearly obsolete farmers. A 2001 USDA report revealed that a mere 150,000 farms produce just about all the food that America eats.[3] Moreover, fewer than two dozen companies do most of the slaughtering of some nine billion poultry birds per year in the United States.[4] And fewer than a half a dozen companies slaughter nearly all of America's cattle.[5]

And finally, where are the animals in all of this? Defenseless. The federal-level Animal Welfare Act does not apply to animals raised for "food, fiber, or production purposes." And state laws are weak to ineffective. Ultimately, if the laws had provided any protection on the animals' behalf, the techniques of modern meat production could never have come into existence.

2 Vegetarian heart

SOUND ADVICE FOR YOUR TICKER

"Vegans have reduced risk for heart disease and stroke due to their high-fiber, low-saturated-fat, cholesterol-free, phytochemical-rich diets."—Brenda Davis, R.D. and Vesanto Melina, M.S., R.D., co-authors, *Becoming Vegan*[1]

The evidence is in. It's been known for well over a decade now. Heart disease, the biggest killer in America by a long shot, can be reversed. It doesn't have to kill you, nor does it have to mean a life sentence of cholesterol-lowering drugs, nor living at the mercy of your cardiologist. All it takes is a nutritionally balanced vegetarian diet (including adequate amounts of omega-3 fatty acids and vitamin B12), regular exercise, and stress management. In the late 1980s, Dean Ornish, M.D., proved that this three-pronged approach is all you need to get your life back. It helped that he had a few cardiac patients—his study subjects—who shared his hunches and were happy to adhere to a diet held by people in areas of the world where cardiovascular disease is rare.

Ornish Zen

Despite its resounding success, the Ornish program is often described in mainstream publications as radical. Yet it turns coronary cripples into functioning human beings.[2] As Dr. Ornish puts it, "I don't understand why asking people to eat a well-balanced vegetarian diet is considered drastic while it is medically conservative to cut people open or put them on powerful cholesterol-lowering drugs."[3] The U.S. Medicare program must agree. In 2000 it announced that it planned to give $7,200 apiece to 1,800 heart patients to enter the Ornish program. In the meantime, dozens of insurance companies have come on board—anything, they must reckon, to cut into America's $370-billion-per-year cost of cardiovascular disease.[4]

Don't blame your genes

We need to remember just how deadly and debilitating this nearly preventable and expensive disease continues to be. Indeed, 2,600 Americans die of cardiovascular disease every *day*. That's nearly two deaths every minute.[5] About 865,000 Americans suffer heart attacks every year, and millions more struggle with chest pain and shortness of breath. One in five Americans has one or more types of the disease at any one time.[6] About 6,700 people below the age of 44 die of heart attacks in the United States every year.[7]

Again, much of this simply does not have to happen. Major population studies have essentially proved that diet and lifestyle, not heredity, have the most bearing on risk. "We've never had a heart attack in Framingham in 35 years in anyone who had a cholesterol level under 150,"[8] declared William Castelli, M.D., of the famous Massachusetts-based NHLBI (National Heart, Lung, and Blood Institute) heart study. It isn't easy to keep one's cholesterol level this low on the standard American meat-centered diet. Moreover, in rural China, where people eat one-tenth the animal protein by calorie intake compared with the average American[9] and where high cholesterol levels equal our nation's lows, heart disease occurs at one-twentieth the rate found in the United States.[10]

Conventional advice: Busted

Regularly eating meat is likely to raise cholesterol and blood pressure levels, as well as body weight—risk factors for heart disease and stroke. In response, doctors tend to prescribe expensive drugs—their long-term effects unknown—and advise diet modifications, such as taking the skin off of one's chicken, rather than wholesale changes.

Enter Dr. Ornish: In the late 1990s, he tested such advice. He brought together 48 heart patients, half of whom were told to go with the part-way measures just described. The other half were prescribed his vegetarian/exercise/stress-management system. The results were dramatic. After a year, those who adhered to the standard regimen did not see their conditions stabilize; in fact, they worsened. Those on the Ornish plan improved.[11]

3 Extreme manure

THE EXCREMENT FILES

"Rail cars from the Midwest carry corn to feed more chickens [on the Delmarva Peninsula]. The rail cars return, but the nutrients [manure and slaughterhouse waste] stay behind."—Peter S. Goodman, for the *Washington Post*[1]

Manure! It's time to dispose of our outdated notions about it. Thanks to today's farming methods, we have gargantuan amounts of it, and land near livestock operations is often dangerously saturated with poisonous amounts of nitrogen and phosphorus, euphemistically referred to as "nutrients." Managing the waste responsibly is an expensive proposition. Tragically, until any meaningful regulation is legislated and implemented, farmers will be wont to dispose of the stuff expediently.

Even with the best intentions, much of the nation's manure ends up in our water, and it gets there by way of a variety of routes. The most insidious occurs when land becomes saturated to excess with nitrogen and phosphorus from farms, which later runs off into waterways with subsequent rainfalls. It's usually impossible to trace this kind of water pollution to its source.

Spills and leaky cesspools are other conduits for manure. These not only foul our waterways but also contaminate our groundwater. And pollution that reaches water tables deep in the earth is essentially impossible to clean out. The worst manure spill on record involved an eight-acre "lagoon" in North Carolina in 1995. Twenty-five million gallons of liquid manure—over twice the volume released by the oil spill of the Exxon *Valdez*—burst forth to befoul local rivers, farms, and highways.

But these are the unintentional releases. Some livestock operators are not beyond constructing gullies to send their discharges directly into nearby creeks and rivers. A *60 Minutes* (CBS-TV) feature in 1996 told of 115 farms that were caught illegally dumping hog waste into local waterways over a four–year period.[2] There have since been numerous examples of operators of so-called confined animal feeding operations, or CAFOs, being found guilty of defying manure-handling rules.[3] Perhaps what is most amazing about these statistics and reports is that anyone was keeping track at all.

Ultimately, whether on purpose or not, our water is becoming befouled by animal waste. According to the EPA and the USDA, one in twenty river-miles surveyed in the United States has been adversely affected by livestock operations.[4]

A Senate report to remember

In December 1997, Sen. Tom Harkin (D-IA) issued an everything-you-never-wanted-to-know report about U.S. manure. It announced that the total amount of manure produced by livestock in the United States comes to a staggering 1.37 billion tons annually, that is, 10,000 pounds for every U.S. citizen per year.[5] The figure dwarfed any estimate that had come before—certainly any that had been issued by the industry itself.

Other reports and surveys have subsequently concurred with the Harkin report.

- Every day the manure from Wisconsin's cows could fill the 76,000-seat football stadium in the state's capital—to the brim.[6] Each cow leaves behind 120 pounds of poop daily.[7]
- Texas produces the most manure of any state: 140 million tons annually, about a tenth of the country's total and twice that of the runner-up state, California.[8] On cattle feedlots, manure is simply allowed to pile up and grow into giant mounds. The animals find refuge atop them during rainstorms as rancid puddles form below into gullies that course their way to nearby ponds. The mini-hills, which may represent several thousand tons of waste, are a serious fire hazard. And when they ignite, they can take months before being extinguished.[9]
- According to the Natural Resources Defense Council, each day "300,000 cows within 50 square miles in Chino, California, generate a football-field-size pile of manure as high as the Empire State Building. Daily, the manure mixes with some 15 million gallons of water used to wash the cows and clean the barns."[10]
- Sun Prairie Farms, though now in the midst of numerous legal entanglements, has negotiated with the Rosebud Sioux to build 232 barns to house 869,000 market hogs per year on 13 farms across the tribe's reservation.[11] If built to capacity, the enterprise would require 600 acres for digesters and open-air evaporation ponds for the excrement.[12] Furthermore, once fully operational, the facility would require nearly 1.7 million gallons of water from the Ogallala Aquifer daily and generate about three times as much fecal waste as the entire human population of South Dakota, where the barns are to be built.[13]
- Six thousand chicken houses on the Delmarva Peninsula confine 600 million birds that produce 750,000 tons of manure per year. Surveys done by the state of Maryland have shown that 70 to 87 percent of all nutrients (nitrogen and phosphorus) reaching the rivers there come from agriculture. One third of all wells in the region exceed EPA safe-drinking water standards for nitrate, a manure by-product that can impede the oxygen-carrying capabilities of the blood, particularly in newborns and children under one year of age.[14]

Manure runoff can have any number of negative consequences. Just one of many examples is the expansion of industrial chicken farming on a plateau upstream from Rochefort, Belgium. It has threatened to pollute the pristine water used at the Abbaye Notre-Dame de Saint-Remy where the highly regarded Trappist beer is still made by monks.[15]

In 2003, environmental groups sued the federal government over rules governing manure management of large-scale farms.[16] They were on to something. Later that year, the government issued two telling reports.

The first revealed that only a quarter of the nation's largest dairies and hog operations were spreading their manure on enough land to mitigate toxic runoff.[17] The second report said that the EPA's own computer systems were grossly inadequate to track down farms lacking manure-management plans.[18] In the end, millions of tons of waste are sent into our waterways, and the government is unable to control it.

Again, the industry doesn't seem willing to pay for the messes it makes. For instance, laws proposed to regulate the treatment of manure in California to reduce choking ammonia emissions from the state's dairy farms—long a problem in the area—were, as recently as 2004, declared by farmers to be prohibitively expensive to their operations.[19] Similarly, that same year, the animal-waste treatment techniques that North Carolina researchers recommended as necessary to neutralize the majority of that state's swine manure pollutants turned out to be five times more expensive to farmers than those already being used.[20]

In the Netherlands, the country with the highest concentration of livestock anywhere, the manure problem escalated to such a point that a bureaucracy—the first of its kind in the world—is now dedicated to tracking and taxing animal waste.[21] The country accounts for manure perhaps more carefully than some countries keep track of their plutonium. What do they know that we don't?

4 Troubled waters

OCEANS IN PERIL

"Fishermen should pay society for the privilege of catching fish, not vice versa."—The Economist[1]

Logic should tell anyone that the oceans are way too vast to succumb to anything man could do to them. And such an opinion has indeed held water for all of human history, that is, until recently. At first the warnings trickled in. By 1998, a major symposium of 1,600 scientists from around the world declared that fishing had put the oceans in peril.[2] They warned that no less than swift action was imperative to prevent irreversible environmental degradation. The alarm is now stuck in perpetual high alert.

While today there is a bit more awareness about the plight of ocean fish—1998 became the UN's International Year of the Ocean—the world remains locked in a state of policy paralysis. It doesn't help that governments continue to send mixed messages. Collectively, $15 billion in annual subsidies continues to be bestowed upon the world's fishers—a quarter of the value of the global fish trade.[3] The world's taxpayers, it seems, are financing the ocean's demise.

And now, between government giveaways distorting people's impressions of the real cost of fish and the industry's technological capacity to efficiently haul in catch, is there any wonder ocean stocks have dwindled?

Stocks stats

- According to the Food and Agriculture Organization of the UN (FAO/UN), 15 of the world's 17 major ocean fisheries are either depleted or overexploited.[4]
- The World Wide Fund for Nature (WWF) declared in August 1998 that nearly 70 percent of the world's 200 most valuable fish stocks are either depleted or overfished.[5] "The global fish catch has stagnated and its quality has declined," according to the FAO/UN.[6]
- In roughly the last four decades, the capacity of the world's fishing fleets has increased fivefold, though productivity of the world's fishing grounds has declined, according to the UN and the WWF.[7]
- Canadian researchers declared in 2003 that 90 percent of the ocean's top predator fish have been fished nearly out of existence.[8]
- Landings of the most commercially valuable species have dropped by a quarter. To make up for the shortfall, fishers are bringing in greater quantities of less valuable species, dangerously depleting fish further down on the food web.[9]
- One percent of the world's fishers (200,000 to 300,000), using the largest boats, harvest the same amount of fish as 90 percent of the world's subsistence fishers (15 to 21 million) using traditional fishing methods.[10]
- Of the 215 stocks the U.S. government tracks, about a third are being fished faster than they can reproduce.[11]
- Industrial countries consume more fish for nonfood uses than India, Latin America, and Africa use for direct human consumption.[12] A third of the world's fish catch goes to feed livestock.[13] The trend is for

increasingly more of the world's 33 million tons of fishmeal per year to feed carnivorous fish on farms.[14]

Bycatch: Indiscriminate and inexact

Since fishing is essentially inexact, much of what causes the damage is collateral. Whatever the method of retrieval—driftnetting, dredging, trawling, longlining, or just "sport" fishing—what comes onto the hook or into the net is often a surprise. So-called *bycatch*, or unintended catch, is typically not worth the cost of hauling in (although this may change with the growth of aquaculture feed needs). Such fish that are caught but are not wanted are usually returned to the water, traumatized, maimed, or dead, with no records of the toll. In other cases, species that may be designated as illegal to land are simply not brought to shore. Again, they will likely be dumped overboard after trauma or death.

A serving of shrimp doesn't tell you that it came your way after some 3 to 15 times the fish in terms of bycatch may have had to die.[16] Shrimp is an extreme case, but, all told, total bycatch amounts to at least 25 percent of worldwide landed stocks.

"Where is the point of no return?" asks Sylvia Earle, the former chief scientist for the U.S. National Oceanic and Atmospheric Administration in a program aired by the National Geographic Channel. "We don't know, but for sure many of the sea's creatures are in trouble."[15]

5 Legal disconnect

FARMED ANIMALS FORGOTTEN

"Every one of us knows a story of animal cruelty, every one of us knows how in one way or another official policies have sanctioned cruelty to animals." —Rep. Dennis J. Kucinich (D-OH), presidential candidate (2004) and ethical vegan[1]

The United States is not a good place to be if you're a farmed animal. Though you are a living, feeling, sentient being, there is little in the nation's laws to protect you from abuse. First, the federal-level Animal Welfare Act has no meaning for you because the word "animal," as legally defined, does not apply to "farm animals used for food, fiber, or production purposes." Consequently, even though the title of this statute implies to the public that the government looks after the welfare of animals destined for the dinner plate, it does not. And by leaving farmed animals unprotected against the onslaught of industrial farm production, the law actually helps to open the floodgates to even more animal cruelty—to a scale, in fact, never before seen. Other federal-level anti-cruelty laws that cover specific conditions during transport, at stockyards,[2] and during the slaughter process similarly lack teeth in their wording and are inadequately enforced.[3]

Of course every state has its own anti-cruelty statute. But, here again, the laws protecting farmed animals are likely to be outright exclusionary or, at best, weak. Curiously, according to David Wolfson, a lawyer and animal-rights law scholar, 30 states in recent years amended their anti-cruelty laws in order to remove protections for farmed animals.[4] As the particularly egregious techniques of factory farming gained ground, agribusiness interests correctly feared that state statutes, as written, could impact their profit-making abilities. So, with little fanfare, the legal dismantling took place behind the scenes. Within a very short time, the laws exempted "accepted," "common," "customary," or "normal" farming practices, thereby allowing what in every other context would be considered cruel acts to be deemed legal as long as they are widely adopted by the industry.[5] Now, with practices fully entrenched, the industry has simply been encouraged to develop still crueler methods of extracting commodity wealth from animals.

On rare occasions farmers and ranchers do get punished for particularly gratuitous acts of animal cruelty.[6] However, it is more likely, when animal protection organizations attempt to obtain legal help for animals, that no laws are found to have been broken, because none had been written.[7] Ultimately, the farming community has come to a uniquely privileged place. It is allowed to define for itself what criminality is in its case—naturally to suit its own purposes.[8]

In the end, we're left with a culture that's numbed into complacency about the plight of farmed animals. It's difficult to convince the general public that there is anything wrong with the system when horrendous conditions are considered entirely legal.

Marketplace versus the courts

In the United States, the marketplace has been the arena for some improvements regarding the plight of farmed animals. The so-called free-range movement, however, is essentially disingenuous.[9] For instance, the rules a producer must abide by in order to label his poultry "free range" are so lenient as to be considered a joke. Producers do have to sign affidavits that their animals can get outside of their holding areas. However, the situation does not have to mean continual or even daily outdoor access. A single small doorway will pass muster, but, according to one farmer consulted for a *Consumer Reports* investigation, the chickens usually have no desire to exit, since food tends to be only indoors.[10]

Even the Better Business Bureau ruled in 2004 that product logos that boast "Animal Care Certified" (used by some egg producers to assure consumers that their hens are raised humanely) are misleading.[11] Furthermore, what have been hailed as sweeping anti-cruelty reforms that McDonald's and others have required of their suppliers similarly merely clip at the edges of industry practices.[12] This is "not an industry that is capable of regulating itself," asserts Bryan Pease, of the California-based Animal Protection and Rescue League.[13] The legal route, which employs rigorous enforcement, is the only true way to protect farmed animals from cruelty.

The European Union is more on track in this regard, as it is scheduled to prohibit a number of cruel farming practices over the coming years: gestation crates for sows (after the first month) by 2012, battery cages for chickens by 2012, and the veal crate by 2007.[14] The World Trade Organization, however, may undermine these initiatives in the name of free trade.[15]

In the end, the only sure way to keep cruelty off your plate is to keep the animals from ever getting near it.

6 Contaminant magnetism

MEAT-MICROBE ATTRACTION

It's hard to remove "surface contaminants from meat because microorganisms hang on tenaciously."—USDA chemical engineer Arthur I. Morgan[1]

It is the peculiar properties found on the surface of meat that turn it into a magnet for microbes. Bacteria are attracted to "high-protein, nonacid foods, such as meat, poultry, seafood, dairy products, and eggs," according to the Economic Research Service of the USDA.[2] Foods of animal origin are identified most frequently as the source of foodborne disease outbreaks reported to the Centers for Disease Control.[3] All the primary foodborne pathogens are tied to animal-based foods.[4] On the other hand, according to the United Fresh Fruit and Vegetable Association, outbreaks of foodborne illness associated with produce are rare. And when they happen, cross-contamination with meat or livestock waste is often shown to be the cause.[5]

The number of kinds of foodborne pathogens has increased fivefold in the last half century.[6] In the United States, 14 people die each day from foodborne illnesses out of a whopping 200,000 daily cases.[7] The Food and Agriculture Organization of the UN estimates that as many as one in three people in industrialized countries is struck by food poisoning every year.[8] Danish researchers believe that actually twice as many people, worldwide, die from foodborne illness than are accounted for by current estimates,[9] since food-poisoning deaths, which can occur even a year after initial infection, are easily attributable to other causes.

Stomach this

Campylobacteriosis is the most common cause of diarrheal illness in the United States.[10] It is inextricably linked to poultry consumption, with 1,000 to 2,000 cases per year leading to Guillain-Barré syndrome, a life-threatening condition that causes paralysis.[11] Salmonella, another common poultry pathogen, causes diarrhea, fever, and abdominal cramps for several days. To those with weak immune systems, it can be fatal. Reiter's syndrome, also caused by these bacteria, brings on inflammation in the joints, eyes, and urinary tract.[12] Both campylobacter and salmonella, along with yersinia, a type of bacteria found primarily in pork, are associated with reactive arthritis, which causes inflammation in the joints. In a sample test conducted by *Consumer Reports* of nearly 500 store-bought, packaged whole chickens in 2002, 42 percent were found to harbor campylobacter, 12 percent contained salmonella, and 5 percent had both pathogens.[13] Incidentally, the government has shown that chicken that is labeled free-range is just as likely to be contaminated with salmonella as is conventional chicken.[14]

Listeriosis, which is associated with cold cuts, tends to attack the fetuses of pregnant women. It has a high fatality rate. And *E. coli* O157:H7, which is associated with hamburgers, is a cause of hemolytic uremic syndrome, a deadly kidney disease.

The ranks of the sickened tend to be filled with children, pregnant women, the elderly, and those with immune deficiencies resulting from AIDS, cancer, or other causes. Death by food poisoning is an excruciatingly painful process in which vital organs break down one by one. Survivors of foodborne illnesses may have to live with neuromuscular paralysis or chronic kidney failure. Parts of their intestines may have to be removed or lifelong dialysis endured. An attack may bring on a stroke or cause brain damage.[15]

Processes, practices hold the key

Investigations by food safety groups, USDA inspectors, and even foreign veterinary experts all point to the same conclusion: Meat in America is dangerous because of the sloppy practices of some producers. In a 1995 summarized report of worst-case "violations of law" caught by federal meat and poultry inspectors in processing plants, diseased carcasses, rancid meat, deadly residues, waste-contaminated puddles, filthy "mixtures," fly infestations, and human waste defilements are discussed ad nauseam. More troubling is the very design of today's processing machinery. Cross-contamination, often on a massive scale, occurs at every step. A group of experts from the European Union observing practices in U.S. slaughterhouses in 1997 found conditions "simply disgusting."[16] Former USDA inspector Rodney Leonard explained in a *48 Hours* broadcast: "I won't eat chicken [or] allow it in my house. It's tragic that chicken is handled so badly that it becomes a major health risk if you consume it."[17]

The untraceables

Ultimately, only 19 percent of foodborne illnesses are ever traced to any identifiable cause, and fewer than 5 percent are even reported.[18] Only extraordinarily dogged sleuthing, record keeping, and persistence bring cases to court, and these tend to be the relatively tiny few that are part of publicized outbreaks. The exceedingly more-prevalent sporadic cases that are suffered by disparate victims invariably go blameless and unprosecuted.

Today, DNA fingerprinting is showing great promise for tracing foodborne infections back to their origins. One day it may routinely lead government food cops to specific producers of filthy food—putting sloppy operations out of business in a hurry. Until that day, and even afterwards, it's a risky proposition to eat meat.

7 Oink!

MODERN PIG LIFE

"Entering, you are greeted by a bedlam of squealing, chain rattling, and horrible roaring from the sows. Row after row, hundreds of the creatures are encased...inside their iron crates."—Matthew Scully, speechwriter to Pres. George W. Bush and opponent of factory farming[1]

They weigh but a few pounds at birth. Yet today's industrial pigs will have grown to 270 pounds when they are sent to slaughter, a mere six months later.[2] Selective breeding and high-protein feed are what allows this to happen. Arthritis and other orthopedic problems frequently set in as skeletal development does not keep pace with the rapid muscle gain. Concrete floors aggravate painful leg conditions all the more.[3]

Today's sow gives birth to about nine piglets per litter, nearly double any natural number she might have brought into the world.[4] Moreover, the industry has reduced the time a piglet has with its mother to two to three weeks,[5] though a piglet would naturally be weaned after about three months.[6] Producers push for early weaning, despite heavy mortalities, because it allows a sow to come into heat within about a week.[7] Not a moment can be wasted in getting this "piglet machine" pregnant again.

Throughout her lifetime, a sow will give birth to more than twenty piglets per year. When her productive capacity wanes, after about eight or nine pregnancies, she will be sent to slaughter.[8] As for the piglets, they will "grow out" in cramped communal pens with no room to root, roam, or carry out normal social behaviors.

Pawing the pavement

A breeding sow will live out most of her four years of life trapped in a crate two feet wide and seven feet long.[9] She will abide in solitary, pregnancy after pregnancy (just short of three per year).[10] Once she gives birth, her body will be pinned in place to expose her teats to her piglets.

The *Handbook of Livestock Management Techniques,* an encyclopedic volume of practical information for the farmer and rancher, tells us, "Sows and gilts [first-time mothers] become restless and irritable immediately before farrowing [giving birth], and some will try to get out of the pen or crate." At this time, sows scrape and paw the concrete in a desperate simulation of nest building.[11]

In nature, swine avoid filth and walk and root over nine miles in a night.[12] Confinement in crates and stalls keeps a sow from even turning around; she will in fact bruise herself repeatedly in attempts to do so. The stench and noxious fumes of putrefying urine and feces endlessly collect beneath her. The floors are hard, cold, and strawless. Straw, if provided, could give a modicum of comfort, but more than this, it could mitigate the oppressive boredom that is fundamental to sow imprisonment. Pigs are highly intelligent and inquisitive animals. Like humans, they can be driven insane by solitary confinement and maternal frustration. And yet the industry blames the sows for what it terms "vices"—neurotic coping behaviors, such as bar biting.[13] It can be argued that for a dairy cow similarly housed, chewing the cud is a source of stimulation.[14] A pig has no such outlet.

Slush cuts

In its unbounded quest for fast-growing ultralarge and ultralean muscle, geneticists have inadvertently bred a stress-syndrome trait into the pigs. Due to the rough treatment typically inflicted on these animals, some of the pork turns to pallid, slushy cuts of meat that become leathery when cooked.[15] According to industry expert Temple Grandin, "If you breed for those superlean big-bubble butts, you tend to breed for a very nervous, excitable pig that's very hard to handle."[16] The industry aims to employ technical solutions to this problem. Phasing out intensive confinement apparently is not one of the options being considered.

8 World water III

TAPPING OUT

"If the wars of this century were fought over oil, the wars of the next century will be fought over water."—Ismail Serageldin, World Bank vice president, 1995[1]

Many of the world's mightiest rivers, including the Ganges, the Yellow, the Nile, and even our own Colorado, routinely run dry before reaching the sea.[2] Aquifer levels everywhere are dropping precipitously. Worldwide, countless smaller streams have dried up. For this we can in large part blame the fivefold increase in world meat production that took place over the last half-century,[3] and the trend has not yet peaked.

Water-hoarding meat

It takes nearly 8,500 gallons of water to produce just one pound of beef, according to a report issued in 2004 by the Stockholm International Water Institute at a meeting of the UN Commission on Sustainable Development.[4] Furthermore, according to the institute, household water needs are minuscule next to those needed to sustain the standard Western diet using prevailing land and water management practices. *Newsweek* once explained: "The water that goes into a 1,000-pound steer would float a destroyer."[5] On the other hand, to produce the flour to bake a loaf of bread requires just 145 gallons of water.[6] Moreover, all fruit and vegetable production in the United States uses less water than what beef production alone consumes.[7]

Total world cereal demand—increasingly for animal feed—is projected to grow by nearly 50 percent within the next quarter-century.[8] In turn, by 2025 about 2.7 billion people—nearly a third of the projected population—are expected to live in regions marked by severe water scarcity.[9] Already, nearly half a billion people in 29 countries face water shortages.[10]

Three quarters of the earth's surface is covered by water; most is undrinkable. Only a tiny portion of all the water in the world is usable by humans, and little fresh water is renewed by nature.[11] Now consider that 70 percent of this precious amount—taken from the world's rivers, lakes, and underground wells—goes to agriculture[12] and that the term "agriculture" increasingly has come to mean "animal agriculture," which uses far greater amounts of water than agriculture that produces foods for direct human consumption. Yet the dwindling of the world's water stores has not warranted anything approaching adequate international concern.

In the developing world—where, in the near term, great increases in population are predicted to take place—demand for meat is expected to grow by 2.7 percent per year up until 2015.[13] Today, 37 percent of the world's harvested grain is animal feed; in the United States, the proportion has climbed to a sobering 70 percent. "If you destroy the animal agricultural industries, you dismantle most of all agriculture," one Midwestern farm writer once tellingly explained.[14]

Going deep

Almost everywhere around the world, water is a concern.

- Australia, for instance, is facing water shortages, yet it has created a net loss for its precious stores by way of its beef exports.[15]
- In the United States, groundwater is being withdrawn 25 percent faster than it is being replenished.[16] In parts of Arizona, the pumping rate is ten times faster than the recharge rate.[17]
- By 2010, irrigated agriculture will probably cease outright in one of China's primary grain-producing regions, halving the country's crop yields.[18]
- With riches in oil, not water, Middle Eastern countries have turned to a solution that would be considered ludicrous anywhere else: desalinization. Salt- and mineral-imbued water is made fresh via energy-intense evaporation processes.
- It is estimated that a half a billion people will be without clean water in Africa by 2025, spurring boundary clashes[19] and leaving farmers unable to grow crops.[20]
- Without government control over the expansion of pumps and wells, Indian farmers have been taking 200 cubic kilometers of water out of the earth per year, with monsoon rains doing little to replenish the drain. "When the balloon bursts, untold anarchy will be the lot of rural India," warned the head of the groundwater station in Gujarat at the 2004 Stockholm Water Symposium.[21]

The stingy earth

Granted, today's water shortfalls are also a product of 45,000 dams worldwide (which can divert as well as direct water where it is needed), pollution, deforestation, urbanization, and general mismanagement.[22] In the United States it is estimated that only half of irrigated water reaches crops; the rest evaporates or seeps away.[23] In any event, adding to such diversions and inefficiencies with the profligate wastefulness of meat is not what the world needs.

People all over the world are in various ways producing foods grown unsustainably—that is, using water that is essentially borrowed from future generations. Every drop that is contaminated or diverted out of reach will eventually return, fresh and clean—this is true—but at earth's own glacial pace. A world transformed to one that favors vegetarianism would take enormous pressure off scarce water supplies.

9 Epidemiologically speaking

THE CHINESE VINDICATOR

"Our study suggests that the closer one approaches a total plant food diet, the greater the health benefit."—T. Colin Campbell, Ph.D., lead researcher, Cornell-Oxford-China Nutrition Project[1]

Want to know just how a diet ranks as a preventer or a promoter of disease? The best way is to examine the dietary habits of separate populations that not only don't eat the same foods but don't suffer from the same illnesses or die from the same causes.

The Cornell-Oxford-China Nutrition Project (the "China Study") ranks as the supreme example of this kind of examination, known as an epidemiological study. In the late 1980s, researchers gathered 367 pieces of data on 6,500 families in 130 rural Chinese villages.[2] The data are particularly reliable, because the subjects were of the same genetic background and tended to reside in their respective native regions for their entire lives; they also consumed locally produced food. Furthermore, because the China Study was designed in a holistic fashion, that is, taking into account a myriad of factors all at one time, its conclusions are considered exceptionally compelling. This study, according to registered dietitian Bob LeRoy-SiBrava, looked at "real populations of real human beings going through their real lives, in order to find out what actually happens to their health."[3]

A comprehensive analysis of the data was at first made over a five–year period, but ongoing interpretations continue to this day. From the 8,000 significant correlations[4] the study brought forth—a bonanza by any measure—we can now feel confident in the assertion that to be human is to be vegetarian.

Calling it like it is: Meat is a carcinogen

The China Study showed that the consumption of foods containing *animal protein*—not fat or cholesterol particularly—is clearly linked to heart disease, hormonal cancers, osteoporosis, and diabetes.[5]

Subsequent studies, according to one of the lead researchers of the China Study, T. Colin Campbell, Ph.D., have strengthened this finding by showing that health benefits do not come to people who simply switch from beef to chicken and fish. Such changeovers merely lower the consumption of fat without lowering the consumption of animal protein.[6]

It bears mentioning that a more up-to-date study of 29,000 post-menopausal women, published in the *American Journal of Epidemiology*, demonstrated the health risks of consuming protein from animal rather than plant sources.[7] The author of the U.S. study, Dr. Linda E. Kelemen, declared in 2005 that the findings should be a concern to those on today's faddish high-protein diets, which push for copious amounts of animal-based foods. "Not all proteins are equal," she stated when the study was publicized.[8] Protein from animal sources specifically can promote artery-clogging plaques. Plant-based proteins simply do not have this effect.

The China Study found that there is virtually no threshold for which lower plasma cholesterol levels do not indicate more protection from disease.[9] Researchers interpret this to mean that even small amounts of animal protein-containing foods in the diet begin to raise risk, not only for heart disease but also for various types of cancers—namely, those of the liver, colon, rectum, lung, brain, blood and bone marrow (leukemia), as well as childhood cancers.[10]

By standards developed in the 1950s, a substance can officially be labeled a carcinogen even if it must be consumed in large quantities to cause cancer. Taking everything into account, Dr. Campbell has concluded that animal protein should be labeled a carcinogen. "In my view, no chemical carcinogen is nearly so important in causing human cancer as animal protein," he asserts.[11]

Other findings of the China Study

- Americans eat proportionally more protein than rural Chinese do, with 70 percent of this derived from animal protein. In stark contrast, only seven percent of the protein that rural Chinese consume is animal-derived.[12]
- Rural Chinese intake of fat is about a quarter to a third of Americans' intake.[13] Reducing fat intake to 15 percent of calories "would prevent 80 to 90 percent of chronic degenerative diseases such as cancer, cardiovascular diseases and diabetes [experienced by Americans] before about age 65," according to Dr. Campbell.[14]
- Osteoporosis is not common in rural China, despite the fact that the inhabitants typically do not drink milk.[15] Calcium is primarily obtained from green vegetables.
- Higher intake of animal protein and lower intake of green vegetables is associated with cardiovascular disease.[16]

- The China Study strongly supported the idea that dietary fiber is essential to human health.[17]
- The rural Chinese tend to have cholesterol levels well below half those considered optimal in the West.[18]

Dr. Campbell has asserted that if China adopts a meat diet to the extent found in the West, the cost to that country in lost productivity, and in treating the extent of degenerative diseases, could soar to anywhere between $300 billion and $600 billion per year.[19]

Ultimately, the epic examination known as the China Study provides a world-class vegetarian vindication. As developing countries become more affluent, they would be wise to take this research to heart by eschewing Western diets and hanging on to their traditional, primarily vegetarian ways of eating.

10 Low rungs

MEAT'S LABORERS

"Automation, which has liberated thousands from backbreaking drudgery, has created a Dickensian time warp for others."—Tony Horwitz, undercover at a poultry processing plant for the *Wall Street Journal*[1]

Slaughterhouse laborer, poultry processing line worker, stock hand, "dairy slave," deck mate: Who would elect to work in these low-paying, inhumane, unhealthy, unsavory, and dangerous occupations? Surely no one who had any choices in life. Recruiters from large U.S. slaughterhouses, for instance, lament that given the low pay scales, keeping employees is a major problem. *The New Yorker* quoted such a recruiter: "Last month, I hired 85 people and 92 left....The biggest problem is...nobody wants to kill cows."[2]

Slaughterhouse human resources departments—if you can call them that—do have to be creative. They might get their employees from prisons or halfway houses. Recruiting from undocumented labor also has its place. *Business Week* reported in 2002 that the government reckoned Tyson Foods, the poultry giant, harbored thousands of illegal workers.[3] In just one raid of an IBP plant, the Immigration and Naturalization Service arrested 142 workers.[4] Periodically, newspaper accounts reveal employee-seeking smuggling rings.[5] Needless to say, illegal immigrants, whose primary worries are about being fired or deported, don't complain much about dangerous working environments, the unrelenting pace, lack of benefits, or poverty wages.

They don't unionize either. Indeed, it was beef giant IBP that first set up the now-common small-town mega-slaughterhouse, far away from the union strongholds of the big cities where 30 years ago a worker could make $18 an hour.[6] A slaughterhouse job was actually a coveted position then.[7] Now, immigrant labor works for $9.50 an hour.[8]

Hell on earth for the humans, too

So what does an industry that slaughters billions of poultry birds and large mammals every year dish up for its mostly unionless workforce? Epidemic incidences of repetitive stress injuries, frigid room temperatures, deafening noise, slippery grease- and puddle-covered floors, fellow knife-brandishing co-workers in tight quarters, exhausting hours, and mind-numbing monotony. Bathroom breaks are afforded to workers grudgingly.

Meanwhile, breakneck conveyor speeds of 91 birds a minute[9] and 400 cattle per hour transform misery into mayhem. When taken together, meatpacking and poultry processing have the highest incidence of repetitive stress disorders.[10] Plant workers may typically perform the same movement 10,000 times per day.[11] One in five packing plant workers experiences a work-related injury or illness every year.[12] The rate of serious injury in a meatpacking plant—that is, getting burned, mangled, sawed, lacerated, caught, doused, gouged, decapitated, pulverized, crushed, stunned, or hanged by machinery or other hazards—is five times the national average.[13] Dizzying line speeds may not allow workers enough time to adequately dispatch the animals, leaving other workers no choice but to butcher them alive. At these times, laborers can be floored by thousand-pound creatures flailing and fighting for their lives.[14]

Hazardous and thankless

Chicken catchers—those poor souls who gather up thousands of chickens from factory sheds for overnight truck rides to slaughterhouses—work 12–hour shifts, but their pay leaves them in poverty.

In general, chemicals and fumes are hazards for those in factory farming's dirty-boot jobs. Poisonous concentrations of dust, hydrogen sulfide, and ammonia from manure eat the lungs. Fifty-eight percent of swine confinement workers have chronic bronchitis.[15] Dairy workers live in constant pain, not only from ailments that are the result of noxious fumes, but from repetitive stress disorders and injuries sustained from cow kicks.[16] Agricultural workers are excluded from the National Labor Relations Act, which gives other workers the right to organize and complain about conditions without fear of employer reprisal.[17]

Down the line at the rendering plant where the industry processes by-product carcass material for industrial ingredients and raw materials, workers likewise suffer asphyxiating fumes in the form of aerosolized fat.[18]

Troubling waters

Finally, there's the plight of the fisher. Worldwide, 24,000 of them die on the job annually, making fishing the deadliest occupation in the world.[19] In one cataclysmic night, 1,400 fishers died in a cyclone off the Indian state of Andhra Pradesh.[20] And probably a year's worth of fisher deaths occurred in just one day as a result of the great tsunami of December 26, 2004. Furthermore, fishing is blighted as a bastion of slavery, with as many as 15 percent of the world's vessels filled with crews in fear of starvation and physical and sexual abuse.[21] Apparently, a harvest of violence nets a sea of exploitation.

11 Hunger/meat connection

IT CUTS LIKE A SCYTHE

"All the world is a birthday cake, so take a piece but not too much."—George Harrison, "It's All Too Much," *Yellow Submarine*, 1968

We humans are eating ourselves out of global house and home. Already, according to the World Wide Fund for Nature (WWF), we need the resource equivalent of 1.2 planet earths to sustain our current rate of consumption—5 planet earths if the whole world lived at consumption levels of Americans.[1] In other words, we are now dipping into our planetary capital, killing off our host, and squandering that which belongs to other people—those who will live after us. Our meat consumption has a lot to do with this.

How, not how many

Most people point to the population pressures that loom over humanity as the slippery slope of man's undoing. Yes, we humans are reproducing ourselves at a galloping pace (7.5 billion projected by 2025 and 8.9 billion by 2050, up from 6.4 billion in 2004).[2] But *how* our growing numbers live may be more pivotal to our fate.

Lester R. Brown warns that if population grows as predicted, the food sector will be the first to unravel. "Eroding soils, deteriorating rangelands, collapsing fisheries, falling water tables, and rising temperatures are converging to make it more difficult to expand food production fast enough to keep up with demand,"[3] he writes. Brown's scenario, however, is dependent upon humanity's carnivorous habits staying the same or, as predicted, increasing headlong: The world is projected to eat 57 percent more meat in 2020 than it did in 1997.[4]

In theory, most of the resultant environmental devastation—and attendant human misery—could be substantially alleviated. According to the Population Reference Bureau: "If everyone adopted a vegetarian diet and no food were wasted, current [food] production would theoretically feed 10 billion people [56 percent more people than alive today]—more than the projected population for the year 2050."[5]

Haves and have nots

Cultivating grain to feed livestock—37 percent of the world's total is handed over to the world's animals—is folly in the extreme. Calculations vary widely, but generally to produce one pound of beef, pork, or chicken you need 7, 6, and 2.7 pounds of grain, respectively.[6] Some calculate the grain/beef ratio at 12:1. The meat industry, of course, works to improve on feed-to-flesh efficiency, but its endeavors come at the expense of the animals via genetic tinkering and growth-enhancing drugs.

For humans to have to compete with any other creature on earth for food might be a regrettable situation if it were something of a natural given. But in the case of industrial agriculture, farmers actually promote this situation by propagating these grain-eating animals by the billions. Meanwhile, 18 million people around the globe actually starve to death every year,[7] and some 840 million[8]—including 150 million children in the developing world[9]—face chronic hunger.

Wars, political turmoil, and greedy warlords contribute to inadequate food distribution, of course. Still, in a tragic irony, there is roughly a direct correlation between the amount of grain needed to eradicate world hunger and the amount of grain fed to U.S. livestock.[10]

The human quest for meat to the degree it has been indulged today inflicts a gouging effect on the carrying capacity of our world. And no planet in the immediate vicinity seems ready to offer any relief.

12 Almost human

ANIMAL INTELLIGENCE AND EMOTION

"When animals are seen as automatons with no emotions, it is easy to treat them as mere property with which humans can do as they please."—Marc Bekoff, Professor of Biology, University of Colorado, Boulder, and Fellow of the Animal Behavior Society[1]

The research is pouring in. Word is getting out. Animals appear to be a whole lot like us. And why not? Could emotion and intelligence in humans have appeared all of a sudden from out of nowhere? Some of our cousins in the evolutionary tree of life—chimpanzees, bonobos, gorillas, and orangutans—share at least 98 percent of our DNA.[2] Our closest relatives use tools, recognize themselves in mirrors, dose themselves with medicinal plants when sick, have diverse "traditions," relay complicated messages using symbolic language, and even, in their way, engage in art, music, and sophisticated politics.[3]

Nor are such extraordinary abilities limited to primates, or even mammals. European jays can recall the locations of more than 6,000 seeds nine months after leaving them.[4] Some ant species farm fungus for food.[5] Beavers engineer precision dams and avoid having to hibernate by creating winter lodges—complete with "refrigerators" to keep the branches they like to eat fresh. "Maid service" is provided by muskrats, who pay "rent" to the beavers by keeping the reed bedding tidy and clean.[6]

To survive, many animals must master lessons that instinct could never cover. For birds, there is the colossal task of committing to memory thousands of miles of migration routes. An adolescent squirrel separated from his mother will die from ignorance of how to live in the wild. Some dolphins learn "proboscis padding" from one another—that is, the technique of spearing sea sponges to help them root around rocky crevasses to scare prey within reach. These behaviors are not merely hard-wired into the animals' brains but are part of what scientists are characterizing as traditions or "culture" passed on from generation to generation.[7]

Animals also express a full repertoire of feelings: Sympathy, devotion, joy, jealousy, grief, anger, embarrassment, and love.[8] Elephants, gorillas, and dolphins mourn their dead.[9] Dopamine, a neurochemical associated with pleasure in humans, is found to be released in the brains of rats when they are at play.[10] Buffaloes apparently like to ice skate and will make sounds of glee as they glide across frozen ground.[11] Whales have been seen doing an alluring "dance" that might be akin to post-coital cuddling in humans.[12] Ravens are said to fall in love,[13] be devious and deceptive, and understand that other beings have thoughts of their own.[14]

And what of animals, such as dogs, pigs, whales, and, in at least one case, a kangaroo, who have rescued a human or another animal from danger? Can we add empathy to the list of qualities displayed by animals? Taken together, the evidence shows our fellow creatures possessing all of these traits, plus probably the most important one of all: Each has the capacity to feel pain and experience fear and suffering.

The animals some call food

A look into the extraordinary traits research has discovered in the animals some people call food is equally illustrative.

- "For me they are as individual as dogs," reports Callum Roberts, one of the world's leading conservation biologists speaking about his favorite animals, fish.[15] "After a while you detect personalities." Fish are very smart, too, Roberts attests, recalling from his younger days that if he missed one with a spear the first time, he didn't get a second chance.
- Chickens that are kept as pets become trusting and lovable companions.[16] They are intelligent, social, protective, compassionate, empathetic, and discerning when faced with a problem.[17] They greet the day with gusto—basking in the sun, stretching their wings, foraging for food, and dust bathing before settling down and engaging in a rich array of social patterns, including a wide variety of calls.[18]
- Pigs are the brainy ones of the barnyard. According to Professor Stanley Curtis of Pennsylvania State University, pigs are creative and innovative, equal in intelligence to the brightest chimpanzees. He taught several of them to understand complex relationships between actions and objects in order to play video games. Once the pigs learned to use the joystick—which took no longer than for any chimp—the pigs figured out the screen games, sometimes within minutes.[19] The pigs were found to possess more ability to focus than chimps. And in other studies, pigs were found to crave attention, becoming depressed if isolated or denied playtime.[20] Psychological distress was found to lead to physical maladies. According to farmed animal welfare specialist Temple Grandin, pigs can form images in their minds, think in pictures, and act by conscious intention.[21]

- Sheep have been found to recognize up to 50 other sheep and up to 10 human faces when presented with flash cards, even after two years.[22]
- Cows produce more milk when soothing recordings are played. Milk production has been shown to increase by 3 percent with slow, stress-reducing music.[23]

We are family

Scientists have discovered 500 perfectly matched DNA fragments among species as unrelated as mice and men.[24] Research now reveals that animals, including humans, share their commonality of form because we all use the exact same set of genes that build the most elementary aspects of our bodies, proving a simple though profound biological fact: We all share a common ancestor.[25] We are all—mammals, birds, amphibians, reptiles, fish, and insects alike—quite profoundly part of the same family.

13 Nitrogen elixir

PETROCHEMICAL TREADMILL

"How are you going to bring things back when you can't see the bottom in six inches of water?"—Chesapeake Bay ecologist Walter Boynton[1]

In the early twentieth century, chemists discovered a way to extract nitrogen from the atmosphere, cheaply and in large quantities. Nitrogen, which constitutes nearly four-fifths of the air by volume, is what allows plant life to grow. Yet the planet's own mechanisms (lightning and certain bacteria are able to fix nitrogen naturally) make this element only sparingly available. The chemists' discovery, therefore, signaled an end to humanity's 10,000-year search for a viable way to boost crop yields—not a small achievement. The consequences of the discovery, however, may ultimately be the greatest Faustian bargain of all time.

Today's nitrogen bounty has become the fertilizer that fueled what has become known as the Green Revolution, an age of crop bounty so monumental that scientists estimate that two billion more people inhabit the earth today than otherwise might have.[2] Just as significant, the world is now able to support populations of meat eaters never before seen, in fact making diseases of excess epidemic in many parts of the world. In any case, this state of plenty—every fourth person on earth is overweight[3]—has kept the dour Malthusians eating their words. (Thomas Malthus was the nineteenth-century philosopher who prophesied that population increases would eventually outstrip food supply.)

Even at current population numbers, which are predicted to rise dramatically in coming years, humans consume 40 percent of what scientists describe as "primary productivity"—or the total amount of plant mass created by earth.[4] And we are just one species among millions. The copious use of man-made fertilizers, which keeps humans supplied with so much agricultural bounty, is sure to eventually catch up to us before we know it, as waterways from the China countryside to the Ohio Valley are already severely polluted by nitrogen runoff. Indeed, just as this life-giving elixir makes crops on land grow lush and green, fertilizer runoff in waterways causes algae to fecundate, robbing fish of oxygen.

Feeding the harvest to foragers

Before the days of cheap fertilizer, no one for a moment would have considered handing over grains, so laborious to produce, to livestock able to forage. But in certain parts of the world today—our own, for one—doing just this has become nearly universal, if not mandatory, in the marketplace. Meanwhile, more commercial nitrogen fertilizer was applied to the soil worldwide between 1985 and 2000 than during all of human history up until this time.[5] Today, waterways in North America and Europe contain 20 times the nitrogen they did before the Industrial Revolution.[6]

Every year, man-made nitrogen inputs exceed the amount of nitrogen the planet itself naturally cycles into the earth.[7] In central China, pig and chicken farms produce more than 40 times as much nitrogen pollution as do all the region's factories.[8] Just a quarter-century ago, harmful algal blooms (HABs), loosely known as "red tides," were relatively rare along U.S. coastlines.[9] Now they heavily dot the national map. Excess nitrogen in the environment is unquestionably behind this phenomenon. In 2004, a particularly monstrous "red tide," the size of Massachusetts, hit the coastline off eastern China.[10] It will not be the last.

Today's mountains of manure—here by the grace of nitrogen-fertilizer-pumped grains—allow the world's excess nitrogen an additional vector into the environment, particularly the water. Approximately one-third of all the agricultural toxic runoff in the United States is caused by animal waste.[11] Even human waste contains more nitrogen than ever before, since people are eating unprecedented amounts of meat.[12] It often ends up untreated in the water as well.

Natural cleansers wiped clean

According to the U.S. Department of Commerce, more than "50 million acres of cropland in the Mississippi River Basin have been drained by tile lines, ditches, and other means."[13] The runoff has become one of the primary sources of nitrate in the Gulf of Mexico.[14] In order to feed society's hunger for meat, vast amounts of feed crops—corn primarily—have not only fouled the environment with nitrogen fertilizer but have replaced the prairies and wetlands that could have otherwise provided vital cleansing mechanisms.

Earth's ecosystems, which evolved using essentially tiny amounts of nitrogen extremely efficiently, are now being poisoned by today's gluts. Ultimately, a world transformed to vegetarianism could go far to stem the toll of excess nitrogen on our planet. To produce a gram of wheat flour, only 3 grams of nitrogen are needed. To produce a gram of meat you need over 15 grams of nitrogen.[15]

14 Genetic integrity

THE ANIMALS' ULTIMATE SACRIFICE

"Genetic diversity is an insurance against future threats such as famine, drought and epidemics."—Irene Hoffmann, chief, Animal Production Service, Food and Agriculture Organization of the UN.[1]

Domesticated livestock have been with us for at least 10,000 years. Yet for nearly all of this epic period, the breeds that man brought forth into existence retained genes that allowed the animals to thrive outdoors—if not in the wild. A radical change, however, took place in the twentieth century with the advent of cheap energy and cheap grain. The ability that livestock always had of being able to forage outdoors on plants that humans cannot eat was no longer a necessity or even an advantage. We are now able to do two things never before imagined: bring the majority of our livestock indoors and produce grain on the animals' behalf. These changes led to the animals being selectively bred for genetic traits with a new set of objectives: improving meat quality and acclimating animals to indoor life.

Mutant genes cultivated in the laboratory

The immeasurable cruelty that farmed animals endure today begins with a supreme indignity, the taking of that which defines the very essence of their being: their genetic makeup. With the historically unique set of givens bearing down with inimitable economic force, genetics has become as important a component of today's intensive farming as drugs and confinement hardware. The animals themselves, right down to their DNA, must stand up to the rigors of the industrial process, both in life and in carcass form. They must produce and reproduce at breakneck speeds and do so on as little feed as possible. And ultimately, the particular output they unwillingly give forth must please our final end user, the consumer, in texture, taste, uniformity, convenience, and price. Today, mutant genes that would never survive in the wild are cultivated in the laboratory to monstrous ends.

Ticky-tacky, all the same

In its quest for productivity, the meat industry has employed the imprudent breeding practice of single-trait selection. With its primary tool, artificial insemination, one bull can sire hundreds of thousands—and in at least one case, millions—of offspring. Indeed, the world's turkeys are supplied by three corporate breeders; the world's broilers (chickens used for meat) are supplied by six transnationals.[2]

Replacing genetic diversity in agriculture with monocultural uniformity threatens food security by bringing on the risk of widespread disease—more of a concern since 9/11. When one animal gets sick, frequently they all do, since they all embody nearly identical genes and their confinement is likely to be intensive. An analogy might be made with dried kindling in a tinderbox: a disaster waiting to happen. Crop monoculture, which is also now fully instituted in the United States, similarly courts disaster from pest outbreaks and blights.

Modern agriculture officially frowns on monoculture and single-trait selection, but it has been hard-pressed to set them aside. Ultimately, the rest of us can send a message regarding this uniformity by rejecting the final products that it creates. Along these lines, commercial meat is a good place to start.

15 Overkill

THE CULL OF THE INNOCENT

"When I went to bed and closed my eyes, I could still hear the chickens screaming. I felt terrible. I couldn't stop thinking about it. Those chickens were innocent."—Hong Kong civil servant, part of bird-flu eradication campaign, 1998[1]

Keep thousands, or even millions, of animals intensively confined on relatively small areas of land, and you substantially raise the risk for disease outbreak or even pandemic. True, animal death from disease is a daily occurrence on factory farms with losses figured into farmers' business plans. Catastrophic mortalities, however, are something altogether different, though not entirely unusual.

Disease can kill off a farm full of animals. A farmer may be forced to destroy his animals if a disease simply makes them less than profitable. Or, if a disease is especially contagious or widespread, whole armies of government workers may be called in to prophylactically exterminate legions of animals—sick or not. Workers called to this type of detail invariably are left psychologically scarred.

The wasting of life: Sick and the healthy alike

As of 2004, the actual number of cattle afflicted with mad cow disease in the United Kingdom was 180,000; 4.5 million animals, however, were eradicated as a buffer.

The number of sheep, cattle, and pigs afflicted with foot and mouth disease (FMD) in England's 2001 epidemic came to a mere 2,030, but more than 6 million animals, mostly sheep, were destroyed just the same.

Governments are invariably saddled with the burden of these types of eradication campaigns—not only in terms of the military personnel they provide for the job, but by way of disaster-relief packages that compensate producers for their losses. According to a news story during England's FMD cull, "Livestock were trucked into the Great Orton airfield and government workers nearby prepared a mass grave the size of two football fields."[2] A post-mortem report described the campaign as "bigger and more complex than the UK involvement in the 1991 Gulf War."[3]

In 1997, Taiwan was also hit with an FMD epidemic. The country slaughtered nearly 14 million pigs to eradicate the contagion.[4] Conscripted soldiers, clad in plastic suits, sent squealing pigs to incinerators and mass graves to the consternation of the nation's television viewers.

Humans in the crossfire

Terrifying, though so far rare, are the instances when an animal disease actually jumps the species barrier to infect humans directly. In Malaysia, in 1999, chaos ensued with the emergence of what became known as Nipah virus. Pigs had directly infected over 250 people. Consequently, nearly a million pigs were herded into pens, shot, and buried.[5] Before the army moved in, panicked farmers had been seen beating their animals to death or dumping them live into mass graves.[6]

It was as recently as 1997 that humans started contracting influenza directly from birds for the first time in history.[7] The strain, H5N1, which has a high death rate, resurfaced in 2003. In 2004 a pan-Asian outbreak of the contagion killed 24 people, and 200 million birds died or were destroyed.[8] People continue to die sporadically from the strain.

Animal disease in America

The United States has not been spared the ravages of animal disease. Sporadic outbreaks are in fact relatively common in America, with some cases affecting entire regions. A major U.S. outbreak of foot and mouth disease occurred in 1929. In 1983 and 1984 an outbreak of avian influenza forced the eradication of 17 million birds in Pennsylvania, New Jersey, Maryland, and Virginia[9] at a cost to the federal government of $60 million. In the fall of 2002 an outbreak of Exotic Newcastle disease in California had the potential to spread to 280 million chickens and turkeys on commercial farms in the state.[10] Total disaster in this case was averted, however, and many fewer—about two million chickens—were eventually destroyed.

Don't forget the fish

Fish farms, as well, are notorious bastions for diseases. Infectious salmon anemia, for instance, has wiped out millions of fish in Europe and North America.[11] In 1995 a shrimp virus ripped through Texas aquaculture pens up and down the state's Gulf Coast. On just one 630-acre farm, nearly all 45 million shrimp perished within days.[12]

16 Cancer connection

THE "BIG C" AND MEAT

"Meat, at most, should be considered as a garnish"—John Potter, head researcher of leading panel review of 4,500 cancer studies, 1997[1]

According to the American Institute for Cancer Research and the World Cancer Research Fund, poor eating habits account for a third of all cancers, the same proportion attributed to smoking.[2] In 1997, these two organizations concurred that those interested in reducing the risk of many types of cancer should consume a diet of little or no meat—at most three ounces per day (about the size of a deck of cards).[3] Fifteen scientists, working for three years, had reviewed 4,500 scientific studies and papers on the relationship between cancer and lifestyle. The diet they recommend consists mostly of fruits, vegetables, cereals, and legumes.[4] Fats, they say, should be limited and come primarily from plant sources. They declared that up to 40 percent of cancers are preventable, with diet, physical activity, and body weight appearing to have a measurable bearing on risk.[5] If people ate markedly less meat and more vegetables, they contend, it could prevent four million cases of cancer worldwide per year.[6] The World Health Organization has more or less seconded these numbers.[7]

Lowering risk with veggies

A State University of Buffalo study in 1985 discovered that not only are poor diets linked to cancer, they appear to negatively impact a person's survival once the disease takes hold. When researchers monitored the food choices of breast cancer patients who were near death, they found that the risk of dying at any point in time increased by 40 percent for every 1,000 grams of fat consumed per month—approximately the difference between the typical American diet and a low-fat, near-vegetarian diet.[8]

Another study published in 1994 in the *British Medical Journal* isolated cancer risk for vegetarians specifically. After researchers had followed the diets of 6,115 vegetarians and 5,015 meat eaters over 12 years, it found that a meatless diet will yield a 40 percent lower risk of cancer and a 20 percent lower risk of dying from any cause.[9]

The National Research Council, an arm of the National Academy of Sciences, declared in 1996 that chemicals such as pesticides and food additives were mostly negligible causes of cancer.[10] A panel study published a year later in the journal *Cancer* suggested that not eating fruits and vegetables because of fear of pesticides was in fact far riskier than eating them.[11]

Heterocyclic, polycyclic

In addition, heterocyclic amines (HCAs) and polycyclic aromatic hydrocarbons (PAHs)—both carcinogenic substances—are created during the process of frying, broiling, barbecuing, charring, and simply cooking animal muscle.[12] PAHs arise when fat from animal flesh drips onto an open flame. The smoke that envelops the meat above contains the cancer-causing substance. HCAs are created in the meat just by extended cooking times.

The National Cancer Institute found that those who preferred well-done rather than rare and medium-rare beef faced triple the risk of stomach and esophageal cancers.[13] Well-done meats are also linked with colon, breast, and possibly prostate cancer.[14] Such information, of course, is at odds with advice that urges thorough cooking in order to neutralize the many deadly bacteria found in meat.

Two broccolis, call me in the morning

On the positive side, fruits and vegetables are packed with antioxidants that fight the daily assaults of free radical damage caused by highly reactive cancer-causing oxygen molecules. Also, fresh fruits, vegetables, grains, and legumes provide thousands of phytochemicals, stimulating enzymes in our bodies that detoxify cancer-causing substances.[15] The blood of vegetarians has even been found to contain 12 times the level of salicylic acid found in meat eaters' blood. Copious amounts of the chemical, which is the active ingredient in aspirin, are contained in fruits and vegetables. The substance acts as an anti-inflammatory agent, which may be an important reason why vegetarians are less likely to suffer from certain cancers and hardening of the arteries.[16]

17 Prescription contamination

ANIMALS ON DRUGS

"Pharmaceuticals should not be recommended or used without good reason."—Handbook of Livestock Management Techniques[1]

Modern farming could not exist as we know it without drugs and chemicals. Factory farmed animals, who would otherwise become ill and even die from the conditions in which they're forced to live, are kept alive with vaccines, antibiotics, sulfa drugs, anti-inflammatories, and vitamins. Hormones and antibiotics speed growth. Medications that induce birth, instigate estrus, synchronize heat cycles, and produce superovulation for embryo transfer will work to micromanage the animals' reproductive systems. And, since the animals today generally spend their lives living in their own waste, disinfectants, antiseptics, insecticides, and medications in general are required to control bacteria, pests, parasites, and worms.[2]

Residue permeating, farm to table

An array of concerns must be tended to when drugs are administered to animals.[3] Precise records must be kept and proper dosages and dosage intervals need to be maintained. Proper administering routes (oral, intramuscular, subcutaneous, or intravenous) must be adhered to. A drug must go to the right species, be applied in a safe manner, and, in most cases, be withdrawn for a designated period of time prior to slaughter. A drug should be legal. All of these requirements need to hold, often for a dizzying number of animals in a single operation. Nationwide, 95 percent of U.S. beef cattle, or 33 millions animals every year, are treated with steroid hormones (just one example)—a logistical nightmare by any measure.[4]

In the factory environment, veterinarians tend to improvise.[5] Mix-ups happen, causing the animals to suffer side effects or worse. Residues in meat can cause consumers to experience allergic reactions or antibiotic resistance to important human drugs.

Drugs can get into end-product meat via overdoses, uneven releases of drugs throughout the animals' bodies (in the case of time-release implants), or because of inadequate pre-slaughter drug-withdrawal periods. Troughs of drug-laced feed are not always thoroughly cleaned before necessarily drug-free feed is poured in,[6] and, since up to 90 percent of certain drugs can survive an animal's digestive tract,[7] manure, which is often a component in feed, can transmit residues.[8]

Criminal and unscrupulous

Most meat and dairy samples are within residue limits, according to the Union of Concerned Scientists.[9] However, critics point to the fact that the government doesn't actually test for all the drugs in the marketplace. Such oversight would be prohibitively expensive. Still, with so many avenues in which drugs are able to taint meat, the lack of oversight might give some consumers pause. People do at times become very ill from drug residues in their meat. They don't always learn the cause of their illnesses, however—such knowledge is often dependent on a trend being spotted when many people become sick.[10]

For all the causes for which drugs can taint meat, not all are accidental or unintentional. Criminal or just unscrupulous mishandling of drugs is always a possibility. In one case, a man who specialized in buying sick, old, crippled, and diseased cattle was caught putting the animals' slaughtered remains into the commercial food supply prematurely, that is, before drug regimens had run their course.[11] In general, so-called fancy veal has been found more likely than other cuts of meat to contain dangerous or illegal levels of drugs. A scandal linking the steroid clenbuterol and "milk-fed" veal broke in 1994. The drug, which is banned in the United States but readily available over the Internet, allows crated calves to gain muscle weight despite inactivity. A federal review of drug-residue violations found veal to be the top offender, which stands to reason: Producers must overcompensate for the severe conditions in which veal calves are kept.[12] Exceedingly more often than pork and chicken, bovine-derived meat, in general, is in violation for drug residues.

Safer, not cheaper

A group of hog farmers who have certified to their customers that the animals they raise are 100 percent drug-free admit that their form of husbandry is very time-consuming. Not surprisingly, the conditions for the animals must be kept immaculately clean—germ-free, dry, temperate, well ventilated, and stress-free. These animals must be kept on a nutritious diet. All told, these things bring farmers' costs up by 20 percent.[13]

In the end, consumers can take their pick about the meat they eat: expensive or potentially drug-contaminated. Or, of course, they can "just say no" to meat altogether.

18 Pandemic in the making

FARMED ANIMAL/INFLUENZA CONNECTION

"In Asia we have a huge animal population, a huge bird population, and two-thirds of the world's people living there."—Klaus Stohr, chief influenza scientist, World Health Organization[1]

The world saw three influenza pandemics in the twentieth century. The worst of them, in 1918, caused perhaps 50 million people to perish over a three–year period.[2] Meanwhile, the conditions that gave rise to this as well as other epic influenza outbreaks are still with us. And animal agriculture is right there behind it all. Indeed, scientists fear the next influenza pandemic is at hand[3] and in fact overdue.[4] The head of the World Health Organization's Global Influenza Program, Klaus Stohr, has said, "There is no doubt there will be another pandemic."[5] As seen with SARS, modern air travel greatly facilitates the spread of infectious disease. A super-mutated version of the influenza strain now putting Asia on edge (see reason #15) could, according to Stohr, conceivably sicken 30 percent of the human population.[6] A billion people could die.[7]

Scientists now have a grasp on how influenza pandemics, such as the one in 1918, take hold: Overcrowded conditions, they tell us, involving domesticated animals, constitute the pivotal element of influenza transmission, although the genesis of the disease derives from migratory birds who pass their illnesses on to farms. Particularly deadly strains that do not survive long in the wild can take hold among intensively confined poultry since so many hosts are available in tight quarters.[8]

From factory-farmed chickens, it is believed, deadly flu viruses can spread to domesticated pigs, who may also harbor human influenza genes in their lungs. Pig lungs at this point provide the perfect mixing bowl for the exchange of genetic material between human and bird influenza viruses.[9] New strains are then able to reinfect humans. Throughout Southeastern Asia—considered the cradle of influenza—it is not uncommon for pigs to share barn space with chickens and for barns to be located in areas heavily populated with humans. Furthermore, most Asian nations lack sophisticated veterinary surveillance systems that could otherwise keep tabs on emerging infections.[10]

Pandemic precursor

The winter of 2003–04 was witness to an unprecedented outbreak of domestic bird influenza that spread rapidly to ten Asian countries. The strain was particularly infectious across the species barrier. Aside from a dozen or so cats,[11] some wild crows,[12] and even 45 zoo tigers,[13] 35 people were infected by this rapidly evolving bird disease, 24 of whom died of the illness—a terrifying 69 percent mortality rate.[14] Moreover, 200 million chickens died or were hastily destroyed,[15] including countless millions incinerated or buried alive by people afraid to touch them.[16] The cull methods were so cruel as to prompt the Food and Agriculture Organization of the UN to make a rare plea for more humane kill techniques.[17]

By late summer 2004, the disease was declared endemic to wide areas across Asia.[18] The emergence of this deadly strain (H5N1)—first seen in 1997—marked the first time in history the influenza virus was transmitted directly to humans. Since then, the lungs of people—not just pigs—are now considered potential incubating vessels for a future pandemic strain. As it happens, in the short span of time between 1997 and 2004, five influenza outbreaks have occurred in which some people contracted their illnesses directly from birds.[19] Even more terrifying, the 2003–04 strain proved to be twice as deadly as the one in 1997,[20] and exceedingly more deadly to the individuals who became sick than the flu pandemic of 1918.[21] It is believed that vaccinations—however selectively used—made the current strain hardier.[22] The fear now is that any future outbreak will not only have a high mortality rate but also will have mutated into a disease with the ability to be transmitted human-to-human. Essentially, a pandemic of H5N1 could make SARS look like a picnic in the park.

Collective indifference

We need to question the acquiescence that is resigning the world to such a tragedy, when simply doing away with intensive animal agriculture would be all that is needed to wipe away the threat. To that end, it might be instructive to review the symptoms of the influenza strain that killed so many in 1918: First, the flu was marked by frenetic coughing that caused abdominal muscles to rupture. Blood would spurt from a victim's nose, ears, and eyes. Air pockets would form under victims' skin, emitting crackling and popping sounds when agitated. Sufferers screamed in pain when they were touched; even eye movements became agonizing. Some victims fell and died on the spot while walking down the street.[23] Most of the victims were young and in the prime of their lives. Sounds like something the world might want to avoid.

19 Indispensable fiber

FOUND ONLY IN PLANTS

"The result of the modern fiber-depleted diet is a whole string of ills, from constipation to colon cancer."—Neal Barnard, M.D.[1]

One of the most beneficial things you can eat has no nutrient value whatsoever. It has zero calories and is not absorbed into the body. You find it exclusively in plant foods, and it is known as fiber—or roughage. The more meat people eat, the less they are likely to get enough fiber. Because of their fiber-deficient, meat-laden diets, Americans on average consume only a third of the fiber they need.[2]

The bulk of the evidence is in

Epidemiological studies have repeatedly shown that pre-industrial populations that typically consume foods high in complex carbohydrates and fiber are free from the killer maladies of the West (heart disease, hormonal and digestive cancers, and diabetes). In fact, when people eat fiberless animal-based foods they are robbing their digestive tracts of an indispensable cleansing mechanism. Fiber acts like both a sponge and a broom to move intestinal waste out of the body. Those who do not eat it risk not only constipation but also the ailments and conditions that constipation tends to cause, namely appendicitis, hemorrhoids, varicose veins, hiatal hernia, diverticulosis,[3] and gallstones.[4] Early fiber researcher Denis Burkitt, M.D., once observed: "The only reason you have a laxative industry is because you've taken fiber out of your diet."[5]

Works like a drug

When a person does not eat fiber, he or she forgoes a nifty benefit. Fiber is filling. It can do a lot to help people on reducing diets control their appetites. Such a mechanism should be particularly welcome to the two-thirds of Americans who are either overweight or obese.

Furthermore, when people with Type II diabetes, in particular, eat the recommended 50 grams of fiber per day (admittedly a hefty amount), they are able to significantly control their blood-sugar levels, according to a peer-reviewed study in 2000.[6] The results were so dramatic that the study's subjects might as well have been taking drugs to control their conditions, researchers found.

Fiber is also good for the heart. An American study looked at nearly 69,000 women between the ages of 37 and 64 and found that fiber is likely the key factor in reducing a woman's risk for heart disease.[7]

A happy ending

In 2001, a study involving over 400,000 people in nine European countries found that a high-fiber diet slashes the risk of developing certain deadly cancers by as much as 40 percent.[8] It gathered data over an eight-year period and showed that fiber was particularly instrumental in reducing cancer of the colon and rectum. Likewise, an American study with nearly 38,000 subjects analyzed the health of people on high- and low-fiber diets. Those who ate the most fiber had a 27 percent lower risk of precancerous colon growths than did those who ate the least.[9]

In some rural areas of China, fiber intake reaches ultra-high levels of 75 grams per person per day. According to the Cornell-Oxford-China Nutrition Project, the most extensive epidemiological study ever done, the higher the fiber intake, the lower the rates of colon and rectal cancers.[10] In some areas of China, researchers found, these cancers—which are epidemic in the West—were almost nonexistent. Moreover, the study's findings challenged the notion of "eating too much fiber." Rural people in China, who adhered to a very high-fiber diet, did not show signs of suffering from mineral deficiencies.[11]

In the end, if the idea of disease in your lower tract—or, for that matter, your heart or any organ susceptible to cancer—sounds particularly unpleasant, keep eating lots and lots of fiber. In other words, go for the whole grains, legumes, fruits, and veggies!

20 Fossil fuel alchemy

THE OIL IN YOUR MEAT

"We have succeeded in industrializing the beef calf, transforming what was once a solar-powered ruminant into the very last thing we need: another fossil-fuel machine."—Michael Pollan, author and essayist[1]

The so-called Green Revolution, which burst onto the world scene in the mid-twentieth century, increased grain yields by two and a half times—nothing short of a miracle.[2] Bombarding the soil with energy-dense petrochemical fertilizers was the doctrine's paramount tenet.

Today's synthetic nitrogen, which requires natural gas for its manufacture, is powerful, compact, and portable—comparable in terms of crop boosting to what the CD-ROM disk has become to the information age. Irrigating the soil with mechanized pumps, tilling crops with motorized farm machinery, and shipping the results via gas-powered trucks are other components of the Green Revolution formula. All told, the system can essentially boil down the backbreaking human-labor equivalent of several weeks into a matter of minutes.[3] The downside is that industrial agriculture amounts to the most inefficient, sooty, and atmospherically disruptive form of food production in all of human history.[4] This "revolution" is really more black than green.

For animal agriculture specifically, this great agricultural transformation has had three components: petrochemicals, mechanization, and genetics (both plant and animal). The first two rest squarely upon the bounty of the oil age. The third is intertwined with oil, because the plants that animals eat are grown with petrochemical fertilizers,[5] and today's animals are bred to be suitable for indoor life and therefore are dependent on heating and cooling systems.

Indispensable ingredient

So energy, and plenty of it, is what the Green Revolution has been all about. And by extension, energy is the indispensable element that allows today's unprecedented (albeit geographically uneven) levels of meat consumption to exist. Indeed, 80 percent of the world's fossil energy is used by the developed world, much of it to produce the inputs of intensive animal agriculture: fertilizers, pesticides, irrigation, and general mechanization and transport.[6]

In America, it takes 400 gallons of fossil fuel equivalent on average per year to feed each citizen,[7] who, at approximately 300 pounds of animal-based foods per capita,[8] consumes 41 times the meat consumed by a person in India.[9] (Four hundred gallons of gasoline could fill the tank of a Ford Taurus about twice a month for a year.)

According to ecology professor David Pimentel, it takes, on average, eight times as much fossil fuel energy to produce animal protein as it takes to produce plant protein.[10] Beef and pork are particularly inefficient users of fossil energy. According to Richard Manning, a critic of modern food-processing methods, it takes 35 and 68 calories of fossil fuel, respectively, to make a calorie of feedlot beef and factory pork.[11]

Not surprisingly, the entrenched use of fossil fuel energy is a fundamental life-support system in every regard. Indeed, according to Canadian geographer Vaclav Smil, without petrochemical fertilizers—if farmers relied only on organic material to add nutrients to the soil—the world could not feed more than three billion people the amount of food to which we are now accustomed.[12] The population of the world is now more than twice that. At the same time, Smil asserts, there are more than enough resources on the planet today to feed everyone without increasing production and destroying the environment—that is, as long as a myriad of conservation techniques are put into place, not the least of which includes having the world shift overwhelmingly to a plant-based diet.[13] It should be noted that it takes ten calories of fossil fuel to produce one calorie of processed foods (such as breakfast cereals, soy burgers, or junk foods).[14]

Ephemeral foundation

All of this is far from academic. The highly evolved version of a world that fossil fuels have given us essentially rests on a deep dependency upon a fleeting support system. Fossil-fuel energy is non-renewable, and the era that it has so totally defined is scheduled to come to a relatively abrupt close starting as soon as 2010, when oil production is predicted to peak and prices start to climb substantially.[15] Moreover, as time goes on, fossil fuels become increasingly harder to obtain. Eventually, the oil gained is not worth the oil required to extract it.

And once the bubble bursts, the world is sure to experience a painful undoing. Already the developing world is buying time by using petrochemical fertilizers in excess to forestall the rising threat of famine[16]—eking out the bare minimum from marginal lands.[17] Yet this is where meat consumption is expected to grow most substantially—2.7 percent per year to 2015, according to the Food and Agriculture Organization of the UN.[18]

Ultimately, we have the power to avert a lot of the suffering. It's just about that time to consider more fuel-efficient foods—that is, whole foods from plants.

21 Fatal entanglements

DREDGERS, LONGLINES, AND DRIFTNETS

"Do we want a world without sharks and giant tunas—some of the most magnificent creatures on earth? Industrial large-scale fishing is making that choice for all of humankind."—Barbara Block, Ph.D., Stanford University marine biologist[1]

Nowadays, fish don't have a chance. It's perilously high-tech out there. Thanks to the advent of a number of sophisticated aids, including sonar, satellite global positioning systems, sea mapping software, radio beacons, sea depth indicators, and even "fish aggregation devices,"[2] much of the guesswork of finding fish is past. And the gear has become breathtakingly efficient: Worldwide, more than 23,000 fishing vessels of over 100 tons apiece, along with several million small boats, constantly scour the seas with destructive trawls.[3] Some nets stretch a quarter-mile across. Longlines gouge out whole populations of tunas and swordfish. Along with the fish slaughter, 800 whales, dolphins, and porpoises are added to the fish casualty list every day.[4] The same gear that is decimating the fish also hooks, slashes, traps, and ultimately dooms these unintended victims to death by shock and exhaustion.

Walls of death

Driftnetting is the supreme example of fishing's mega-kill techniques. Gigantic gill nets are suspended curtain-like in the water with floats and weights. Ninety percent of what gets pulled up is unintended catch, much of which will be discarded, already dead.[5] In their ignoble heyday of the 1970s and 1980s, the aggregate length of the driftnets launched every night amounted to 30,000 miles worldwide—some nets stretching as long as 90 miles. Driftnetting is considered to be the most destructive fishing practice ever devised. Moreover, since nets are cheaper to replace than to repair,[6] they may conveniently be dumped overboard to "ghost catch" indefinitely. Eventually, they ball up and sink under the weight of the dead marine life they ensnare.[7]

In the early 1990s, it was determined that driftnetting was threatening the fundamental ecological balance of the entire ocean.[8] Though a

1991 UN moratorium on the most destructive kinds of driftnetting has effectively reined in much of the devastation, enforcement of this relatively stringent rule continues to be lax.[9] Italy, France, Turkey, Morocco, and probably other countries as late as 2002 were believed to have significant numbers of boats equipped for driftnets, according to the World Wide Fund for Nature (WWF).[10] Further, there is evidence that most of the northern African countries are currently expanding their driftnet fleets.[11]

Longlines: Arbitrary and deadly

These days, fishers don't just hook one fish at a time. Thousands of hooks, or longlines, will be baited to dangle behind a single boat. The lines can extend as long as 80 miles, snagging unintended species just as easily as targeted ones.[12] Longlines have been implicated in the near annihilation of the ocean's top predator fish around the world. They also hook and drown an estimated 300,000 albatrosses per year[13] and have, in part, caused the population of Pacific Ocean leatherback turtles to plunge by 95 percent in just 22 years.[14]

Dredging to eco-oblivion

Dredging has been compared to clearcutting the forest, with yearly destruction amounting to twice the surface area of the United States.[15] Imagine a ton of gear dragging across the bottom of the ocean, whisking up in a plume of sediment every living thing that dwells there and amassing it into a cone-shaped net. If it were just the fish that were depleted by this method it would be bad enough. But the gear that takes the fish also wrecks lush ocean-floor habitats. Most tragically, deep-sea, cold-water corals are also leveled by the dredgers. Going back 8,000 years in some cases, the corals could possibly be the oldest living organisms on the planet.[16] They provide regenerative habitats for rich outgrowths of biodiversity. Their yearly rings, like those of trees, offer scientists a virtual Rosetta Stone for deciphering the ocean's history.[17] "Without intact coral reefs...you will not be able to restore fish stocks fully," warns Klaus Töpfer of the UN Environmental Program.[18]

Kill to chill

By being able to stay out for months at a time, the world's supertrawlers have become the world's indomitable fish predators—packing and flash freezing their catches as they go or just processing the fish of a nearby fleet of smaller boats.[19] The largest of these leviathans have nets large enough to engulf the Statue of Liberty and can bring in 600 metric tons of fish in a day. By the time the ship gets to port, the haul may already have been sold to customers via the Internet.

Collapse of the commons

Perhaps to the greatest extent anywhere, the ocean is the victim of what has become known as the "tragedy of the commons." There is no convincing incentive for any individual fisher to choose conservation. The oceans have historically always been free and open to all, but we've come to a place where the ethic of share and share alike is not compatible with the survival of ocean life.

To end the devastation, the remedies put forth by conservationists are as unequivocal as they are illustrative: Not only does the world need to end dredging, longlining, and driftnetting, it needs to enforce international agreements, end all subsidies, decrease the number of boats, set fewer traps, and begin government-sponsored vessel buy-back programs. Vegetarians would add one more item to the list: Stop eating fish.

22 Swallow this

MARKETING TO THE MINIONS

"[Children are] virgin ground as far as marketing is concerned."—confidential operations manual, McDonald's Corporation[1]

Can't anyone stop them—those playground pushers of salty, sugary, fatty, nutrient-void, and no less addictive[2] fast-food burgers—as they go about infecting the minds of impressionable youth? With toys, gimmicky packaging, blockbuster movie tie-ins, interactive Web sites, and cartoon characters of every deliciously colorful stripe, Big Food has infiltrated every conduit to every prepubescent neuroreceptor in the nation via Ronald McDonald, Winnie-the-Pooh, Beanie Babies, Simba, and Bugs Bunny. The heavy-handed messages are in our kids' faces, in their own language, at school, and in Saturday morning television cartoons. Logos adorn everything from Barbie dolls to video games to book jackets[3]—all to mold, shape, and monopolize young, pliable minds.

British activists distributing a leaflet tallying criticisms against McDonald's needled the burger giant into going after them in court. What became known in the mid-1990s as the McLibel case ended up backfiring on the company, not least because the final verdict, made in a London court, sided with the defendants' assessment that McDonald's exploits children with its promotions.[4]

Billions at stake

For what purpose all this cranial colonization? That's easy: money. Every year, U.S. kids not only spend $30 billion on their own but influence the direction of $600 billion in purchases by their parents.[5] "A child who loves our TV commercials and brings her grandparents to a McDonald's gives us two more customers," McDonald's founder Ray Kroc once beamed.[6] With four out of five food ads marketing products attractive to children,[7] the logic behind the $40 billion funneled to food advertising every year worldwide becomes clearer.[8] Some of these food dollars go to targeting children as young as two years old.[9]

For every dollar spent by the World Health Organization preventing the diseases caused by Western diets, more than $500 is spent by the food industry promoting these diets.[10] Periodically the industry, even by its own mercenary standards, oversteps common codes of conduct. In 2004, the FTC (Federal Trade Commission) successfully pressured KFC, the fast-food chicken franchise, to pull ads that deceptively characterized fried chicken as healthful.[11] However, the California Milk Advisory Board (CMAB) could not be shamed into pulling its obfuscating "happy cows" TV commercial once a judge ruled, on a technicality, that truth in advertising laws did not apply, because the CMAB is a state entity.[12] Apparently, the advisory board may deceive the public as freely as the government does with legal impunity.

Animals: Love 'em or eat 'em

Fast food is so ubiquitous, we don't always notice how complicit society is with its designs. Children's TV programming will suffer if you disallow kid-directed fast-food advertising, assert junk-food apologists.[13] School operations will collapse without fast-food revenues, others explain. A fifth of U.S. school lunch programs offer brand-name fast food.[14]

Meanwhile, kid-targeted advertising conditions youngsters to accept bizarre incongruities: A movie character named Babe, at first dismayed that he may have "no purpose except to be eaten," is then employed hawking McDonald's Happy Meals with his barnyard pals. No less preposterous are the hot-dog ditty "I Wish I Were an Oscar Mayer Wiener" and Charlie the Tuna, who longs to taste good.

Stealth elixirs addict

Finally, artificial and "natural" flavors remain the active ingredients in today's enticing fast and processed fare. They infuse apparently tasteless raw material—whether French fries or "spent" layer hens and dairy cows—with intoxicating olfactory sensations, colonizing unsuspecting minds from swing set to grave.[15] Author and investigative journalist Eric Schlosser explains: "The flavors of childhood foods seem to leave an indelible mark, and adults often return to them without always knowing why."[16] If the tastes of our youth shape our food choices for life, all the more reason to keep kids away from fast-food burgers at the very minimum—and, if we're smart, junk food in general.

23 Nagging conditions

ABOVE THE BELT

"A quick look along the aisles of your local drugstore or in the neighborhood supermarket will show you...a lot of people are hurting."—John A. McDougall, M.D.[1]

It's well known that eating meat is linked to the big killers of the Western world: heart disease, cancer, stroke, and diabetes. But daily meat consumption is also linked to pains, maladies, disorders, and nagging ailments that impact one's daily quality of life.

The following represents just a smattering off an extensive list of conditions brought on by meat-based diets. These center on parts of the body *above* the belt. (See next reason for those *below* the belt.)

Girding for GERD

Heartburn, or gastroesophageal reflux disease (GERD), should really be dubbed esophagus burn. Ingesting fatty meat stimulates an overproduction of stomach acid, which, not unlike battery acid in its caustic properties, can painfully slosh onto the under-protected esophagus. Assaulted over time, the esophagus can develop scar tissue or even a patch of altered cells that may become cancerous.

Heading off the migraines

Much is still unknown about migraine headaches. Yet it is believed that almost anything can be the cause of one: sleep disorders, chemical sensitivities, changes in weather, and stress, just to name a few.[2] Certain foods can also trigger an episode as well, with meat, dairy, and eggs being some of the worst offenders.[3] Aged cheeses, meats, and red wine contain tyramine, a compound that in some people can increase blood pressure and dilation of blood vessels in the brain, leading to head pain.[4]

Calcium and magnesium are important minerals that have been found to keep migraines in check. These are best obtained from vegetarian foods: collard greens, oatmeal, and fortified orange juice for calcium; barley, navy or white beans, and Swiss chard for magnesium. Figs and tofu contain both nutrients.

Roller-coaster estrogen shifts during a woman's monthly cycle can also bring on a migraine. To mitigate the peaks and valleys, women should avoid animal fats completely and keep vegetable oils to a minimum.[5]

This is your brain on meat

Research conducted at the University of California, San Diego, and published in the *Archives of Neurology,* found that women 65 years or older with elevated cholesterol levels had decreased mental function.[6] In much the same way that cholesterol damages the heart, elevated levels of this waxy, fat-like substance are believed to impair the mechanisms that bring vital blood flow to the brain. Fatty meat diets, which tend to be low in complex carbohydrates, are not only associated with diabetes but are linked with the impaired ability to learn new tasks, studies show.[7]

A four–year study conducted by researchers at Rush-Presbyterian-St. Luke's Medical Center in Chicago found that people who consumed the most saturated fat—primarily found in animal-derived foods—had 2.3 times the risk of developing Alzheimer's disease compared with those who consumed the lowest amount of saturated fats.[8] Study subjects who ate the kind of fats found in non-animal sources reduced their risk of Alzheimer's disease by 70 percent.[9]

Researchers publishing their results in the journal *Neuron* in 2004 discovered that one of the omega-3 fatty acids, DHA (docosahexaenoic acid), is especially protective against Alzheimer's disease.[10] Vegetarians can obtain adequate supplies of this nutrient, (for which nonvegetarians often turn to fish) by consuming ground flax seeds on a daily basis.

Seeing is believing

Macular degeneration is a condition caused by hardening of the blood vessels behind the lens of the eye, leading to vision impairment and loss for a quarter of the U.S. population over 65.[11] The same meat diet that hardens the arteries in the rest of the body is a cause of this condition as well.

24 Nagging conditions

BELOW THE BELT

"Unfortunately, we live in a modern society where suffering from preventable illness and chronic disease is the norm."—Joel Fuhrman, M.D.[1]

In a continuation of the theme begun with the last reason, here are some *below*-the-belt ailments linked to the meat-based diet.

Let's not get stones

Adhere to a diet high in fruits and vegetables and low in animal protein, and you can lower your risk for one of the most excruciatingly painful disorders known: kidney stones. Eliminating meat from the diet will reduce the amount of oxalate, calcium, and uric acid excreted in the urine, a welcome protection for many people predisposed to getting them.[2] A vegetarian diet provides ample amounts of citrate, magnesium, and potassium as well, which also tend to reduce stone formation. A high-fiber diet—one necessarily consisting of whole vegetarian foods—has also been shown to be instrumental to kidney health.

Reducing calcium consumption was once thought to be the proper therapy for the elimination of recurrent kidney stones. But more recent research has proved that animal protein intake, excessive salt, and low water consumption are the real culprits. Eliminating animal protein from the diet also has the added benefit of reducing risk of renal disease caused by diabetes and hypertension.[3]

Rheumatoid arthritis

A Brigham and Women's Hospital (Boston) study found that women with rheumatoid arthritis have twice the risk of heart attack—a clue, it surmised, that inflammation is a common catalyst for the two conditions.[4] The question naturally arises: How to forestall the inflammation? A vegan diet is a good place to start: A study in 2003, headed by

John McDougall, M.D., showed that all measures of rheumatoid arthritis were reduced significantly in 24 closely monitored subjects who adhered to a low-fat vegan diet for four weeks.[5]

Uncramping your style

The trick to reducing menstrual pain is the same one that reduces the risk for breast cancer: decreasing the volatility of blood estrogen levels. The amount of estrogen in the bodies of women in their childbearing years rises and falls twice during the month. Normally, estrogen will regularly leave the body via natural waste-removal systems. Vegetarians tend to have more sex hormone binding globulin (SHBG), a protein that binds and inactivates estrogen. Fiber in the diet, also key, functions as a ready-made sponge for waste estrogen coming from the liver.[6] Estrogen that has no fiber with which to bind will be recycled back into the body. Excessive estrogen also causes the endometrial cell layer that forms once a month to be larger than it needs to be.[7] The smaller this layer, it is hypothesized, the less likely that mechanisms will be put into place that cause nausea, headache, and cramps.[8] A study of 33 subjects sponsored by the Physicians Committee for Responsible Medicine showed that a low-fat vegan diet will grant relief from menstrual cramps in most women.[9]

Down south

One of the greatest benefits of the vegetarian diet is its curative power over constipation. If one keeps his or her non-meat diet unprocessed and rich in variety, plant-based foods automatically bring copious amounts of fiber—the substance that acts like a sponge (soluble fiber) or a broom (insoluble fiber) in the digestive tract. Every day a person needs 30 to 40 grams of fiber, yet most people in America, partly because of high volumes of meat in their diets, consume only half this amount.[10] People who suffer frequently from constipation, and who use laxatives regularly, have been found in clinical studies to be four times as likely to develop colorectal cancer as those who do not.[11] Meat, it bears repeating, contains no fiber.

A low-fiber diet can put a person, particularly over the age of 50, at risk of developing diverticula—small pouches in the inner intestinal layer. Because of the stress of strained, constipated bowel movements, these pouches can bulge out through weak points in the muscle layer in similar fashion to an inner tube distending through a tire. The condition, known as diverticulosis, requires drainage and intravenous antibiotics.[12]

Hemorrhoid horrors

If you live in the fiber-deprived Western world, you know about hemorrhoids, the nettlesome condition best described as varicose veins of the anus and rectum. Constipation and hardened stools, resulting from meat-based diets, are clearly linked to the malady. Sufferers must endure periodic pain, bleeding, and itching, as well as doctors' admonitions to eat more fiber! Extreme cases require surgical removal.[13]

The cow-Crohn's connection

A person with Crohn's disease suffers what can become a lifelong daily battle with "profuse urgent diarrhea, nausea, vomiting, and fevers,"[14] according to Michael Greger, M.D. The intestines of sufferers can become so ulcerated as to require incremental surgical removal of the bowel—until, in some cases, there is nothing left to take out.

The precise cause is unknown. However, the disease is found most often in the United States, the United Kingdom, and Scandinavia.[15] Like other inflammatory diseases involving the lining of the intestines, Crohn's disease is prevalent in the developed world where processed and animal-based foods are common.[16] There is now strong evidence that a bacterium called mycobacterium paratuberculosis (MAP), which is found in cows suffering from Johne's disease, could also be responsible for producing Crohn's disease in humans who drink cows' milk.[17]

Real men eat their fruits and vegetables

It makes sense: Eat meat and face a higher risk of impotence. According to Ronald W. Lewis, M.D., president of the International Society for Impotence Research, "A large part of erectile dysfunction is due to vascular (blood vessel) problems"—those associated with a high-fat, carnivorous diet and lack of exercise.[18] A study of 440 impotent men, which was published in the *Lancet* in 1985, found that risk factors associated with heart disease were present far more often in impotent men than in men in the general population.[19] Impotence, in fact, can be the first sign of heart disease and diabetes, both tied to the rich Western diet.[20] It's ironic that meat eating is associated with virility in the popular mythology, since this is often exactly what impairs a man's sexual function.

25 Modern mutant

E. COLI O157:H7

"To me, the 'E' in E. coli stands for 'evil'."—Nancy Donley, founder, Safe Tables Our Priority (S.T.O.P.), a citizens' food-safety group[1]

In 1982, the deadly *Escherichia coli* bacteria strain O157:H7 was first identified. A little over a decade later, the pathogen caused a watershed disaster in the Pacific Northwest, changing forever our view about sanitation. In 1993, the ingestion of under-cooked "Monster" hamburgers infected with E. coli O157:H7 sickened over 700 people, put 171 in the hospital, and killed four in the infamous Jack in the Box outbreak.[2]

By 1994, the head of the U.S. Food Safety and Inspection Service (FSIS), Michael Taylor, attempted to regulate the bug out of existence and, in the process, stood the meat industry on its head. Jim Hodges, the president of the American Meat Institute Foundation (AMIF), responded at the time: "It's like saying 'We're going to pass a law that it's illegal to have a car accident.' "[3] But where collisions are inseparable from moving vehicles, there is nothing about E. coli O157:H7 that is intrinsic to meat. This bug is a creation of the modern feedlot—a cross between bacterial evolution and greed.

Mutant of industry

E. coli O157:H7 is a mutant bacteria that evolved to survive conditions in the gut of modern feedlot cattle, which, over the years, has been made particularly acidic by a highly unnatural diet of corn and other grains. By extension, O157:H7 is able to survive the acidic environment of the human stomach.[4] Whereas the bacteria has no adverse effects on cows,[5] every year, Americans experience tens of thousands of O157:H7 illnesses, and from these 60 people die terrible, painful deaths.[6]

On feedlots, the cattle live on mounds of their own waste, and in the summer the deadly strain is especially prevalent, present in the intestines of half the nation's cattle.[7] It has been proved that the bug is dramatically diminished in its poisonous effects when cattle are fed a more natural diet of hay. But hay is not nearly as effective as corn in bulking up the animals, so producers cannot afford to use it.

By the time most cattle arrive at the slaughterhouse, their hides are caked with dried manure. From here, or via intestinal spillage, the

O157:H7 bacteria can migrate during the slaughter process to the meat.[8] Slaughterhouse line speeds are notoriously swift and carcass evisceration is often sloppy. Butchering is a highly skilled operation but is often done by novices, due to high turnover rates.[9] Down the line, inspectors typically give their okay to three hundred cattle carcasses per hour.[10]

The USDA revealed in 2003 that about 60 percent of the largest U.S. packing plants failed to meet federal food safety regulations for preventing E. coli from getting on meat.[11] The USDA found 1.8 percent of sampled carcasses still testing positive for O157:H7, despite sprays, washes, steams, and other treatments.[12] Later, at the grinder, meat from up to 4,000 carcasses can be pooled together in one lot,[13] and one ground-beef burger can consist of hundreds or even thousands of different animals.[14] Due to this pooling process, the average American samples an estimated 5,200 to 10,400 cattle in a year.[15] Finally, modern distribution methods put potentially contaminated beef into the hands of consumers within days, anywhere in the world, and long before recalls, if found to be necessary, can be implemented.

Ruining it for the rest of us

Manure is nothing short of hazardous industrial waste,[16] loaded not only with E. coli, but also with giardia, salmonella, cryptosporidia, and chlamydia, as well as wormy parasites and viruses.[17] More than 40 diseases can be transferred to humans via animal excrement.[18] So, meat-eater or not, we are all affected by today's mountainous deluges that overflow into the environment from cattle operations. Everyone from backyard gardeners to organic farmers to produce merchants and consumers must take extraordinary precautions to protect themselves against these now-ubiquitous poisons.

26 A big problem

THE VEGETARIAN SOLUTION

"In three states [Louisiana, Mississippi, and West Virginia] 25 percent of adults are obese—not overweight but obese. It's a catastrophe in our country."—Julie Gerberding, director, Centers for Disease Control and Prevention[1]

Abundant fat cells[2] and the so-called thrifty gene have each served humankind well throughout the ages when finding food wasn't quite so effortless as SUV-ing to the supermarket. In today's food environment, however, these traits—which in the past worked so well at conserving caloric energy—are a liability. They're now important reasons behind the great increases in the ranks of the obese and overweight—legions of people whose numbers now roughly match the number of people on earth victimized by hunger: 1.2 billion.[3] Today's "malnutrition of excess" doesn't kill nearly as many as does paucity. Yet obesity has become a significant cause of death just the same. Along with attendant "poor diet" and "physical inactivity,"[4] the condition kills approximately 365,000 Americans every year, according to the Centers for Disease Control (compared, for example, with 435,000 American deaths each year from smoking—a mere 20 percent difference).[5]

Over two-thirds of Americans are either overweight or obese.[6] Fifteen percent of American kids, ages 6 through 19, are severely overweight or obese.[7] Our fatness is linked to certain cancers,[8] heart failure,[9] heart attack,[10] birth defects,[11] and especially diabetes. One in five U.S. hospitalizations in people over 45 uncovers an attendant diagnosis of diabetes,[12] a disease that results in 87,000 amputations in the United States every year.[13] Obesity threatens to cancel out health gains older Americans are making through early disease detection with cholesterol screenings, prostate exams, mammograms, and blood-pressure checks.[14] And it costs the nation about $75 billion every year.[15] Not surprisingly, the Centers for Disease Control has declared our weight problems a top health threat.[16]

Sedentary lifestyles and high-fructose corn syrup-packed junk food brimming with trans-fatty acids, tempting people through advertising and availability, certainly have a lot to do with this epidemic. However, animal-derived foods are also to blame. The meat of today's corn-fed factory animals—the kind most people are eating—is much higher in girth-promoting saturated fat than with grass-fed or wild-game meats.[17]

The hamburger—that American staple, which is derived from spent dairy cows—starts as something quite lean. But to give consumers consistent fat content, beef fat is added—a whole day's worth in each burger.[18] In addition, Americans are getting at least twice as much protein as they need. The excess is turned into midriff, thigh, belly and neck blubber.[19]

Recipe for losing

It would take talent, so to speak, to get obese on a diverse, whole-foods vegan diet. A diet of nutrient-rich fresh fruits and vegetables, beans, and whole grains naturally provides abundant satiating fiber, an imperative in keeping body weight safely in check. Vegetarian diets, of course, lack the dangers of ketosis, the primary component of the carbophobic and meaty Atkins Diet, which brings its own form of satiety through gobs of fat, saturated or otherwise. Fiber, which is absent in meat, is a natural component of an all-plant diet. It facilitates the slow absorption of carbohydrates[20] and prevents calories from being turned into fat.

Fiber stands in the way of blood-sugar build-ups and suppresses appetite-stimulating insulin responses.[21] Some Type II diabetics have been able to reduce or quit their medications after committing to a low-fat vegan diet.[22]

The proof is in the registry

Most people listed with the National Weight Control Registry (which keeps data on people who have lost weight and kept it off) report that the secret of their success is regular exercise and maintaining a low-fat, high-carbohydrate (read: veg-friendly) diet—this, and reducing their fat intake to 25 percent of calories.[23] Less than one percent report adhering to an Atkins-esque, high-fat, low-carbohydrate plan.

27 Desertification

HOW DRY WE'RE GETTING

"We should bear in mind that almost a billion people are threatened in their very existence by desertification and recurrent droughts."—U.N. Secretary-General Kofi Annan, conference on desertification, Havana, 2003[1]

Farming is to some extent or another destructive to the environment. It takes the land out of equilibrium in terms of plant diversity, and over time erosion inevitably sets in. If we could keep our farming to a minimum and/or farm organically and still obtain all that we need, the world could be the better for it. But thanks to the historically recent phenomenon of feeding the harvest—much of it anyway—to livestock, the world ends up overcultivating itself, and desertification is the result.

Desertification, which refers to land degradation specifically caused by human activities, is indeed spreading at an alarming rate. According to satellite photos, maps, and other data, erosion and nutrient depletion have degraded 40 percent of the world's agricultural land.[2] Fertile areas amounting to three-fifths the size of Alaska are lost every year to soil degradation across the globe.[3] An estimated 250 million people worldwide have been directly affected by desertification so far, and about a billion are at risk.[4]

Using up the land

About 37 percent of the world's grain goes to feed animals. And a meat eater, by extension, requires two to four times more farmland than a vegetarian.[5] A vegan needs still less. The world is currently able to produce about two billion tons of grain per year,[6] thanks largely to the ongoing, though faltering, Green Revolution. With expected population growth and increases in meat consumption, however, 40 percent more grain will be needed by 2020.[7] Unfortunately, land productivity worldwide, as represented by per-capita grain production, peaked long ago in 1984.[8] Any near-term increases in yield will come from intensified crop cultivation, exacerbating current trends.

Other forces that degrade land include overgrazing, deforestation, overfertilizing, the planting of monocultural crops, and aquifer overpumping.[9] Again, the engine behind all these environmental stresses is livestock production.[10]

The degradation often begins with deforestation.[11] Worldwide, the annual net loss of forest land equals an area the size of Indiana.[12] It ends with erosion. With less topsoil—the earth's sponges—the land loses diversity and becomes less fertile.[13] According to agricultural ecologist David Pimentel of Cornell University, between 1955 and 1995 the world lost nearly a third of its arable land,[14] largely because of aggressive farming practices. On lands where feed grain is produced, soil loss averages 5.25 tons per acre per year.[15] Each pound of meat, poultry, eggs, and milk represents five pounds of topsoil loss.[16]

Furthermore, livestock themselves dry out the land when they graze in places that cannot stand up to them. Former cattle rancher Howard Lyman explains: "Overgrazing leads to more dust and drier air (as less water transpires from vegetation), leading to less rain, resulting in still less plant life." Topsoil is bared to the elements and "tends to experience greater extremes in temperature, destroying root systems and soil organisms."[17] Twenty percent of the earth's rangeland has lost productivity because of overgrazing.[18]

The Green Revolution, which allowed today's great yields along with today's great degradation, put current trends in motion. Animal agriculture was able to get a foothold, and the human costs along the way were enormous. According to *The Economist,* "the way the Green Revolution was implemented in some countries caused considerable upheaval as large numbers of peasant farmers—most of them women—found themselves replaced by the contents of a bottle [of chemicals]."[19] Alas, desertification is not just an issue of environmental cause and effect. It's a symptom of an unjust world—the result of globalization, cash-crop colonialism, and the desperate pressures of Third World debt.

Poor cry for help

At a major meeting on desertification in Havana in 2003, world leaders proposed that $25 billion be spent to undo some of the damage.[20] Nowhere near this amount was forthcoming from rich countries. For the moment, desertification is a problem of the world's poor. The rich are so far able to finance their penchant for meat by spending away the multibillion-dollar costs of some of its symptoms: soil erosion, drought, floods, and falling water tables. Eventually, however, desertification will catch up to all of us, either directly or from the fallout of a wretched horde waving flags of desperation. All around, a vegetarian world offers a far more civilized alternative.

28 Habit forming

ANTIBIOTICS ON THE FARM

"The irresponsible misuse of antibiotics on the farm is unilaterally disarming our species from our precious last line of defense, and devastating epidemics may be the legacy of hunger for inexpensive meat."—Emanuel Goldman, Ph.D., Professor of Microbiology and Molecular Genetics, New Jersey Medical School[1]

The antibiotic is a miracle tool, fighting countless diseases that have plagued humanity for millennia. Yet it is being compromised by drug abuse on the modern industrial farm. Tests on nearly 500 random chicken purchases sampled by *Consumer Reports* in 2002 found two common harmful bacteria (campylobacter and salmonella) significantly more resistant to antibiotics than in a similar test five years earlier.[2] Other studies concur that antibiotic resistance in the bacteria that infect meat is on the rise.

As this trend progresses, people who get sick from these food bugs today could have a much harder time overcoming their illnesses than in years past. One U.S. government study even suggested that up to 5,000 Americans within one year might have suffered more lengthy bouts with food poisoning because they ate chicken filled with antibiotic-resistant strains of bacteria.[3]

Don't use them, don't lose them

There's a wise saying when it comes to antibiotics: "If you use them you lose them." Yet, according to the Union of Concerned Scientists, about 40 percent of all antibiotics in the United States are used in animal agriculture.[4] For two short-term profit motives, farmers are squandering these crown jewels of medicine on livestock. They're countering an endless syndrome of animal disease, born of unhygienic, crowded conditions, and they're imposing unnatural levels of growth on to the animals.

Feeding antibiotics to livestock puts people, and ultimately everything in the environment, at risk for untreatable disease.[5] Curiously, farmers need no prescription when they administer these drugs to their animals. They come as part of the feed that farmers are compelled to use. Thanks to the rising phenomenon of contract farming—which concentrates control in the hands of the large processors—farmers have no say over what feed they must use.[6]

Up against the resistance

When a bacterial strain is about to do harm or even kill its host, antibiotics can immediately provide a last-ditch, heavy-handed defense. Unfortunately, both good and bad bacteria are wiped out. Two concerns immediately arise: Were the harmful bacteria eradicated? And how are you going to reinstate the beneficial (probiotic) bacteria? Any harmful bacteria left behind may be drug-resistant. And the presence of beneficial bacteria is crucial to crowding out harmful bacteria.

Since the primary purpose of antibiotics on the farm is not therapeutic but rather growth promotion via sub-clinical doses, a number of dangers arise. According to Stuart B. Levy, the director of the Center for Adaptation Genetics and Drug Resistance at Tufts University, this purpose forms "the perfect formula for selecting increasing numbers of resistant bacteria in the treated animals."[7] He further points out that these drug-resistant bacteria can be passed on to the animal caretakers, to the people who prepare raw meat, and even to those who eat undercooked meat. In the case of poultry, spurring growth with antibiotics allows farmers to bring their birds to market just one day sooner.[8]

But the story is still not over. Bacteria are capable of sharing antibiotic resistance.[9] So having any antibiotic-resistant bacteria around anywhere presents a danger. That resistance may migrate to harmful bacteria off the farm, including bacteria that cause disease in humans. For example, serious human illnesses resulting from now-antibiotic-resistant forms of *Staphylococcus aureus* and *Streptococcus pneumoniae* are on the rise.[10] Could these bacteria have acquired their drug resistance from the factory farm? We'll never know. In any case, according to Levy, "the exchange of [bacteria] genes is so pervasive that the entire bacterial world can be thought of as one huge multicellular organism in which the cells interchange their genes with ease."[11]

It doesn't seem worth it to continue to incubate antibiotic resistance on the farm. The first step is to take these drugs off our plates.

29 Toxic trickle

KILLING US SOFTLY

"There is far too much [chicken manure] to use on Delmarva without damaging water quality."—William C. Baker, president of the Chesapeake Bay Foundation[1]

What should we picture when we hear the word *agriculture*?—a pasture? acres of alfalfa? a row of organic vegetables? a factory? With a huge proportion, about 70 percent, of all U.S. grain being grown to feed livestock or fish, much of that which we view as "agriculture" actually represents *animal* agriculture. Those glorious miles and miles of corn stalks you see from your car window on that Midwestern road trip are not likely to be corn flakes in the making but rather pork chops and beefsteaks. The EPA has declared that "farming" is behind 70 percent of waterway pollution in the United States, overtaking sewage treatment plants, urban storm sewers, and pollution deposited from the air. Because of *agriculture*, the agency further asserts, 173,000 miles of waterways have been contaminated with animal waste, chemicals, and erosion.[2]

Of those U.S. rivers and lakes the EPA has surveyed, toxic runoff from *agriculture* is the leading source of water quality impacts.[3] Forty percent of America's surveyed rivers, lakes, and estuaries are, in fact, not clean enough to meet basic recreational uses,[4] and more than half of the nation's 127 coastal bays are befouled.[5]

When it rains, it trickles

By physical area, 70 percent of the continental United States is in private hands, and 80 percent of this is farmland.[6] According to former USDA deputy secretary Rich Rominger, speaking at a 1999 conference on animal residuals management, "Odds are good that your water, whether you're from New York City or Cumming, Iowa, has passed through agricultural land."[7] Even worse, perhaps, two-fifths of the continental United States is within the Mississippi River watershed—precisely where most of the nation's intensive feed-grain production takes place. A toxic trickle in fertilizers, manure, herbicides, and pesticides moves down creek, down stream, and down river to the Gulf of Mexico from the nation's vast breadbasket.

Other key areas around the nation that are poisoned by manure and runoff include the cow-fouled Chino Basin in California; the manure-caked feedlots of the Texas Panhandle; the nitrogen-rich Raccoon River that runs past Des Moines, Iowa; and the hog-manure-saturated coastal plain of North Carolina.

And let's not forget that symbol of our national heritage, the Chesapeake Bay, now 40 percent oxygen-starved.[8] It's befouled, in large part because of poultry farms on Maryland's Eastern shore and Virginia's Shenandoah Valley,[9] as well as dairy operations in Pennsylvania's Susquehanna River watershed.[10] By some estimates, Chesapeake Bay cleanup is projected to cost $19 billion.[11]

Enviro-legislation wanting

When the Clean Water Act of 1972 was being written, *non-point-source* pollution, or toxic runoff, was not seen as an ecological threat. In the years since, however, this kind of pollution, which is by and large caused by farms, has become a primary one. According to the Pew Oceans Commission, an independent government-policy watcher, feedlot and fertilizer runoff are among the fastest-growing sources of ocean pollution that can often come from thousands of miles away.[12] Collectively, the nation's small livestock operations can add up to be just as destructive as the big ones.

Meanwhile, the EPA struggles to gain authority in the face of a legal tangle. It wasn't until 2000 that limits on runoff from farms were even set.[13] And this occurred only after a test case made it all the way to the Supreme Court. Ultimately, states have the final authority about land use. Unfortunately, they are typically more easily swayed by big farm interests.

Finally, many farm operations can in fact be characterized as *point-source* polluters, that is, emitting animal waste that does more than just trickle into the environment. Massive spills, or deliberately gouged-out gullies that allow waste into waterways, are not unheard-of abuses. Despite such blatant breaches of federal law, culprits are often able to slither past inadequately funded enforcement.[14]

30 Cluck!

MODERN BROILER LIFE

"Chickens can be profoundly mistreated and still 'produce.' Like humans, chickens can 'adapt,' up to a point, to living in slum conditions. Is this an argument for slums?"—Karen Davis, Ph.D., United Poultry Concerns[1]

In the "broiler" business, where chickens are processed into meat, systems are as thoroughly intensive and highly evolved as any in agriculture. Precise input costs are paired off against measured volume output. The animals' needs and desires are inconsequential. Their bodies are treated as if they were inanimate production units—to be understood only to be better exploited. No industry practice is deemed off limits, no matter how much suffering it may cause.

Fully automated poultry barns, which typically hold 20,000 to 25,000 birds, are designed to run themselves with minimal labor input—the animals meriting little care or comfort. How else could you process the bodies of nine billion chickens per year in the United States alone? This is a numbers game with profit per bird measured in fractions of a penny—although the industry often quantifies the birds not as individuals but by the pound.

Growing pains

Activists have filmed poultry operations littered with dust, manure, filth, and decomposing carcasses.[2] The animals suffer from untreated sores, abscesses, and walking disorders. Chicken deaths, or "mortalities" as the industry describes them, are a major part of this business—essentially the result of freakishly efficient feed conversion, a key genetic trait that has been inflicted on the birds.

Over the last quarter-century, the time it takes for a broiler to grow to slaughter weight has been cut in half[3] to a mere six weeks. Weight gain occurs so fast that the birds' eyes will still be blue at slaughter time, a sign that these animals are still only babies.[4] At this age they would normally be sheltered under their mother's wing, but of course, these birds never know their mothers.

Fast muscular weight gain occurs without commensurate skeletal development, causing a host of orthopedic problems. A Danish study found that 30 percent of broiler chickens had leg problems of a degree likely to lead to chronic pain.[5] In the United States this proportion represents billions of animals. In any event, if any one of these birds that is bred for rapid growth is allowed to live beyond its industry-designated years, it will naturally become obese. Indeed, breeder birds for the broiler industry must be maintained continuously on severe reducing diets, since they, unlike their offspring, live long enough to become overweight.[6]

Furthermore, heart and lung development also do not keep pace with the growth of the rest of the birds' bodies. Two percent of chickens die from heart failure.[7] And veterinary care for any one of them is nonexistent, since an animal doctor's time far outweighs the worth of any one bird. All told, the industry plans for 10 percent of the birds to die before reaching slaughter. Producers see early mortality as a disposal problem.

Gobble, gobble, quack!

For the most part, factory-raised turkeys and ducks share the same dismal fate as chickens. Orthopedic problems in turkeys, however, are especially pronounced. By the eighth week of life, a commercial turkey's breast has already grown to the point that the animal is unable to walk.[8]

Ducks are waterfowl with strong instincts to swim. In a factory setting they are forced to live in oppressively crowded, windowless sheds where the only water is in a narrow trough.

31 Biosecurity

A-SCRUBBING AND A-SCRAPING WE WILL GO

"Terrorists wouldn't need sophisticated biological weapons to bring the livestock industry and the related export business to a halt."—National Research Council report, 2002[1]

Livestock producers don't like people near their herds and flocks. Animal activists snooping around, wielding video cameras and sending footage of cruel conditions to local media are particularly unwelcome. But there are other, far more important reasons why "no trespassing" signs greet visitors to farms these days. Operations need to keep contagions away from the animals. There's even a name for these efforts: biosecurity.

Animal constitutions: Delicate and vulnerable

Thousands of pigs or tens of thousands of chickens today not only share intensively crowded conditions inside typically unsanitary climate-controlled housing; they also share nearly homogeneous genes. The beef cattle and dairy cows corralled in outdoor manure-soaked yards also share similar genes.

Such stressful conditions are why the first threat to the modern factory farm and feedlot is disease. On the farms of old, animal immunity came from exercise, sunlight, and the freedom to peck or root in the soil. But given that the industry breeds the animals for consumer- as well as producer-driven traits—rather than for robust lives in nature—drugs and vitamin supplements must come to the rescue to prop up the animals' health.

An entire litany of illnesses plagues animals on farms today. The most potentially devastating of them include foot and mouth disease (FMD), avian influenza, swine fever, and Exotic Newcastle disease.[2] Poultry producers, in particular, estimate that disease eats up at least 10 percent of their total production costs.[3]

Scrub for your life

Vaccines and medication go just so far to combat infections. Meanwhile, antibiotics continue to lose their efficacy from overuse. In the end, if you want to raise animals with modern systems, you'd better be something of a clean freak. Cleanout regimens between production cycles are intense episodes of pressure washing, scrubbing, scraping, disinfecting, fumigating, and fogging.[4] Ultimately, just one negligent producer can bring catastrophic mortalities not only to his own farm but to those of his neighbors.

Farmed animals can be infected by workers, visitors, dust, poultry litter, water, air, feed, vaccines, insects, rodents, pets, wild birds, parasites, and the animals themselves. Those whose job requires them to go from farm to farm may be asked to drive their cars or trucks through antiseptic rinses, scrub up in the shower, don plastic suits, and walk through foot dips before being allowed near the animals.

Agroterrorism, a real threat

Since September 11, 2001, the U.S government has indicated that animal agriculture could be a perfect target for terrorists. According to the National Research Council, "The U.S. livestock industry...is extremely vulnerable to a host of highly infectious and often contagious biological agents....These agents can easily be obtained and can readily be released, given the general lack of security on farms and fields and their formidable size." Former U.S. secretary of Health and

Human Services Tommy Thompson exclaimed a day after his resignation in December 2004 from President Bush's cabinet, "For the life of me, I cannot understand why the terrorists have not attacked our food supply, because it is so easy to do."[5]

Anthrax spores are still emanating from the graves of infected cows along nineteenth-century cattle trails.[6] Salmonella, which is as accessible as a trip to the grocery store chicken display case, can be reconstituted in the laboratory to be a lethal weapon of great proportions.[7]

Livestock shows and state fairs are increasingly potential bastions for animal disease. Poultry of all sorts are regularly banned from them. The stringent precautions of biosecurity may be necessary to protect against virulent contagions such as foot-and-mouth disease (FMD).[8] The stakes are high. An FMD outbreak in the United States could cost the nation $24 billion, according to the Government Accounting Office (GAO).[9] Perhaps 10 million animals would have to be destroyed.

Meanwhile, the U.S. food-safety network operates ineffectively as a crazy quilt of loopholes and redundancies. Security breaches in 2003 at Plum Island, New York—the animal-disease research center where the U.S. government holds repositories of some of the most potent animal pathogens—have been symptomatic of the chaos, according to a GAO report.[10]

Okily locally

Ultimately, decentralized, local, and seasonal food production and distribution systems remain best. These provide the only defense against a myriad of catastrophes.

32 BSE

THE COWS ARE MAD AS HELL

"What is surprising is that we actually found a case of mad cow disease in the United States at all, given the inadequacy of our surveillance program."—Michael Greger, M.D., advisor, mad cow disease, Organic Consumers Association[1]

What did forced cannibalism in the cattle industry bestow upon the world? You guessed it: mad cow disease. But while animal-carcass recycling might have been regarded as frugal at one time, it eventually ushered in a brain-rotting menace. And since the disease has a multi-year incubation period, the worst of its consequences may yet be felt.

Mad cow: The genesis

Mad cow disease—the graphic nickname for Bovine Spongiform Encephalopathy (BSE)—is believed to have a mystifying misshapen protein, called a prion, as its infectious agent. A major UK inquiry into BSE's causes concluded that the disease probably originated spontaneously as a result of a genetic mutation and was later amplified by the industry's feed practices.[2] Renderers—those enterprising folks who process livestock remains into such things as glues and lubricants—have long taken the virtues of their recycling techniques too far. By including animal remains in cattle feed, they transformed the herbivorous cow into a cannibal and an agent in the spread of this dreaded disease.

Curiously, before mad cow's human connection became an official working theory, England, over an eight–year period,[3] exported over a million tons of BSE-infected meat and bone meal to 80 countries, including the United States.[4] The exports were made even while the British government prohibited its farmers from feeding the potentially poisonous mix to their own animals.[5]

Stanley Prusiner, a Nobel Prize-winning neurologist and authority on prion diseases, asserts today that a home-grown American version of BSE is festering under the radar screen. It's only a matter of time, he says, before the disease fully manifests itself throughout the nation.[6] A primary fear is that these prions will eventually lodge themselves in the environment.[7] Some contend they already have.[8]

Prions are seemingly indestructible—standing up to extreme temperatures and harsh solvents.[9] In country after country, the industry has fought regulation at its own peril. American meat producers have been no exception. Still, in some respects, BSE has so far amounted to little more than a giant nightmare for the world's meat producers. Relatively few people (approximately 153) have died from or contracted the human version of the disease, Creutzfeldt Jakob Disease (vCJD). The millions of cows and sheep that have been destroyed because of it were essentially doomed animals anyway.

In any case, even though vCJD has infected only a small number of people, its horrors amply justify the public's fear of the disease. Victims literally lose their minds as their brains turn to sponge-like latticework. This always-lethal, generally year-long illness begins with insomnia, depression, and confusion. Balance, speech, and memory soon slip away.[10] Then, bizarre involuntary movements and erratic behaviors begin to take hold. Victims may hallucinate such things as bugs crawling all over them. Finally, coma. It makes "ebola look like chickenpox," opined *Newsweek*.[11]

USDA: Protecting an industry

It seems the U.S. government was caught off guard when a single mad cow was found within the country's borders in 2003—twenty years, nearly to the day, after the first mad cow was detected on an English farm.[12] Fifty countries halted $3.8 billion in U.S. beef imports and have since been reluctant to reinstate them. The public quickly learned that U.S. testing is statistically minuscule and voluntary[13] (possibly invalid, according to the USDA's own inspector general),[14] surveillance is corrupt,[15] viable livestock-tracking systems are years away,[16] and prion research is paltry at best.[17]

United Press International uncovered USDA records in 2004 that showed that the agency failed in 2002 and 2003 to test nearly 500 suspect animals, "including some in categories considered most likely to be infected."[18]

Officially, the USDA now merely sample-tests what it considers high-risk older and downer cows. But the policies, it seems, do not cast a wide enough net. The sole U.S.-found mad cow was by all accounts ambulatory—culled because of complications in pregnancy.[19] Also, testing in Europe has found young cows to be infected.[20]

Since testing costs up to $50 per cow,[21] the industry rigorously continues to fight comprehensive surveillance.[22] Meanwhile the United States promotes a stance that essentially amounts to "don't look, don't find."

33 Number's up

CHOLESTEROL AND BLOOD PRESSURE READINGS

"This opens up the possibility that diet can be used much more widely to lower blood cholesterol and possibly spare some individuals from having to take drugs."—David Jenkins, lead researcher of a Canadian study that proved the vegetarian diet can lower cholesterol as well as drugs[1]

From the human body's point of view, modern life sure is a killer. It's shock and awe daily as we damage our bodies with rich foods and sedentary habits. The human frame—finely tuned for bare-bones survival on a lean diet and regular physical challenges[2]—begins to rebel. The damages, as assessed by one's doctor, come in the form of numbers:

high blood pressure (hypertension) and high cholesterol readings. Still, people's habits keep getting worse. Meanwhile, the major health organizations keep shifting the goalposts that define what is considered healthy[3]—each time pressing more people into the ranks of the unfit. Many are suddenly forced to reassess not only that desk job but also those daily meals of meat.

Drugs or diet: You choose

Our doctor's cajole us to keep our cholesterol and blood pressure numbers in check, since no outward signs tell us we are at risk. When we fail, we're usually prescribed powerful and often expensive drugs that can cause muscle pain,[4] sexual dysfunction,[5] or reduced mental ability.[6] Some of the drugs may effectively lower cholesterol but not necessarily lengthen our lives.[7] Our doctor might tell us to improve our diet, that is, cut out animal products. But don't count on it, since he or she probably had little to no training in nutrition.[8] Indeed, studies have shown that a vegetarian diet can lower cholesterol levels as well as drugs can.[9]

Sure, cholesterol is essential in forming certain hormones, membranes, and other necessary tissues. It helps a person digest fat and manufacture vitamin D. But the human body is fully capable of producing all the cholesterol it needs without any extra coming from food. Indeed, excess cholesterol, as most people know, is plainly associated with cardiovascular disease.

Only animal-based foods have cholesterol. And though chicken is lower in saturated fat than beef, it contains as much cholesterol.[10] On the other hand, all plants are cholesterol-free. In fact, phytosterols, or plant sterols, are beneficial to the body.[11]

The silent killer: Hypertension

High blood pressure also has its own mechanisms, which start with high cholesterol levels that stiffen and narrow arterial pathways with plaque. Add to this increased blood viscosity from regular meals high in saturated fat[12]—the kind that is solid at room temperature, found primarily in meat. Throw in sodium—also plentiful in meat[13]—which increases the amount of blood flow in the arteries. The extra pressure against arterial walls that these factors combine to produce causes even more plaque buildup.[14]

Ultimately, you have the makings of hypertension and pre-hypertension, which together afflict 95 million Americans.[15] Nearly a third of these people are unaware of their debilitating, often fatal illness. The final stages of the malady cause kidney or heart failure, dementia,[16] blindness, stroke, and heart attack.[17]

A whole-foods vegetarian diet that keeps excess salt intake in check and includes regular intakes of vitamin B12 (by supplementation) and ground flax seeds (two tablespoons per day), will substantially reduce the risk for these ailments. In general, vegetarians have one-third to one-half the incidence of hypertension that meat eaters suffer.[18]

Furthermore, vegetables and fruits are rich in potassium, a proven corrective in the fight against high blood pressure. The nutrient works as a natural relaxant for the arteries.

In the end, if you want to beam rather than wince when you and your coworkers compare cholesterol and blood-pressure numbers at the water cooler, get with the program—vegetarian style.

34 Row upon row

AMBER WAVES OF FEED

"Corn is actually a huge, inefficient, polluting machine that guzzles fossil fuel."—Michael Pollan, author and essayist[1]

In their vast and superabundant corner of the world, farmers in the Midwest have over the last century endeavored with great industry to transform the earth's crust. By draining more than 105 million acres of this region's wetlands—half of all that once existed[2]—they uprooted a lush slice of biodiversity and replaced it with tidy row crops particularly good for feeding animals. Iowans stand out as especially proficient in this regard. Of the state's original 3 million acres of wetlands, only 50,000 acres survive intact.[3] And of the prairies that once covered 80 percent of the state, only .01 percent of their original acreage remains.[4] *New York Times* editorial observer Verlyn Klinkenborg brought home the devastation when he wrote, "Biological complexity and diversity sound like abstractions, until you see a patch of prairie beside the monotony of a [cultivated] field."[5]

The side with the prairie, as opposed to the side with the crops, will perhaps jut up above the ground the full height of a man.[6] It remains rich with biodiversity, and its soil level grows a bit higher with each passing year. Some 200 species of plants on the prairie side will work in concert—each in its way doing its part in promoting water retention, wind breaking, fertilizing, or attracting beneficial birds and insects.[7] In the end, both plants and soil are kept grounded. On the other hand, the side with the row crops is left increasingly depleted by topsoil erosion. If the farmer did not rigorously intervene year after year, the land would revert to biological complexity. Today's farmer who feeds into America's meat culture essentially contributes to the transformation of earth's lush ecosystem into the proverbial parking lot.

Prairies and wetlands are self-sufficient and cleansing ecosystems. Not so the areas planted with the nation's primary feed-grain, corn, which requires not only 4,300 gallons of water per bushel[8] but also more fertilizers and herbicides than any other crop.[9] The chemical infusion pumps U.S. corn output on 79 million acres to 138 bushels per acre,[10] which is nearly seven times the yield of unfertilized land.[11] According to the National Research Council, however, only one-half to two-thirds of the fertilizer is ever utilized by the plants.[12] The rest either contributes to acid rain in the form of atmospheric ammonia or inflicts environmental havoc downstream in the form of nitrate that is leached into rivers and streams.

The latter has occurred most destructively in the Gulf of Mexico by way of the Mississippi River.[13] Between the nitrogen from the petrochemical fertilizers, the methane from decomposing vegetation, and the nitrous oxide from acidification, the modern cornfield emits a global warming effect not unlike a Los Angeles freeway—this despite the oxygen-creating and carbon-dioxide-neutralizing effects of the plants themselves.[14]

Oily food

But pollution is only part of the story. The world's most cultivated plant is unnecessarily dependent on supplies of oil, at least indirectly. Every acre of corn essentially gobbles up 140 gallons of petroleum, because this is what is required to produce the synthetic fertilizers to make the crop grow.[15] By extension, when you eat foods derived from corn-eating animals you might as well be guzzling gas yourself.

Every 1,250-pound steer embodies 283 gallons of oil[16] or, according to *National Geographic* magazine, three-quarters of a gallon per pound of meat.[17] Far less would be needed, of course, if producers allowed their animals—cattle and other ruminants in this instance—to do what came naturally to them, that is, eat grass. The bovine, in case some of us have forgotten, comes equipped with its own 45-gallon rumen, an extraordinary organ designed to digest fibrous plant material that is inedible to humans. Modern cattle producers essentially pour intense concentrations of solar energy into these animals in the form of corn kernels to make them grow at extraordinary rates—a very expensive practice when examined from the point of view of the environment.

Indeed, those who produce grass-fed beef are quick to tout their methods of animal rearing as *more* planet friendly, and they're right. However, one needs to bear in mind the operational word here: "more." Because of the grazing factor (see reason #52), grass-fed beef cannot be described as environmentally friendly when employed in any kind of excess—let's say if it replaced feedlot beef to fulfill today's demand. But we digress.

Cows on the corn dole

At first glance it makes no sense to feed corn to animals. That is, until one takes into account the farm subsidies and cheap oil that allow farms to grow it to such excess. A bushel of corn (56 pounds) costs the livestock operator the artificial price of about $3.[18]

Meanwhile, thanks to the high-energy starch and portability of corn—it's been equated with fattening the animals on Snickers bars[19]—a steer that once took four to five years to grow to slaughter weight on the range now lives only 14 months, birth to butcher. Appetite enhancers make double sure the super-growth system works. The economics are irresistible to the modern rancher who faces slim profit margins. Sadly, the overly fortified feed often causes bovine heartburn, diarrhea, ulcers, bloat, liver disease, pneumonia, or feedlot polio in the animals.[20] These diseases will be countered with antibiotics and other medications.

But corn-fed beef has what consumers have learned to crave: marbled cuts of meat, brimming with saturated fat. That's the kind, of course, that raises the risk for hardening of the arteries, which leads one down the road to heart attack, stroke, hypertension, diabetes, aortic aneurysm, macular degeneration, and so on and so on.

35 Meat and poultry inspection

WHERE ARE WE NOW?

"I eat very little to no meat."—Delmer Jones, federal food inspector for 41 years, president, National Joint Council of Meat Inspection Locals[1]

Thanks to the advent of factory agriculture and industrial processing of meat over the last generation, novel and tenacious pathogens have been on the rise in the slaughterhouse. At one point it became clear that microbial testing, not just visual carcass examination, had to make its way into the inspection process. A quality assurance system called HACCP (Hazard Analysis Critical Control Points)—which is based on prevention rather than detection—was federally instituted in 1998. Meat and poultry inspectors from the old school of "poke and sniff" initially welcomed the innovations as a natural augmentation to their work.[2] But overzealous HACCP advocates from both industry and government have combined forces to take away inspectors' authority. In a survey of inspectors in 2000, 84 percent said they are generally compelled by the system to oversee paperwork rather than carcasses.[3] It wasn't long before HACCP acquired an alternative name: "Have a cup of coffee and pray."

Today's federal meat inspectors, who often don't have much more than a high school education, have expressed confusion and frustration with HACCP. Moreover, they are increasingly on the front lines of a bitter battle with recalcitrant meat plants more concerned with pumping out product than keeping food safe.

At a "listening meeting" in 2000, nearly a quarter of the inspectors in attendance indicated that they had been physically abused while on the job.[4] The meeting was an impromptu gathering after an incident where a sausage-factory owner, at his wits' end, gunned down three meat inspectors who were trying to enforce food-safety rules in his filthy plant.

Bacteria in the cafeteria

Food-safety watchdog groups voiced initial skepticism about HACCP. They said that under the system the industry would not be able to police itself. To appease them, the Clinton administration instituted the so-called salmonella test, which would serve as a standard, or objective measure, for processing plants to live up to. The belief was that if salmonella were present, other bacteria probably were, too. Part of the agreement allowed the government to shut a plant down if it repeatedly failed the test.

Only once, however, did the USDA dare to use its plant-closing power. The target: a germ-ridden ground-beef plant and supplier to the national school lunch program, which had failed the salmonella test three times. Suddenly, the USDA was confronted with a ferocious court battle, which it eventually lost.

Meat industry trade groups have all along been behind the elimination of the salmonella test, despite the fact that only a small percentage of plants fail it.[5] Their reasoning is telling. The salmonella test does not necessarily indicate the overall cleanliness of a plant as food-safety advocates assert. A ground beef plant, in particular, can be perfectly clean, they explain, but fail the test, because contaminated carcasses can enter from the outside at any time—something plant personnel have no control over. The dirty meat will also likely carry the USDA stamp of approval. And besides, they say, salmonella has not legally been declared an adulterant. It is considered intrinsic to meat and, for this reason, up to the consumer to neutralize via cooking. The meat industry's argument, of course, leaves out the fact that salmonella kills hundreds and sickens over a million Americans every year.[6]

The logic of the argument eventually comes full circle. By rejecting the salmonella test, are opponents of it inadvertently touting the point of view of animal protection organizations and factory farming opponents? Might they be suggesting that the USDA direct its attention to the intensive confinement of animals, the ubiquity of animal waste, and the dispensing of antibiotics, all of which hold the key to why so many pathogens have come to infect ground meat in the first place? Perhaps so. In any case, the USDA has no jurisdiction over pathogen contamination on farms.

36 Franken-farmyard

THE FREAKS ARE HERE

"Pigs [genetically] selected for large amounts of lean meat are so nervous that they often have heart attacks and die during handling or transport. . . . Cattle with double-muscle traits cannot birth normally and must undergo Cesarean sections. . . . Chickens bred for rapid weight gain often develop . . . weak legs and peck other chickens."—Temple Grandin, farmed animal welfare specialist[1]

Farmers have always had to optimize to stay in business. Today, however, this can mean fractions of a penny on the unit. With profit margins slim, today's livestock—through carefully selected genes—are, more than ever, compelled to do specific things and do them impeccably well. Fall down on the job as an egg layer or a lactator, and it's off to the slaughterhouse, pronto. The same goes for breeder stock. And animals that get sick? If no drug can get them going again soon, they're landfill, dead meat, or feed.

Until recently, the same breed of chicken provided both eggs and meat. Now we have two distinct birds, though still the same species. Broilers (chickens raised for meat) literally flesh out in a brisk 42 days.[2] And layers lay 12 times the number of eggs this species ever produced as a wild Southeast Asian fowl.[3] Weak skeletons in young turkeys do not stand up to the excessive weight of their modern-bred breasts. But, worse, huge turkey front quarters make the toms unable to copulate on their own. Reproduction is induced via artificial insemination.

Making pork makers

With the help of high-tech genetics, top pork producers get 25 to 29 piglets per sow per year—although the industry average is more in the range of 18 or 20. As sows are pushed to piglet limit, geneticists have worked to breed in more teats.[4] Meanwhile, the weaning age for pigs has been steadily shortened to as little as two to four weeks, down from eight weeks just a couple of decades ago, thus allowing sows to become pregnant increasingly earlier.[5] Also soon in the offing is the use of non-surgical, laboratory fertilization of superior-trait sow eggs that are later designated for implantation into surrogate sows, perhaps ones bred for good mothering.[6]

Kowtowing to profits

Thanks to artificial insemination and embryo transfer, twinning in beef cattle is holding "promise" for the industry. In one selection program, twinning increased from 4 percent to 31 percent of pregnancies over a 14-year period. However, difficult births became twice as frequent.[7] The project was deemed a success, just the same.

In general, today's prize beef calf will have wide hindquarters and broad shoulders in order to hang a lot of meat. In only 14 months, the animal grows from 80 pounds at birth to 1,250 pounds at slaughter, albeit aided by a corn-fed diet, hormones, and antibiotics.[8] British science journalist Colin Tudge gets to the essence of today's agricultural ethic: "To the farmer, muscle is meat and fat is succulence or 'finish,' while bones are a dead loss."[9] Muscle growth has come without attendant skeletal development, causing chronic orthopedic pain for those animals bred for their flesh.

The modern dairy cow must likewise "put out," or it's off to hamburger heaven. Geneticists have boosted the milk yield of at least one breed to 3,000 gallons per year,[10] about nine times the amount that might have been produced naturally.[11]

Over-breeding has metamorphosed animals into skittish, high-strung beasts. Bred for fast growth and lean meat, both pigs and chickens are more likely to experience heart attacks during handling or transport.[12] Likewise, animals bred to grow quickly must be slaughtered early in life, or they will grow obese. Furthermore, the mothering instinct can be bred right out of an animal, which may or may not be a problem for a producer.[13]

Finally, in a demonstration that not one aspect of the modern poultry bird is sacred, a breeding project out of Israel recently created a featherless chicken to save producers money on feather disposal.[14] The breed is destined for developing countries in hot climates.

37 Roots to nuts

NEW FOUR FOOD GROUPS

"Why do we have a milk group? Because we have a National Dairy Council. Why do we have a meat group? Because we have an extremely powerful meat lobby."—Marion Nestle, Director of Public Health Initiatives for the Steinhardt School of Education, New York University[1]

Meat and dairy are associated with risk for disease. Yet the USDA promotes these foods using its iconic food pyramid. As everyone knows from school days, meat and milk are well represented on this chart. Indeed, they each get their own food group! The disconnect between scientific finding and nutritional recommendation has everything to do with the influence of industry on the people who sit on the agency's advisory panels. After all, the USDA's primary mission is promoting American agricultural goods.

All the more reason to be grateful for the Physicians Committee for Responsible Medicine (PCRM). In 1991, it issued the *New* Four Food Groups. Meat and dairy, it contends, are "optional" foods at best. Here are the final four—drum roll, please.

Fruits are packed with potassium, which helps regulate heartbeat, prevent strokes, and negate the effects of salt, thereby keeping blood pressure levels in check. Fruits are rich in vitamin C, which has too many benefits to list.[2] Beta-carotene, which the body converts into vitamin A, is abundant in many fruits. This phytochemical has antioxidant properties that work to neutralize highly unstable and destructive molecules called free radicals, which are believed to accelerate the aging process and are implicated in up to 60 different health conditions, including cancer and atherosclerosis.[3] One serving of fruit may contain hundreds of other health-giving phytochemicals as well.[4]

Vegetables. Eat your vegetables and greatly reduce your risk for the big killers: heart disease and cancer. Vegetables are, in just about every case, low in calories and fat and rich in just about everything needed to keep you healthy: vitamins A, B, C, E, and K; calcium; potassium; and iron, as well as voluminous varieties of phytochemicals. Eat your vegetables to reduce your risk of diabetes, hypertension, and cataracts. They even help to lower your cholesterol level.

Studies have shown that diets high in fruits and vegetables—the more colorful the better[5]—lower the risk of stroke,[6] slow brain aging,[7] and ultimately could cut the death rate by 20 percent.[8]

In general, diets high in animal proteins and processed foods and low in fruits and vegetables tend to flood the body with sodium and starve it of potassium, two conditions that together have causal links to high blood pressure, heart attacks, strokes, kidney stones, and osteoporosis.[9]

Legumes, better known as beans, are valuable for dieters and diabetics because they are low in fat, high in fiber (higher than any other food), and prevent blood sugar levels from rising too rapidly after a meal.[10] They are a primary source of protein. Beans are rich in B vitamins and complex carbohydrates. A cup of beans will provide more potassium than a banana and more calcium and iron than 3 ounces of cooked meat.[11] They are a cancer and heart-disease fighter and have been shown to lower cholesterol levels.[12]

Whole grains (as opposed to refined ones) reduce the risk of heart disease. Because they are rich in fiber, both soluble and insoluble, they aid digestion.[13] Both the bran and the germ are rich in B vitamins, iron, and zinc. The germ also contains vitamin E, magnesium and phosphorus.[14] The endosperm is packed with complex carbohydrates, protein, and fiber. Whole grains—which include barley, brown rice, oats, wheat, rye, quinoa (technically a fruit), buckwheat, bulgur, and millet—are naturally low in fat, and so are a dieter's friend. Processed grain foods (junk, in other words) are a dieter's enemy, because they tend to be stripped of their nutrients and laden with hidden sugars, fat, and salt.

38 Feces fiasco

OPERATION CONTAMINATED CHICKEN

"Poop is poop. I can't see how it is tolerable to have fecal material on any meat coming off the line."—Carol Tucker Foreman, Consumer Federation of America[1]

Chicken slaughter in the United States burgeoned during the twentieth century, rising from 143 million birds in 1940 to an unfathomable nine billion birds in 2000. By the mid-1970s, super-efficient automation was instituted to meet demand. Soon, the industry was arguing that the requirement to trim off visible fecal matter from bird carcasses—accidents do happen—was slowing down the line, and that merely washing affected parts with rinses, or simply cooking infected meat, was just as good.[2]

In 1978, the U.S. government, with the blessing of the top USDA food-safety official at the time, Carol Tucker Foreman, went along with the industry's line of reasoning.[3] Ever since, Ms. Foreman, now a food-safety advocate, has regretted giving in. A number of studies have proved that rinsing bird carcasses, even up to 40 times, is not effective in eliminating bacterial contamination.[4] According to the Agriculture Research Service of the USDA, many bird carcasses "escape hot-water washes or sprays containing bactericide and surfactants....An impossibly high water pressure would be needed to overcome the capillary pressure in a pore just large enough to house a bacterium."[5]

In the meantime, the chicken industry has no incentive to provide a wholesome product. In fact, one in every 100 birds that passes government inspectors is contaminated with feces or signs of disease, according to the USDA itself.[6] Down the line, diseased birds end up in the school lunch program, but they "do not pose a food-safety issue," the agency at one time assured the public, despite the "sores and scabs."[7]

Follow that poop

So how do bacteria and disease end up in packaged chicken in the first place? Let us count the ways. First, right from the start, chicks can be hatched infected with salmonella, either from their mothers or from contaminated shells.[8] Later, in the chicken sheds, which typically hold about 20,000 birds, the animals peck at everything, including each other's feces. Feed can harbor salmonella as well. In transit, pathogens can be spread between agitated birds, who are packed solid in cages.

After slaughter, bird after bird is submerged into a scald tank so feathers can be loosened for removal. Since the water may not always be kept hot enough to kill bacteria, the tank becomes a breeding ground for cross-contamination. Later, the violent motions of defeathering rubber fingers not only work to squirt feces out from the chickens' bodies[9] but can permanently act to embed bacteria deep into crevices of birds' skin.[10] Then, on to degutting. At this point, poorly calibrated mechanical entrails scoopers may occasionally puncture intestines, bringing feces onto edible parts.[11] Later, bird carcasses are dunked by the thousands into an icy chill tank to lower their temperature for final processing. Inspectors have dubbed this the "fecal soup."[12] Here, the industry norm is for only one carcass of every 22,000 birds to be microbially tested for generic E. coli.[13] Meanwhile, government inspectors get all of two seconds to check carcasses for defects, such as lesions and other signs of disease, as well as visible signs of contamination.[14] In transit to the supermarket, there is little regulatory oversight to make sure chicken parts stay properly refrigerated at all times.

Treachery at the meat counter

At the store, other commercial practices also put consumers at risk. A comprehensive undercover TV investigation by Dateline NBC showed that re-wrapping and re-dating packages of meat is commonplace across the nation. Investigators found that there are no laws to force stores to be honest about their product dating; it's considered a courtesy.[15] So, even insignificant colonies of bacteria have the chance to grow into significant ones. If bacterial counts are already high, they can grow inside packages into counts of hundreds of millions, and at these levels no piece of meat can be considered safe, even after thorough cooking.[16]

39 Blue pastures

AQUACULTURE'S FLOATING FEEDLOTS

"There are some fjords in Norway where 90 percent of the fish have escaped from farms."—The Economist[1]

One in three fish that ends up on dinner plates worldwide never knew freedom in the wild. It was raised in confinement on a farm. In some places, aquaculture is practiced using more sustainable methods thousands of years old. But the overwhelming trend today is toward factory production. Fish that are raised in these modern systems will be crammed together in cages or tanks as tightly as one foot-long fish per gallon of water.[2] And indeed, every terrible thing you can say about factory farming on land—cruelty, wild traits bred out of the animals, a profusion of waste, disease, drug use, and predator control—you can say about the new feedlots of the sea, but worse. Since fish farms exist in fluid environments, usually adjacent to or submerged in wild settings, a host of additional problems arise.

Pigments, pellets, and droppings

The droppings of farmed fish have become a major threat to environments near modern fish farms. In the United States, the provisions of the Clean Water Act have yet to be applied to aquaculture operations.[3] In China, 30,000 aquaculture cages are packed so solidly along one stretch of coast across from Taiwan that the fish have at times become poisoned on their own waste. In 1998, toxic algal blooms wiped out 90 percent of that bay's caged fish.[4] On China's coasts and throughout Asia, toxic "red tides" due to aquaculture have become a perennial problem.

But excess manure is only one negative aspect of fish farming. Uneaten, highly concentrated protein pellets can smother the sea floor and rob oxygen from bottom-dwelling creatures.[5] Oily fishmeal, used as feed, can form a scum on the surface of the water; at low tides it stinks up beaches.[6] Drugs (antibiotics and hormones), pigments (that turn gray salmon flesh pink), pesticides, and herbicides are used on the fish or in their pens.[7] In addition, sulfates are used to keep nets free of algae.[8] All of these chemicals freely suffuse the surrounding waters.

Enviro-havoc of the escapees

Today's lab-bred farmed fish are the aquatic version of broiler hens, bred to grow fat fast under tightly controlled conditions. Because they've been selectively bred for captivity and fast growth, any escapees become invasive species. Once in the wild, they spread disease and compete with native fish for habitat, mates, and food. When they mate with the natives, they weaken the genetic vigor of wild stocks.[9] A study in 1996 found that a quarter of the spawning salmon in Norwegian rivers and streams were escapees of fish farms or their descendants.[10] In 1975, the Norwegian government was forced to use poisons to destroy all the wild fish in 38 rivers and streams when a deadly parasite from nearby aquaculture operations infected them.[11]

In the Pacific Northwest, a million Atlantic salmon are believed to have escaped through storm-wrecked nets.[12] Sadly, with nearly 20 wild salmon species in the region listed as endangered for one reason or another, the domesticated, transcontinental interlopers are the last thing the fragile situation needs. Fish farmers, however, are not required to report fish escapes.[13]

Specious solution to extinction of the seas

Eighty percent of farmed fish are fed grain[14]—an inefficiency from the start since such grain could go to sustain consumers directly. But the trend today is toward something far more wasteful. Market forces increasingly favor farming carnivores—until recently an anomaly in the world of rearing animals for human consumption. (Some have equated the cultivation of the carnivorous salmon to raising tigers for food.) Meat-eating animals not only tend to be lacking in delectability, but their cultivation has always been considered supremely inefficient. In the case of salmon, up to five pounds of wild fishmeal is required to grow one pound of fish flesh.[15] During the six-month fattening period, caged bluefin tunas consume 10 to 17 pounds of wild fish per pound of flesh yielded. Furthermore, those species typically used for fishmeal—herring, mackerel, and sardines—are now threatened under the strain of industrial harvesting. The disappearance of these species could severely disrupt marine food webs.[16]

Finally, biomass fishing—a technique that employs tightly wrought nets—indiscriminately harvests marine life for a mash to feed farmed fish. Everything and anything gets scooped up with this technique, including juvenile fish that have not had a chance to breed, as well as endangered species.[17]

Other eco-invasions

Some farmed-fish species, such as grouper, milkfish, and eels, cannot be bred in captivity. Therefore, juveniles, which never get a chance to replenish their numbers, are essentially kidnapped from the wild to be farmed. Furthermore, mangrove forests, which provide fish with a refuge from predators, nurseries for offspring, and places to spawn, are summarily cleared away to build coastal aquaculture pens. Fish farming is the primary reason that half of the world's mangroves are gone.[18]

40 The slurry slope

THE COW IN YOUR ASPHALT

"The capacity to turn a cow into fabric softener is a kind of industrial farming...we all participate in, whether we know it or not, whether we choose it or not."—Verlyn Klinkenborg, editorial observer, *The New York Times*[1]

It might seem that the ubiquity of consumer goods that contain animal-derived elements exists just to irritate the sensibilities of vegans. But these days, anyone, meat eater or not, might have concerns about those leftovers from the slaughterhouse being simmered, distilled, and centrifuged down in order to be remade into every kind of commercial product.

Most Americans don't think about it much. The 47 billion pounds of animal remains our nation generates annually[2] (mostly through the meat industry) usually don't reveal themselves in the open air as decomposing sludge in the town dump—although this is always a possibility. They are more likely to be rendered into ingredients for lipstick, cake mixes, crayons, gummy bears, linoleum, antifreeze, tires, photographic paper, glue, asphalt, or soap. For those with a stomach for it, the British government has in fact compiled an exhaustive list of cow-part ingredients. In any case, to make a vast tangle of putrefying entrails, beaks, hooves, snouts, bones, feathers, tendons, and milk sacks both usable and safe for the by-product market is a monumental task.

Cheaper by the million

Simple economics dictates the ever-presence of animal-based ingredients: The raw materials are plentiful simply because we have such an immense meat industry. Furthermore, hundreds of millions of farmed animals die every year before making it to the slaughterhouse. Their bodies need to go somewhere.

Manufacturers would no doubt use non-animal-based raw materials if they had to, or if they were cheaper. But as it stands, few restrictions apply, and plenty makes cheap, so animal by-products are used. When describing the source of vaccine ingredients, an FDA document once candidly stated, "Cow components are often used simply because cows are very large animals, and thus much material is available."[3]

It is worth noting that the meat and the animal by-product distillation industries grew in tandem over the last half-century—one might say symbiotically.[4] Neither could have grown so great on its own. A corollary to this: Animal by-product sales have long allowed the meat industry to charge consumers less for its meat.[5] Indeed, the money a producer makes on by-product often becomes the sole source of profit.

Mad-cow snag

Then there was mad cow disease, or Bovine Spongiform Encephalopathy (BSE), and everything changed for the by-product industry—certainly when it comes to cattle feed. BSE is linked to the feeding of infected cow and possibly sheep parts to cattle. International trade has been disrupted over confusion and contention about what constitutes infectious material. While it is agreed that cow brain and spinal cord should be off limits for ruminant feed, the rules are murky for cow blood, tonsils, adrenal glands, placenta, nasal mucosa, sciatic nerves, bone marrow, livers, and thymus glands.[6] Each has been considered a BSE risk.

Numerous products, in fact, derive directly from some of these questionable parts. Brain-power supplements, contact lens care products, steroids, anticoagulant drugs, and cosmetics, for instance, are made, respectively, from brains, liver enzymes,[7] adrenal glands, mucosa, and placenta[8]—all derived from high-risk fluids and tissues of the cow. Since bovine central nervous system tissue is no longer allowed in meat products consumed by people, such material has increasingly been relegated to pet food. No need to waste 100 pounds per cow of good skull, brain, and spinal cord, explains Dan Murphy of the American Meat Institute.[9] Unfortunately, there is evidence that some animals can be silent carriers of BSE.[10]

"We can use eyeballs from the cow, as well as their brains, pituitaries, intestines, and stomach," Allen Kramer told the Associated Press in 2001. He's the founder of a biotech company that uses cow parts for pharmaceuticals,[11] and his work has no doubt become more complicated since the United States became, in 2003, a nation that has officially harbored at least one mad cow. The United States can no longer claim to be BSE-free, a critical designation for trade in products that contain cow-derived material.

Several days after the discovery of America's first mad cow in Washington, a spokesman for the state's agriculture department revealed: "We have nearly 100 percent utilization of the animal. But when you have so many niche markets, it makes it incredibly challenging to trace where this one cow may have gone."[12]

Indeed, even low-risk consumer cow parts, such as gelatin—a ubiquitous ingredient—could be dangerous from a cow who actually had mad cow disease.[13] A scientific study made public in 2005 revealed that the prion, the infectious agent believed to cause mad cow disease, may be able to migrate to any organ in a cow's body, suggesting that no part of an infected cow is safe to eat.[14]

41 Large-mammal slaughter

INEXACT AT ANY SPEED

"You cannot begin to know what the conditions are...unless you have worked on the kill floor and seen them for yourself."—a slaughterhouse worker's letter to his supervisor[1]

Slaughter *can* be made somewhat humane. If a cow on the way to her doom is herded down a serpentine chute that doesn't allow her to see what lies ahead, if her pathway does not betray anything different from every other ramp she's ever been on throughout her life, if odors of freshly butchered cows are not detected (this may be the most difficult to achieve),[2] if she is pinned inside the knocking pen for a brief moment and brought to insensibility in an instant by way of a captive bolt to the head from a properly powered and well-maintained cartridge-operated device—then the rest of the process of hoisting, throat slashing, flaying, eviscerating, and butchering will be like going to surgery in a state of oblivion.

This is the way it's supposed to be—and not just legally—according to celebrated slaughter expert Temple Grandin, who actually devised a scoring system that ranks slaughterhouses by how much the animals moo or squeal, slip and fall, get zapped with electrical prods, and are scalded to death or butchered alive. Many slaughterhouses are more humane because of Dr. Grandin's work, which, since 1999, has been supported by McDonald's.[3] But can anyone really keep tabs on a slaughterhouse when it is audited only once a year[4]—particularly when the public is not privy to the audit results?[5]

Slaughterhouse of horrors

Firsthand accounts from the people who actually do the stunning and slaughtering day in and day out are surely a better way to assess the conditions of the animals.

"I have seen thousands and thousands of cows go through the slaughter process alive since I have been at the plant"[6] is one assessment from the slaughterhouse front lines. "The chain goes too fast, more than 300 cows an hour....If I can't get the animal knocked [stunned] right, it keeps going....The chain doesn't stop. It keeps running. It never stops. The cows are getting hung alive or not alive. They keep coming, coming, coming," explains another.[7]

In any case, a lot of things have to go perfectly, every day, every hour, every animal, to keep a slaughterhouse humane. Killing animals is unwieldy under the best conditions, but with several thousand animals passing one worker in just one shift, inevitably the situation is going to get sloppy. Some animals will go to the rail partially stunned, repeatedly stunned, or even without being stunned at all. Animals not stunned are shackled, bled out, flayed and eviscerated while still conscious. Some animals get caught in the machinery. Others fall off the line. According to a 2001 *Washington Post* exposé, one beef packer that was repeatedly caught with insufficiently stunned animals on the rail resisted USDA warnings by saying "its practices were no different than others in the industry."[8]

Since the late 1970s, conveyor-line speeds have doubled while wages have plummeted. Non-English-speaking slaughter workers have become a new exploited class in dangerous environments with extremely high turnovers. The advent of a new federal inspection system, called HACCP, added to a high-stress situation, as it worked to lock out inspectors concerned with humane issues from the areas where stunning and slaughtering take place.[9] The animals have paid the price, as have the workers. Today's slaughterhouse employees may complain that they're forced to work on terrified, thousand-pound creatures, inadequately stunned, fighting for their lives.

According to *Slaughterhouse* (1997) author Gail Eisnitz, today's HACCP "self-inspections...are meaningless. They're designed to lull Americans...about what goes on inside today's slaughterhouses."[10] The USDA "has never taken its humane slaughter mandate seriously," she asserts.[11] Indeed, several media exposés prompted Congress to appropriate $5 million so the USDA could hire 50 full-time inspectors to oversee humane violations specifically. A 2004 audit, however, revealed that the agency had simply used the money to up the hours of meat-contamination inspectors already on staff.[12]

42 CAFO in town

GAGGING FOR SANITY

"A smell so thick you can taste it."—Barbara Dunham, who lives near 7,200 sows[1]

There are a lot of absurdities about eating meat, but few tip the scales so completely as the issue of factory-farm odor. Here's something that is as unnecessary as it is awful for the people who have to endure it. These are *not* the smells our grandparents knew—the everyday odors that rural people have been accustomed to since livestock were domesticated. These smells could, so to speak, make a maggot gag, although they actually do a good job of attracting flies and other flying and crawling pests.

Assessing the new neighbors

Imagine waking up to find that thousands of hogs had just moved in next door. Adjacent to the barns that hold the animals is likely to be an open-air pit of urine and feces. A hog-manure cesspool can be up to 25 feet deep and 18 acres in size.[2] Periodically it will be emptied over "sprayfields" nearby. The effluvium will from time to time be trucked out of town. When you're downwind, the stench hammers you—perhaps only intermittently, like being tortured by water slowly dripping on your forehead. You'll find you can no longer open your windows. Everything porous on your property, indoors and out, becomes imbued with a festering, pungent stench, and if you go outside, your clothing, hair, and skin become impregnated with odor-permeating dust.

People who live near hog farms experience more headaches, diarrhea, burning eyes, and respiratory problems, such as coughing, than those who do not, studies have shown.[3] If mega-farm odor affected everyone, it would be a national crisis. For now, you'll mostly have to go to the inner pages of your newspaper to read the frustrated words of its victims.

There's Larry Guffey, for instance, who is within whiffing distance of a half million factory-housed hogs that are now resident in three northern Missouri counties. He says, "Sometimes in the night, in the summer, when they start pumping effluent, it wakes you up. You're gagging."[4]

Karen Hudson describes the smell from a seven-acre "lagoon" containing 40 million gallons of manure on the brink of overflowing near her Illinois home: It had a "decaying smell of a dead body."[5]

Bonnie Dancy, who is the neighbor to a million gallons of hog excrement from 4,000 hogs in Maryland: "It's like you're being gassed....Even with the windows closed, it can come into your house."[6]

And Jerry Taylor, who lives near 35 chicken farms on the Delmarva Peninsula: "I think our county has sold us out."[7]

And, of course, businesses can be ruined by livestock odor. For instance, 75 wineries in the picturesque region of the Finger Lakes in New York state, which depend on walk-in tourists for up to 90 percent of their business, have been threatened by 20,000 hogs pent up nearby.[8]

Just get out of town

Perhaps the best place for a livestock operator to be is just so far away from civilization that nuisance laws do not catch up with him. Essayist Michael Pollan has described such a place: Poky Feeders in Kansas. The runoff from this feedlot of 40,000 cattle is so concentrated with nitrogen that it cannot be used as fertilizer; the potent infusion would burn crops yellow.[9] The slurry is simply left to linger in lagoons until it eventually breaks down. In the meantime, the ponds emit an acrid "bus station men's room smell" that carries even in the open air, Pollan attests.

Nearer to civilization, complaints about livestock odor are usually categorized as simple nuisances, not serious air-quality infractions. Laws that protect households nearby from bad smells are generally grossly inadequate or loosely enforced. In 2005, large livestock operations were granted exemptions from liability for past violations by the EPA while the government sets out to establish standards for air emissions on their farms.[10]

In any case, measuring odor is subjective and therefore difficult to regulate. Victims nonetheless often turn to the courts, but face drawn-out fights, handicapped by having nothing but ephemeral evidence to back them up. But in at least one case, in Illinois, the odors of industrial animal agriculture were perceived as so noxious that a lawsuit reduced property-value assessments on nearby homes by 10 to 30 percent.[11]

43 Dairy, be wary

LOSING TOLERANCE FOR MILK

"In most Asian countries, where dairy is generally eschewed but soy products and sea vegetables are abundant, calcium deficiencies are virtually nonexistent."—Lisa Turner, for *Vegetarian Times*, March 1998[1]

It sure is odd. The apologists for dairy foods are always saying there's something wrong with *us* that our bodies cannot digest cows' milk. Lactose "intolerance," they call it—known for causing cramping, flatulence, diarrhea, and bloating. It's like saying there's something wrong with your gasoline engine after you fill it up with diesel fuel. A full 75 percent of the world's population has some trouble digesting lactose, that is, dairy sugar.[2] Non-Caucasians tend to be least adapted.

Where there's an ill, there's a whey

But human "intolerance" to dairy is only just the beginning of the story about cows' milk. Epidemiological examinations have long been clear about its ill effects.[3] Indeed, clinical studies have likewise amassed gallons of damning evidence: Cows' milk is not only a suboptimal food in terms of nutrition, it is in fact associated, perhaps even causally, with various cancers, cardiovascular diseases, diabetes, a number of allergy-related diseases,[4] arthritic symptoms, cataracts, and asthma.[5] Cornell University professor T. Colin Campbell, who was a lead researcher for the China Study, has said, "Cows' milk protein may be the single most significant chemical carcinogen to which humans are exposed."[6] A physician, Robert M. Kradjian, took it upon himself to review 500 articles in the scientific literature, each distinguished by showing conclusive evidence of milk's effects on human health. "They were only slightly less than horrifying," he concluded.

Mucilaginous baby food

Cows' milk is much more suitable for nourishing a calf than a human being. Baby bovines grow to 650 pounds in just eight months.[7] Cows' milk has twice the protein of human milk[8]—some if it coming in forms that cause allergic reactions. Cows' milk is also overly rich in certain vitamins and minerals that stress the kidneys.[9] Two mechanisms put into motion by this foreign substance can lead to anemia: Cows' milk causes microscopic intestinal bleeding and is low in iron, a nutrient vital for infant development. The American Academy of Pediatrics recommends parents avoid giving it to their babies.[10]

Brimming with saturated fat and cholesterol, cows' milk is now recognized as a problem even for older children. It is also devoid of the essential fatty acids that today's diets need but too often lack. Furthermore, studies show that over two-thirds of children can be relieved of the symptoms of constipation simply by switching from cows' milk to soy milk.[11] Some evidence links the white stuff to pimples!

Hold the bone

Though cows' milk is offered as the pat remedy for the growing incidence of osteoporosis, some experts actually see it as instrumental in the *cause* of the bone-crippling disease. The nations with the highest consumption of dairy products are in fact the same ones plagued by brittle bones.[12] It's becoming clear that osteoporosis is caused not merely by calcium deficits but by nutrient imbalances. Excess animal protein tends to make the blood more acidic, which results in the body taking calcium from the bones to balance the pH.[13] Americans are ingesting so much animal protein these days that their calcium needs have shot up to unattainable levels.[14]

In a study of 70,000 American nurses, it was found that the women with the highest calcium consumption from dairy products actually had more fractures than did those who drank less milk.[15] According to a study by the Agriculture Research Service of the USDA "bone formation was significantly less in omnivore women than in vegan women...even though the omnivore women had a higher calcium intake than did the vegan volunteers."[16]

Isn't it time we started weaning ourselves from the baby food of other species and going for the fortified orange juice, kale, collards, broccoli, blackstrap molasses, and tofu for delicious, absorbable, plant-based calcium?

44 Pork for pork and other meats

INDUSTRIES ON THE DOLE

"If people had to pay the free market price for meat, they'd eat beans instead."—William Harris, M.D., director, Kaiser Permanente Vegetarian Lifestyle Clinic[1]

The meat, dairy, and fishing industries are subsidized, propped up, pampered, assuaged, coddled, and otherwise indulged in every way imaginable by the U.S. government. Favors come to these industries overtly, obscurely, or invisibly, by way of tax breaks, price floors, bailouts, commodity support purchases, and emergency aid; as exemptions from animal welfare and environmental laws; and in the form of operating costs—such as food safety, research and development, consulting, trade negotiations, and international public relations.

By hook or by crook, these industries endeavor to slough off their costs onto the rest of us. And our government's behind them all the way. Meanwhile, the more they get, the more they grouse. And they never, ever seem to get enough.

Meat-industry subsidies emerge from what one would think was an impossible dilemma: how to remake what has always been a luxury good—with its high production costs—into one that is universally consumed. It simply cannot be done without an extremely effective public relations engine that sees to it that this industry's costs are externalized onto society as a whole. The heavy burden is transferred to several victims that quite conveniently are unable to fight back: the animals, the environment, and the taxpayers.

Jaw-dropping giveaways

Animal agriculture long ago eclipsed fruit and vegetable farming in the United States in importance.[2] While U.S. government support for produce growers is nothing to speak of, the cup runneth over for those who stick with the major commodity crops, which include several feed grains. The bigger your operation, the bigger your government checks—direct payments that, over a span of only a few years, can amount to over a million dollars.[3] With this kind of money, a farmer can buy out his small-farmer neighbors for whom the subsidies, way back when, were designed to help. "Any person engaged in small business in America would be amazed....Their jaws would drop at the money farmers receive," explains Keith Collins, chief economist at the USDA.[4]

For feed crops, annual government handouts amount to double-digit billions. The unnatural support creates oversupplies of both grain and livestock, engendering gluts that eventually require their own government bailouts with expensive price tags. For instance, to appease farmers besieged by historically low hog prices in 1999, the U.S. government forked over $250 million to producers.[5]

What happens to those who try to fight the system? In 2001, the newly appointed USDA secretary, Ann Veneman, naively questioned the wisdom of farm subsidies prior to the passage of the big Farm Act of 2002. The Congressional committees on agriculture, which dispense the farm-subsidy largesse, promptly let loose their attack dogs.[6] Not long afterwards, the president obediently signed the bill.

Line-item pork barrel

The following is a list of a few exemplary items one regularly finds in USDA budgets. Most are enough to make any taxpayer fume, vegetarian or not. (Numbers in parenthesis are approximate, total annual costs.)

Commodity purchases ($500 million): The government regularly makes food purchases of beef, chicken, eggs, cheese, fish, pork, turkey, lamb, goose, and, of course, milk. Buffalo and salmon have graced the list in years past. They're deemed "surplus removal programs," and they're designed to shore up prices for producers. The USDA buys up so much powdered milk it literally cannot give it away fast enough. Storage costs come to $20 million per year for the $1 billion perpetual stockpile.[7] In the end, all this high-fat fare goes to prisons and the school lunch program. When surpluses are dumped on foreign markets as aid or as underpriced food items, they disrupt local economies and cause obesity in recipient populations.[8]

Food Safety and Inspection Service (FSIS) ($800 million): This program primarily oversees the safety of meat and poultry. Notwithstanding the fact that the program is inadequate to handle the job properly, the question remains: Why can't the industry reimburse the government for its trouble via user fees as do other industries that similarly require government oversight? Proposals to require any payback to the government get voted down in the Congress every time.

Conservation Reserve Program (CRP) ($2 billion): This program rents from farmers strips of land that lie between farmland and waterways. The government then seeds the areas with foliage to buffer toxic runoff created by the farm. The program does not stop the pollution from flowing in the first place. And even if the CRP were the way to solve the problem, the farmers should pay for the buffers themselves, passing their costs on to their consumers and ultimately raising the price of meat to a level that reflects the cost of production.

Environmental Quality Incentives Program (EQIP) ($1.3 billion): A farm operation can receive up to $450,000 for conservation expertise and assistance over the six–year life of the current federal farm law (ending in 2007). Critics assert that this program essentially dispenses money to the biggest farms so they can better tackle their industrial-sized manure problems.

Ranching subsidies ($500 million) consist of general support to ranchers on public lands. A study commissioned by the Center for Biological Diversity discovered that when indirect costs are added in, the total is closer to a billion dollars per year.[9]

Disaster relief (special appropriations in the neighborhood of $2 to $4 billion): These sums are distributed to people who raise livestock in areas where they shouldn't be in the first place. See reason #52.

Research ($1.1 billion, for all purposes): Livestock research comes to roughly $275 million per year and tends toward projects that aim to solve meat-pathogen problems. Other projects may seek practical uses for a by-product material, such as feathers, which amount to four billion pounds per year.[10] Genetics research has worked to determine the sex of embryos or to develop a semen extender to aid in artificial insemination. Many other research dollars end up benefiting animal agriculture indirectly, such as the development of a certain kind of corn feed that mitigates the polluting effects of hog waste.

Market Access Program (MAP) ($125 million, total, for all commodities): This program gives the U.S. Meat Export Federation over $10 million, the U.S. Dairy Export Council over $2 million, and U.S. Livestock Genetics Export, Inc., over $700,000 every year to expand markets in foreign countries.[11] These are just a few specific examples in this category.

Dairy Export Incentive Program (DEIP) ($53 million) helps exporters of U.S. dairy products meet prevailing world prices in foreign markets.

Separation of meat and state

Producers of animal-derived food possess a rare sort of chutzpah when it comes to asking the government for bailouts. In 2000, Long Island Sound lobstermen asked and received $50 million to make up for losses they incurred because a parasite lowered yields on the luxury food they harvest.[12] In 2004, the Bush administration proposed funding of $441 million for programs to fight mad cow disease and other threats against the U.S. meat supply.[13] And in what may take the cake, dairy farmers in 2000 asked the government for $1.3 billion to eradicate Johne's disease, a bovine scourge that costs the industry $200 million per year.[14]

Intangible burdens

Subsidies to support the production of animal foods are not only a disaster in economic terms, but they speed the destruction of the environment and cause unhealthful foods to flood markets. There is no way to put a dollar figure on it all.

Outside of specific cleanup projects—$19 billion for the Chesapeake Bay, for example—overall environmental costs of animal agriculture cannot be measured. Who could, for example, put a dollar figure on the exemptions this industry enjoys from the Clean Water Act and the Clean Air Act?

Health costs due to poor diets have been estimated at $250 billion per year in the United States alone.[15] Surely, this does not tell the whole story. Heart disease alone costs $370 billion every year. According to *Vegetarian Journal*, a study of California Seventh-day Adventist vegetarians and non-vegetarians indicated that vegetarians use fewer medications, have fewer surgeries, and use fewer health services.[16]

And finally, what's the true value of the Animal Welfare Act to the meat industry? As written, nothing short of indispensable, invaluable, and incalculable, since the law exempts animals raised for "food or fiber." Essentially, factory farming only exists at all because of this exemption.

Lesson from down under

Farm subsidies were ended in New Zealand in 1984, despite an even higher percentage of subsidization and relative importance of agriculture to the country's economy than in the United States. Today, New Zealand's farm economy is healthier than ever.[17] The next step for them and everyone else should be not merely to end farm subsidies, but to tax meat![18]

45 Operation ocean plunder

JELLYFISH RULES

"There are a lot of people out there willing to fish the last fish."—Dr. Jeremy B. C. Jackson, professor, Scripps Institution of Oceanography[1]

The world's overbuilt fishing fleets employ high-tech tools. Not surprisingly, fisheries are crashing one after the other. Consequently, fishers do what comes naturally to them as they are stripped of adequately profitable catches: with devastation behind them, they simply pack up and move on.[2] This may mean turning to "trash fish" that previously might have been rejected, fishing down the food chain, robbing the harbors of poor nations, or hunting the deep sea. According to Reg Watson, a scientist who took part in a major Canadian study about the state of our oceans, "If you look at those prime table fin fish: In the 1960s, we had about 21 pounds per person, now we're down to a third of that. If you extrapolate the linear trend, within 10 years we'll be talking about fish as if they were a myth; as if they were fond memories."[3]

Trash in, trash out

With a boat-to-fish ratio severely strained across the globe, fishers are desperate enough to consider just about anything to stay in business. The transformation of so-called trash fish into viable, marketable species is just one telling trend marking fishing today. Sea urchins from Maine are the perfect example of the modern-day trash-fish Cinderella story: a worthless nuisance to fishers one day, the rage in Asia the next, and a crash in population soon after. Regulators in the state have become so sensitive to the problem that they have instituted the Emerging Fisheries Act, designed to forestall the scenario from happening again. And none too soon: The sea cucumber as a target species is threatening to fall into the same pattern. One can understand why this invertebrate came to bear the trash-fish epithet. Only two morsels of its body can be considered edible: a small ring of pink muscle and a patch of dark skin.[4] By weight, these pieces come to less than five percent of the animal.

Catch as catch can

As fishers move down the food chain after depleting species higher up, fish become more abundant, though much less valuable per pound. Fishers must extract larger catches to keep their incomes the same. In the 1980s, five of these less valuable species made up nearly 30 percent of the world's fish catch but accounted for only six percent of its monetary value.[5]

In the end, fishing down the food chain may allow some fishers to stay in business, but their lease on life cannot last long. Meanwhile, the original depleted species, which relied on these lower-trophic-level fish for food, become further depleted as they are deprived of an adequate food source. The ultimate disaster of this strategy is that once all the prey fish are gone, you've killed an ecosystem. As conservation editor Ted Williams puts it, "As you destroy each descending link, you reduce biodiversity, until you literally hit jellyfish."[6]

Third-world deception

When industrial countries deplete their own fisheries, they pressure poor ones to open up theirs.[7] Approximately 85 percent of internationally traded fish originates in developing nations.[8] "There's not enough fish left in European waters, so our boats go to the waters of developing states to overfish there," explained a WWF (World Wide Fund for Nature) spokesperson in 2003.[9] At the same time, rich countries have increasingly come to protect their own fish through regulation and fishing moratoriums.

Deep-sea fish: The final frontier

Finally, there's the deep sea. Here—6,000 feet below the water's surface—is a place where even plants don't exist. Exotic creatures do, however, despite the darkness and the incredible pressure, which for a fish is the equivalent at the deepest levels of 50 jumbo jets weighing down on a human.[10] At thousands of feet down, you would think that land-dwellers would be forced off limits. But think again. Deep-sea fish have suddenly had to face a predator never before seen and never so ravenous: man.

Before its population collapsed, the orange roughy, a deep-sea inhabitant, was the rage at every trendy restaurant. Tragically, since this New Zealand fish does not come to sexual maturity until age 30—not atypical for denizens of the deep—the gold rush on its flesh quickly became a recipe for near extinction. In terms of impact, people who eat it—or any of the other deep-sea varieties, including crab, royal red shrimp and spiny dogfish—might as well be eating the flesh of Bengal tigers. In ecological terms, the removal of even one species from such delicate food webs is highly disruptive.[11]

46 Slumgullion stew

UNFIT FOR MAN OR BEAST

*"There are over 100,000 cows a year that are fine at night and then found dead in the morning. They are rounded up, ground up, turned into feed, and fed right back to other cows."**—Howard Lyman, celebrated rancher turned vegetarian activist, *The Oprah Winfrey Show*, April 16, 1996

If you only got your information about what livestock eat from a child's story book, you'd assume that cattle and cows live on grasses and hay, hogs on leftover table scraps, and chickens on corn kernels. As it stands, today's livestock are grown out on cultivated grains laced with industrial waste, dead animals, and chicken manure. Modern industry has plenty of these additives, which all in fact facilitate growth.

So much offal, so little time

Farm "mortalities"—about a billion animals per year in the United States alone—comprise much of the visceral mix. Road kill, euthanized pets, and expired circus and zoo animals may also augment this corpse-filled brew. Moreover, a third of a cow and a fifth of a pig is considered by-product or offal,[1] forcing the industry to dream up uses for the excess.[2] One of the reasons why the U.S. meat industry has been able to swell to a $100-billion dollar business is that it has had a handy repository for its colossal accumulation of dead animals and parts of dead animals—all told, 47 billion pounds every year in the United States (approximately the weight of an average-sized man for every citizen).[3] Carcasses are conveniently carted away, and the intensive farm conditions that cause so many animals to die before slaughter in the first place remain unchallenged.

Feed makers and renderers liken what they do to recycling. Animal remains are reconstituted into blood meal, hydrolyzed feather meal, fishmeal, meat and bone meal, and poultry by-product meal that other animals can eat. Indeed, the alternatives to augmenting livestock feed with animal protein—carcass burial, incineration, and composting—arguably pose even greater dangers to the public. Burial and inadequate composting can leach pathogens, such as E. coli, into the groundwater, and incineration can release dioxins into the air.

* It is no longer legal in the United States to feed ruminant remains back to ruminants.

A solution with problems

Meat and bone meal (MBM), derived from the remains of cattle, is not only especially flammable when stored, as it often is in great quantities, it is always potentially contaminated with prions, the infectious agent for mad cow disease.[4] Since the European Union severely curtailed the feeding of animal by-product back to livestock,[5] warehouses are overflowing with MBM, and stockpiles of the moist and smelly red powder are now posing a public health threat. Much of this material has become an additive in cement.[6] In addition, the handling and storing of MBM has become expensive as well as logistically daunting for EU governments.

In the United States, most forms in which ruminant remains have traditionally been fed back to ruminants were banned in 1997 as a preventive measure against mad cow disease. Beef blood, chicken litter (which might include beef protein residue in spilled feed), restaurant table scraps, and downer cows were added to the list of banned bovine-feed additives as late as 2004.[7] Government reports, however, have revealed that the industry is wont to defy,[8] be confused by, or simply be unaware of such rules.[9] The FDA itself has asserted that an estimated 350,000 U.S. cattle (about one percent of all) that people end up consuming every year are fed beef by-products.[10] The Government Accounting Office asserted in 2002 that the "FDA's failure to enforce the feed ban may already have placed U.S. herds and, in turn, the human food supply at risk."[11]

According to former feedlot operator Howard Lyman, now a vegetarian advocate and spokesman, ranchers are generally disdainful of regulatory agencies and basically operate with impunity.[12] "The consequences of getting caught are one in a million," he explains, and repercussions for defiance are essentially nil.[13] In any case, rendered chickens and pigs fed on cow protein are regularly fed back to cows.[14]

Feed dangers lurking

Feed filler of by-product from the food industry—such as cooking grease, cannery and bakery waste, liquid whey, candy, or rotten cull potatoes—may seem harmless by comparison, but even these may transmit contaminants if not carefully processed.[15] Otherwise, dioxins, drug residues, and pesticides are also periodically found in poisonous concentrations in batches of feed, prompting sometimes massive recalls.

And what about chicken manure in animal feed? Except for batches destined for cattle, no U.S. restrictions are in place. In any case, farmers may not always allow enough composting time to kill the bacteria inherent to the waste.[16] Poorly treated chicken manure could contain deadly pathogens. Otherwise, heavy metals are there too—not unlike human sewage, which, according to some reports, also finds its way into feed from time to time.[17]

Bon appétit.

47 Passage to extinction

HUNTING AND FISHING FOR "SPORT"

"Laws and institutions must go hand in hand with the progress of the human mind. As that becomes more developed, more enlightened, as new discoveries are made, [and] new truths disclosed...institutions must advance also, and keep pace with the times."—Thomas Jefferson

Early humans, with a voracious appetite for meat, and armed with nothing more than spears, fire, and other simple but effective hunting techniques, eradicated more than half of the megafauna in what was to become the Americas in just one cataclysmic millennium. A similar scenario took place in Australia.[1] Giant woolly mammoths, marsupials the size of Humvees, and armadillos the size of baby elephants were among the victims. Scientists suggest that bloodlust and gratuitous overkill are likely to have been factored into the extinction.[2]

But why would humans kill to excess? The surplus killing in these early humans was apparently beyond simple food requirements. One theory proffered by a few scientists these days has been, because they could. And once techniques were perfected, the killing became a habit. The behavior, though rare, is found in other animals.[3]

Much later, in thirteenth-century New Zealand, 11 species of the giant Moa (a 440-pound flightless bird) were wiped out within a space of about 60 years.[4] Centuries later, rapacious hunting killed off the dodo bird and passenger pigeon and nearly annihilated the buffalo. Countless other creatures have been hunted to extinction throughout our reign as earth's dominant large mammal. Apparently, a few people who get comfortable with atrocity can do a lot of damage.

Humans, essentially harmless

With the advent of farming about 10,000 years ago, the practical need to hunt animals for food largely disappeared.[5] Some believe "sport" hunting emerged in Mesopotamia as an avocation among the privileged classes. Today, multibillion-dollar hunting and angling outfitters continue to indulge an intense primal need. A journalist who covers today's hunting industry once observed, "Man with his bare hands is a pretty harmless creature."[6] But augmented by today's array of space-age and military technologies, he's instantly transformed into a coolly precise and efficient killing machine. Multiplied out, his ilk can undermine an entire ecosystem without even trying. Scientists have in fact determined that the hunting of marine life worldwide over the past thousand years or so has been far more detrimental to coastal marine habitats than has pollution and global warming.[7]

Today, a riotous trade in bushmeat is rapidly sending Africa's gorillas, chimpanzees, and bonobos to extinction. Wielding automatic weapons, hunters (in some cases with huge commercial enterprises behind them) are moving into forests on roads newly cleared by loggers. The animals don't have a chance.[8] Similarly, "sport" fishing is now so popular that its collective adherents—10.5 million strong and wielding high-tech gear[9]—are for certain species beginning to vie with commercial fishing in terms of ecological impact,[10] although the aggregate impact of "sport" fishing compared with commercial fishing is still relatively negligible.[11] Ironically, Atlantic salmon and trout may now enjoy a reprieve from "sport" fishers, since these species were recently found to contain dioxin in their bodies.[12]

Chronic culling

Chronic wasting disease (CWD) is now prevalent among North America's deer and elk populations. Like mad cow disease, it has the prion as its infections agent. Scientists blame the spread of the disease on the growth of game farms that raise these animals to be sold to restaurants and to people who provide areas for canned hunts. Now that CWD has infected wild deer and elk, traditional hunters have been afraid to eat the game that they kill for fear of ingesting "mad elk" or "mad deer" disease.

There is some talk of shutting down the entire game-farm industry, although this has yet to happen. Instead, both the U.S. and Canadian governments have facilitated massive culls to eradicate the disease. In the United States alone an estimated one million wild deer and elk may eventually be hunted down over the current decade.[13] What gives these governments the right to perpetrate wholesale eradication measures upon wildlife on behalf of ranching and hunting interests remains an unanswered question. In any case, killing off healthy as well as sick animals serves to reduce the chances that this disease will ever be allowed to run its course.[14]

A vegetarian mind

Thomas Jefferson, as we see above, expressed unabashed optimism that with "new discoveries" and "new truths" the "human mind" would naturally "advance." And with this, "institutions [would] keep pace with the times." Certainly much is known that squarely incriminates hunting as a threat to the natural world that sustains us. Surely that knowledge should count as "new truths disclosed." Indeed, now that we have this knowledge, it is time to "advance" to the next step: that of instituting vegetarianism into our daily lives.

48 Fruits, nuts 'n' other morsels

PHYTO-HEALTH APLENTY

"Behold, I have given you every herb bearing seed...to you it shall be for meat."—Genesis 1:29

Fruit is richly imbued with health-giving phytochemicals, antioxidants, vitamins, and fiber. Fruit is indeed synonymous with life. Our own hands are dexterous appendages fashioned by nature to perfection for picking, holding, pealing, and conveying fruits, as well as nuts and seeds, to the human mouth. The following fact morsels should bring a new appreciation for these foods, although the list below is but a tiny sampling.

Apples. Eating apples regularly has been found to improve lung function.[1] Both their skin and their flesh are associated with inhibiting the growth of colorectal cancer and in neutralizing tissue-damaging free radicals.[2]

Avocados are one of the most nutritious foods you can eat, with more potassium than a banana and a good amount of iron, beta-carotene, and vitamins, including B6, C, and E. They contain folic acid and copper and pack as much fiber as a slice of whole-wheat bread.

They're high in monounsaturated fat, which lowers cholesterol in the same way as olive oil.[3]

Blueberries. These bulbous, indigo fruits are believed to counteract the problems of aging; in particular, they may improve short-term memory, reverse loss of balance and coordination, and reverse nerve dysfunction.[4] Studies by the USDA have discovered that half a cup of wild blueberries delivers as much antioxidant power as five servings of other fruits and vegetables such as carrots, apples, squash, or even broccoli.[5] Other studies credit blueberries with lowering cholesterol levels as well as guarding against cancer, heart disease, and diabetes.[6] So what don't they do?

Cranberries. These tart red berries have the ability to prevent E. coli from adhering to the cells lining the walls of the bladder. This makes them good at blocking urinary tract infections. Their anti-adhesion mechanism may also be instrumental in the fight against ulcers.[7] Cranberries have also been shown to prevent kidney stones and to remove toxins from the blood.[8]

Flax seeds are a nutritional substitute for fish because they contain alpha-linolenic acid, which enables the body to manufacture omega-3 fatty acids—one of the nutrients often difficult to obtain in a vegan diet. Vegans need to ingest two tablespoons of ground flax seeds per day to overcome generally poor omega-3/omega-6 ratios. Other important sources for omega-3 fatty acids include walnuts, pumpkin seeds, and hemp seed oil. Flax seeds are also believed to improve the condition of nails, hair, and skin, as well as boost energy levels and strengthen the immune system.[9]

Grapes and red wine consumption are associated with a lower risk of heart disease. A substance in the skins of grapes called *resveratrol* is believed to be a potent cancer inhibitor as well, thanks to its apparent ability to cause pre-cancerous cells to revert to normal. Moreover, studies have also found that resveratrol lowers cholesterol levels and acts as an anti-inflammatory substance.[10]

Kiwi. A comparative analysis of 25 common fruits found kiwi to be the most nutritionally dense. Runners-up were papaya and mango.[11]

Nuts (tree seeds) are high in fat per calorie, but this is far from a reason to avoid them, even—one might say especially—if one is on a reducing diet. Eaten in moderation, they satiate quickly and cut the cravings for empty calories that put the pounds on.[12] The fat in nuts is considered heart healthy. In a famous study among Seventh-day Adventists, those who consumed nuts at least five times a week were found to have 50 percent less risk of coronary heart disease than those who ate no nuts.[13] Other studies have shown that nuts help prevent diabetes.[14] Some nuts are high in vitamin E, a powerful antioxidant. They're also a great source of calcium and magnesium.[15] Brazil nuts are the preeminent source for selenium, a potent antioxidant.

Prunes. When researchers working with the USDA ranked the antioxidant abilities of various fruits and vegetables, prunes (dried plums) came out on top. Next on the list were raisins, blueberries and blackberries, kale, strawberries, and spinach.[16]

49 Vegetable kingdom

OF CABBAGES, ROOTS, STEMS, AND LEAVES

"Eat your vegetables."—Grandma

Roots, stems, and leaves, just like fruits, are sources for antioxidants and phytochemicals, the powerful compounds that provide a virtual fountain of youth in health benefits. Ongoing research is showing how these substances not only fight disease but also provide specific health benefits. Antioxidants generally prevent the body's deterioration at the hands of oxidation. Phytochemicals, which evolved to protect plants from disease and the elements, pass their benefits to people who consume them.

A word of warning: Antioxidants and phytochemicals are best ingested as part of their original packaging—foods—and may even be toxic when taken in excess in supplement form. They work best in concert as part of a balanced vegetarian diet. Now for a bit of vegetable appreciation.

Broccoli: How do we love thee? Let us count the ways! Numerous health studies placed this cruciferous veggie at the top of the list as a cancer fighter, particularly cancers of the colon, breast, and prostate. In addition, broccoli has been found to be protective against stroke and cataracts.[1]

A serving (half a cup) of broccoli is packed with more vitamin C than an orange, more calcium than a glass of milk, and more fiber than a slice of wheat-bran bread. It is considered to be one of the richest sources of beta-carotene.[2] It is also packed with selenium, an essential trace nutrient that helps keep the immune system strong and damaging free radicals in check.[3]

Broccoli is part of the cruciferous family of vegetables, which includes arugula, Brussels sprouts, cabbage, cauliflower, kale, radicchio, and radishes. These vegetables are all rich in vitamins A and C, as well as potassium and fiber.[4] They contain four powerful phytochemicals that have been found to reduce cancer risk (*indoles, dithiolthiones, sulforaphane,* and *isothiocyanates*). One study found that men who ate cabbage once a week had 66 percent less colorectal cancer than men who never ate it.[5] Sulforaphane has been found to kill helicobacter, a bacteria found in areas of the world where sanitation systems are inadequate.[6]

Carrots. This veggie is rich in beta-carotene, which, in food form, is not only a cancer fighter but also believed to improve lung function and reduce complications associated with diabetes.[7]

Garlic. Just as phytochemicals in other fruits and vegetables manifest themselves with a rainbow of colors, the healthful substance in garlic makes itself known with scent and flavor. In these odoriferous veggies, a substance called *allicin* works to fight colds and flu and acts as a powerful anti-cancer agent.[8]

Greens (salad). The green leafies are some of the most nutritious vegetables of all—the darker the better. Aside from their many other pluses, they contain folic acid in abundance, which has been found to prevent fetal brain and spine deformities in newborns[9] as well as combat the onset of Alzheimer's disease.[10] They are rich in vitamin K, which fulfills a critical role in blood clotting and activates at least three proteins involved in bone health.[11]

Spinach and kale. These dark leafy greens are particularly associated with eye health. When people over 55 eat a small serving of kale every day, they suffer only half as much from age-related blindness as those who shun this vegetable.[12] Diets rich in *lutein*—found in dark green vegetables—are in fact curative for people with age-related macular degeneration. Corn, which contains *zeaxanthin,* is believed to have the same effect. Furthermore, the folic acid in spinach is believed to reduce symptoms of depression.[13]

Sweet potatoes. Rich in beta-carotene—necessary for the body's manufacture of vitamin A—this root vegetable made the short list of *Vegetarian Times'* 13 most-nutritious vegetarian foods.[14]

Tomatoes. Strong evidence exists that tomatoes protect against cancer, heart disease and the aging process itself. Though technically considered a fruit (it bears seeds), this "garden veggie" contains the antioxidant *lycopene,* believed to be a powerful combatant against prostate cancer. Lycopene is also found in ruby-red grapefruit and watermelon.[15]

50 Conveyor of tears

MODERN CHICKEN SLAUGHTER

"Every time you miss one you hear the awful squawk it's making when you see it flopping around in the scalder, beating itself against the sides. Damn, another 'redbird'."—Virgil Butler, former poultry hanger, Tyson Foods[1]

Vegetarians don't need to slaughter their food. They don't need to anesthetize their grapefruit before sectioning it out. To stun a broccoli spear or a flax seed and bleed it out and butcher it—not necessary. An artichoke does not foam at the mouth—it does not have a mouth, or a mother, or a face—or fill up with adrenaline out of fear or look at you in panic before you cut it. Plant foods do not wail in pain when you prepare them. What a great feeling of solace to know these things, when all you eat is plants!

Such solace quickly evaporates, however, when one considers the transformation of living creatures into pieces of chicken. About 25 *million* chickens are slaughtered in the United States every *day.*[2] And no federal laws protect a single one of them during the process, or at any other time, for that matter. Poultry death comes by whatever means is most convenient for the producer, despite minor appearances to the contrary. Birds are not provided a swift death such as one that is legally, though not always in practice, afforded large mammals. And, not surprisingly, concerns about cruelty are essentially absent from the minds of the designers and operators of poultry slaughter machinery.

Billions of a feather shocked together

At the chicken slaughter plant, birds will flail and vocalize for a time. But, if all goes according to plan, the fluttering will subside, just as soon as an electrified brine bath transforms the blur of winged animation into a steady line of drooping chicken heads.

But what appears as relief for the birds is not what it seems. The stunning trough is not there for humane reasons. It exists to minimize all that inconvenient flailing—nothing more. The electric current is set at voltages just high enough to immobilize the birds. Higher voltages, which might knock the birds unconscious, tend to hinder efficient bleedout, break bones, and cause product-damaging hemorrhages.[3] So birds are not afforded this amenity. Indeed, a second charge may be administered just after the chickens' throats are slit—this one to "calm" the birds a bit for easier de-feathering.[4] Essentially, the birds bleed to death fully sentient—flaccid and unable to express any protest.

Boiled alive

Bird-killing mechanisms require regular oversight and maintenance. When systems are down, chaos quickly ensues for both birds and workers. Indeed, when chickens miss the throat-slitting machine, because they also missed the electrified trough that is meant to keep their bodies limp, they go to the scalder alive. Every day the USDA condemns 30,000–60,000 broiler chickens, because their carcasses did not get a chance to properly bleed out before scalding.[5]

Virgil Butler, a former poultry worker who is now an advocate for more humane slaughter methods, has attested that every fifth bird at his station at one of the smaller Tyson Foods plants where he worked, was not properly stunned.[6] His job when necessary was to catch struggling birds and slit their throats in order to keep them from going to the scalder alive. Some always got past him. Industry lingo refers to live-scalded birds as "redskins."

In a signed account in 2003, Butler wrote: "The chickens flop, scream, [and] kick, and their eyeballs pop out of their heads [when they're live in the scald tank]....They often come out the other end with broken bones...and missing body parts because they've struggled so much in the tank."[7] Butler describes an atmosphere of disarray and consummate abuse of the chickens at the hands of rickety equipment that frequently breaks down. Callous factory workers and negligent managers add to the mistreatment, he has asserted.

Butler maintains that when certain machinery broke down at the plant where he worked, the birds would invariably be caught in every haphazard position in which the apparatus might put them. This could mean hanging in painful positions for hours. Depending upon the mishap, death for the birds might come by drowning, freezing, suffocation, or dehydration.[8]

Activists go to the videotape

Undercover video footage of a West Virginia Pilgrim's Pride slaughter plant, made public in 2004, confirmed Butler's assessment of the wanton abuse that such settings bring out in poultry-slaughter workers. Employees were caught on camera violently stomping on birds, drop kicking them like footballs, and lobbing them against a wall apparently for fun. The footage clearly indicated that the workers did such things with little thought and as a matter of course.[9] According to the *New York Times,* the investigator who shot the videos "saw 'hundreds' of acts of cruelty, including workers tearing beaks off, ripping a birds' head off to write graffiti in blood, spitting tobacco juice into birds' mouths, plucking feathers to 'make it snow,' suffocating a chicken by tying a latex glove over its head, and squeezing birds like water balloons to spray feces over other birds."[10] According to the story, workers inflicted the tortures out of boredom. Neither employee orientations nor the company manual made any mention of animal welfare.

51 Disaster developing

POOR NATIONS CLAMOR FOR MEAT

"We want people in China eating U.S. beef."—Pres. George W. Bush, speaking to the Cattle Industry Annual Convention, Denver, Colorado, February 2002[1]

It's no secret that the affluent nations of the world have lost their battle of the bulge and likewise have been ravaged by our era's ignoble diseases of excess: heart disease, stroke, diabetes, certain cancers, and constipation.

What is less known is that the world's have-nots are themselves quickly losing their defenses against these scourges. Health-promoting native diets of beans, rice or tortillas, and plenty of fruits and vegetables, combined with regular exercise—usually in the form of physical labor—have given way to chicken nuggets, oily corn chips, and automobiles.

It seems that the slightest uptick in prosperity for a country can transform it overnight from a nation fending off famine to one plagued by diabetic amputees, although many countries find themselves wavering between a perplexing combination of the two. And worse, people's attitudes are not turning around fast enough to comprehend the dangers of the new diet. Indeed, pudginess is still associated with prosperity in many places.

The cost of globesity

Emerging economies today that are raring to grow are suddenly being saddled with coffer-breaking angioplasties and heart surgeries.[2] Developing countries simply do not have the luxury of forking over dearly earned cash on the consequences of obesity-generating diets. Yet, noncommunicable diseases already have become the dominant cause of death around the world, with the majority of chronic disease problems now occurring in developing countries.[3] Cancer cases worldwide are expected to increase by 50 percent from 2003 levels by 2020, partly because poor nations are adopting unhealthy Western habits. And 80 percent of cancer patients in poor countries die, compared with 50 percent in rich countries.[4] Heart disease kills men in Russia at five times the rate it kills men in America.[5]

In Singapore, the incidence of diabetes has doubled every decade since 1970, and it is predicted that a third of the world's diabetics will reside in China and India by 2020. Sadly, the slightest bit of flab on the generally smaller Asian physique can be particularly detrimental. Obese Asians are in fact two and a half times more likely to develop diabetes and hypertension than Caucasians.[6]

Devitalized processed foods—albeit often vegetarian in makeup—combined with newly adopted sedentary habits, are acting to fuel what's now known as New World Syndrome.[7] But the influx of fatty dairy products and meat surely provides the engine behind it all. Between 1983 and 2000, developing countries increased their meat consumption by 50 percent. China led the transformation. With increased meat, dairy, and farm-raised fish in their diets, the Chinese doubled their protein and tripled their fat consumption.[8]

Grain used for feed in China surged up from 14 million tons in 1960 to 100 million tons in 1997.[9] Mexico feeds its livestock nine times more grain than it did in 1960, Egypt, ten times.[10] Though U.S. per-capita meat consumption is four times that of China's, the differential is sure to narrow as China vies with Europe and the United States in the coming years to become the world's largest economy.

Protein overflow

The developing world is quite willingly adopting the Western style of eating. But surely the developed world is happily globalizing it for them. "We are exporting more corn and soybeans, but in the form of meat and poultry," the USDA boasts.[11] "We're part of a global protein market. I'm growing corn for meat that will be sold in China," a Midwestern farmer explains.[12] What is not readily acknowledged is that $10 billion in taxpayer money goes to corn growers each year in the form of subsidies,[13] later fueling surpluses that must be exported. Corn is the consummate feed grain of industrial agriculture. Two-thirds of America's agricultural exports go to feed livestock abroad.[14] Meanwhile, McDonald's operates more than 540 restaurants in 23 Chinese provinces.[15]

Traveling gonads

The trend today is for high-tech, industrially bred livestock—or just the semen, ova, or embryos—to be exported to developing countries, presenting particularly acute risks for them. First, according to the Food and Agriculture Organization of the UN (FAO/UN), the recipient countries soon find they cannot afford or sustain the high-protein feed, medication, and climate-controlled housing that the super-breeds require.[16] Also, without modern infrastructure and communication systems, poor nations more easily fall prey to livestock-disease outbreaks. Finally, the introduction of industrially bred animals in the Third World has begun to threaten indigenous breeds of livestock, thereby jeopardizing general food security in remote parts of the globe. Local "vernacular" breeds that have long carried site-specific disease resistance and adaptations to local parasites, pests, and climates are being eclipsed by the new-fangled super-breeds. Local breeds are lost to extinction as recipient countries cross-breed their animals with the high-tech varieties or replace them outright. According to the FAO/UN, 1,350 domestic animal breeds are considered at risk for extinction.[17] Already, last century, a thousand domesticated breeds were lost worldwide.[18]

52 Harm on the range

EXTINCT IS FOREVER

"Ranching is the number one source of water pollution, soil erosion, and species endangerment in the West."—George Wuerthner, outspoken opponent of public-lands ranching[1]

In the late nineteenth century, settlers began in earnest to seed America with cattle.[2] With the bison herds by this time annihilated, the white man was having his jerky and eating it, too. The desire for beef aplenty, however, came at an enormous environmental cost. Not native to this hemisphere, the new bovines never did fit in ecologically. Today, an area in the West, four times the size of California, has been degraded, primarily by cattle.[3] Indeed, this interloping species demands a far hardier habitat to stand up to it—similar to those in which its predecessor, the forest-dwelling aurochs, evolved.[4]

Hooves of destruction

Today's cattle in America's West are particularly hard on riparian zones, the fertile areas along rivers and streams where 75 percent of the region's wildlife species congregate and regenerate.[5] The Government Accounting Office has said that grazing is responsible for 70 percent of the damage to riparian areas on federally owned lands.[6] These delicate ecosystems, which act as natural purifiers of the water, are summarily trampled flat and contaminated by cow manure. A herd of cattle will easily graze a stream bed—once teeming with insects, fish, and cooling shrubbery—into a barren bank of dried mud.[7] Unlike the native elk or bison, if cows are not herded along, they will denude the foliage down to the nub.[8]

In addition, grazing cattle are directly or indirectly responsible for much of the soil erosion in the United States; 54 percent of U.S. pasture land is being overgrazed.[9] Furthermore, cattle grazing is the number-one reason why species are placed on the endangered species list.[10]

Frequent fire program

Range scientists today argue that the frequent incidence of massive, destructive forest fires, particularly in the nation's Southwest, is the result of cattle grazing.[11] Historically, "cool" grass fires were an annual event in this area. They stayed low to the ground, rarely getting a chance to reach the canopy of the trees. Frequent fires kept the saplings of smaller trees from getting a foothold and also kept the forest floor free of too much fuel that could kindle more destructive fires.[12]

From the time of the early settlers, however, these "cool" fires were regularly suppressed on behalf of cattle. A tinderbox of dense foliage was allowed to build up below the taller trees. Moreover, the fire cycle was disrupted by the animals themselves eating the grasses away.[13] Extremely dense forests eventually grew up in the void. Where 100 trees per acre might have been the norm in a historic Ponderosa forest, today, because of cattle, many sites exceed 2,000 trees per acre.[14] Insect infestations and destructive fires take hold more easily under these conditions.

Besides these scenarios, we need to factor in an invasive Eurasian plant nicknamed cheatgrass, now covering millions of acres across America's West. It never would have gotten a foothold but for the cow-degraded landscape. This dense interloping weed germinates early, crowding out native grasses for land space. It then dies out early, providing a vast abundance of papery kindling when the weather is still hot and dry. Major forest fires now occur at the rate of one every three years, where such a conflagration would normally have happened once in a century.[15]

Corporate cowboys

Roughly 90 percent of government-managed land and 69 percent of government-managed forest is leased to livestock producers. This includes areas cordoned off as national parks, wildlife refuges, and other nature preserves.[16] Yet cattle grazing, we find, is the primary cause of widespread habitat destruction on America's 260 million acres of public lands. And in exchange for all the ecological disruption, only 3.8 percent of the nation's beef cattle come from these lands.[17]

Meanwhile, ranchers continue to be heavily subsidized by the U.S. government, grazing their animals at the rock-bottom rate of $1.43 per month for each cow and calf.[18] Market rate for the same thing is over $10. And more than a few of the "welfare ranchers" using these commons for their own private feedlot can in fact be counted as millionaires or large corporate entities. According to a Freedom of Information Act investigation conducted by the *San Jose Mercury News*, the richest, top 10 percent of grazing-permit holders control 65 percent of the livestock on Bureau of Land Management property.[19]

53 Life of the hen

CRUELTY IN THE EGGS-TREME

"My purpose is to shoot a documentary. As for raising awareness, it seems to be working. It's getting incredible amounts of media attention."—Rob Thompson, Ottawa video artist, who in 1997 paid two people $1,800 each to live like battery hens for a week[1]

Commercial egg-laying hens probably take the prize for the most abused farmed animal—quite a statement considering the cruelty that abounds in modern agriculture. Cold, hard economics dictates as farmers pack sentient creatures by the hundreds of thousands into huge buildings filled with so-called "battery cages"—rather mini-prisons—for anywhere between 10 and 18 months. The birds are cheap, but the cages are expensive, so the farmer essentially charges his inmates rent—the currency being eggs.

A commercial egg-laying hen lives her entire life in a volume of space just bigger than the space taken up by her body. Essentially immobilized for months at a time, her claws may actually grow to permanently clutch the wire floor. She never gets to run, build a nest, enjoy a cleansing dust bath, mate, forage in the sun, perch, fly, shelter a chick, or even lift a wing, though her every instinct will yearn to do so. Her life will consist of thwarted urges as she spends her time crouching and fending off the frantic "feather pulling" of cage mates. And though her life is dedicated to creating potential life, every egg she lays will roll away out from under her and out of reach because of the slope of the wire floor that also cripples her legs and feet.

Incarceration

It is not uncommon for millions of hens to be kept on a single farm. Multitiered hen houses may hold 250,000 birds each.[2] The ammonia-saturated air from manure pits below causes lifelong respiratory problems for the birds. Historically, this species foraged a varied diet; in confinement, automated feeders dispense a monotonous gruel. Lighting is manipulated: first dim to reduce fighting, then bright for many hours to mimic egg-producing spring days.[3] Rubbing against wire cages wears away the birds' feathers. In some poorly designed systems a bar encumbers the eating process, further resulting in painful abrasions over time. Many birds will be afflicted with a myriad of grotesque diseases, born of the unnatural conditions they are forced to endure.[4]

Caught in the clutches

The wild ancestors of the modern hen laid only two clutches of a dozen eggs apiece per year. In the 1950s, hens were bred to produce about 70 eggs over the same amount of time.[5] Now, 300 eggs are a normal annual yield.[6]

No feed is nutritionally adequate to the demands that egg laying puts upon a hen's body. The bones of the hens will become brittle as calcium is taken for the eggshells. Deficiencies do not impact the eggshells, however, only the bones, which are easily broken, usually during rough treatment at the end of the bird's life.[7]

Meanwhile, tight living quarters often cause frustrated birds to fight. Once started, so-called "cannibalism," an industry term, is hard to control. So, producers debeak all birds as a matter of routine to head off potential damage.

Otherwise, male chicks are considered a liability to the egg farm, as they have little or no commercial value. Their genes do not yield a bird worth raising for meat, either, so they become a disposal problem—an expense. Chick "sexers" pick out the males, just hatched, who are then expediently destroyed. Humane methods are not required by any law. So the chicks are dumped in trash bins to die by crushing, suffocation, starvation, or exposure.

Finally, the torture of egg laying for a confined hen is not merely physical. Laying, according to the late ethologist Konrad Lorenz, is in fact a most private act. He equated laying eggs in full view—as a battery hen must—with humans being forced to defecate in each others' presence.[8]

The end

When a hen no longer yields eggs at the rate her captors require, her only value may lie in her body's use as feed for the next flock. There are no restrictions on using the remains of dead chickens as feed for animals, including chickens. She is not even worth a trip to the renderer, and so she becomes an expense. No method of disposal will be cheap enough. She may be packed in a crate and buried alive. Or, if lucky, she will be gassed. But with this method, again, she may not be dead before she is buried.[9]

54 Antidotes to filth

HIGH-TECH BATTLE OF THE BUGS

"Our greatest weapon in the battle to ensure food safety is new technology."—former USDA secretary Dan Glickman[1]

The meat industry has made one fine mess of things, polluting our food and our environment with newly emergent killer bacteria. Just 25 years ago people did not have to worry about listeria, E. coli, or campylobacter—each a major poisoner of animal-based food.[2] The Economic Research Service of the USDA estimates that the cost of foodborne disease in terms of human illness amounts to nearly $7 billion per year for just five foodborne pathogens—including the above three—all associated with animal-based foods.[3] Lawsuits resulting from food-poisoning victims using DNA traceback methods are forcing the meat industry to amass an arsenal of technical fixes to wash away bacteria. And what they can't wash they try to kill. The 50 million Americans who live with compromised immune systems[4] have made this endeavor particularly urgent. However, keeping microbes off the product isn't always easy, and some of the technologies may carry more risks than they are worth. In any case, developing antidotes to pathogen-prone meat has become an industry in and of itself.

On the farm. A process known as competitive exclusion works by misting newly hatched chicks with specially designed cocktails of benign (friendly) bacteria, or probiotics, in an effort to crowd out bad bacteria.[5] Some fear the merged-in bacteria may themselves initially or eventually become dangerous.[6] The mixtures contain 65 different species in concentrations of 10 billion bacteria per gram.[7]

Other processes remove pathogen-laden dust from animal sheds with air-ionizing electrostatic energy.[8] Cherries[9] and hay[10] are added to cattle feed in an endeavor to reduce E. coli O157:H7 in the bovine gut.

In the slaughterhouse. Carcasses go through steam/vacuum chambers or are sprayed or rinsed with saline, acidic, chlorine, and/or ozone-infused solutions. A substance derived from whey, called lactoferrin, may similarly be applied to meat as a surface antimicrobial.[11] Other carcasses may be treated with a stream of energized electrons in a process known as electronic pasteurization.[12] Some packing plants may inject the carotid artery of freshly slaughtered bovines with a cold sugar-and-salt solution, pushing out pathogen-attracting bacteria.[13] Liquid nitrogen, at a temperature of –320°F, is used to "contact-freeze" bacterial growth stone dead.[14] Oysters are cryogenically purified for safety and longer shelf life.[15] Vaccines, ultra-high pressure,[16] and anti-microbial packaging are also part of the meat industry's growing bug-fighting weaponry.

Various bacteria-testing technologies have likewise been brought into use. At one point the Agriculture Research Service of the USDA announced it was working on a fluorescent fecal contamination detector, dubbed a "scat scanner."[17]

Food irradiation. And what of FDA-approved food irradiation—the nuke-based slaughterhouse-bacteria fighter? Despite public uneasiness, the technology is increasingly, though haltingly, being adopted by food companies. Opponents have warned that food irradiation reduces nutritional value and produces a number of carcinogens in the meat.[18] Its greatest hazard, however, both for workers and the public, probably lies in handling and transporting the risky fuel source.[19] Moreover, consumers of irradiated foods still end up eating the fecal filth anyway, albeit in neutralized form.

Off to market. Time/temperature detection tabs monitor food's spoilage thresholds.[20] Other detection devices include fiber-optic pathogen sensors that use vibrating quartz crystals.[21]

In the kitchen. A silver-coated cutting board kills food bacteria. But, since it tends to work like an antibiotic, some fear its use will engender resistant bacteria.[22]

In your body. Now, if after all of this you still get sick, you can take a sugar-derived toxin receptor—a drug to absorb the poison.[23]

Finally, none of these technologies is 100 percent effective, and their use tends to give consumers of meat a false sense of security. The antidotes help us to ignore the main reason we are inundated with so many killer bacteria in the first place: the intensive confinement of animals on farms and feedlots.

55 Heavy petting

LET'S TALK ABOUT SEX

"The artificial insemination of birds and other animals removes humanity further and further away from any possibility of establishing a civilized relationship with the rest of the living world."—Karen Davis, Ph.D., United Poultry Concerns[1]

If you have even the slightest vestige of a Victorian sensibility about sex, you'd better get over it fast if you want to survive as a farmer today, particularly if you want to involve yourself with breeding—now a specialty operation. It's positively pornographic out there—no, perverted. A good measure of bestiality, it seems, takes place for the sake of animal-based food production. The animals have no choice but to join this tawdry world that humans have devised. The uncooperative are shipped straightaway to feedlots or to the slaughterhouse.

Collecting the prize

Few bovine males get to keep their testicles in America. If they do, they become breeding stock for either beef or dairy operations, reduced to their fundamental essence: sperm. Since livestock sex brings the dual hazards of disease and injury, today's operations use artificial insemination—now nearly or completely universal on dairy, hog, and turkey farms. Animals used exclusively for breeding purposes—whatever the species—are nearly always produced by artificial insemination.

Every day, the following scene takes place at points all across America, initiated by what most would consider entirely legitimate businesses. An elephantine-sized stud bull with strikingly huge genitals is led by the nose into a ring.[2] He's sniffing, moaning, and feeling eager. His ears are propped up. His nearly two-foot-long penis is getting ready to emerge via its able retractor muscle.[3] In the arena, all there is besides the stock hand is either a steer (a castrated bull) or even an uncastrated bull like himself. No other creatures are in view, least of all a cow. A female simply would not be able to hold up under him. Venereal disease is another concern. Beyond view, rookie bulls, shall we say voyeurs, may be gazing on from behind a gate, getting hot and turned on also.[4] They're learning the ropes, because soon they too will be doing the same thing.

Suddenly, the big bull mounts the "jump stock," but just before he ejaculates, a collection technician reaches underneath him and grabs his penis in order to sheath it, apply pressure to it, and direct the flow of semen into a three-foot-long tube, or "artificial vagina."[5] Thus goes ranch life for a sex machine. Indeed, this super-sire will never accomplish a natural service at any time in his entire life. Just the same, he will father thousands, and perhaps hundreds of thousands, of offspring.

Meanwhile, bull sperm is kept viable indefinitely in "straws," preserved by liquid-nitrogen refrigeration. Breeders are able to ship specimens anywhere in the world. The remote-control servicing of cows generally costs about $15 per dose. Whatever the species, artificial insemination is not only easier, it's an amazing bargain, and the efficiency is irresistible.[6] Prize bull semen, of course, can be bid up into the hundreds of dollars per dose.[7]

Rendezvous with a dairy-ère

Down the line, techniques that implant the sperm into cows are equally bizarre. As stock hands stand watch, heat (fertility) detection is accomplished by nearby animals who cannot be allowed to penetrate. This may be done by other cows who tend to mount cows in heat.[8] Other systems work with bulls who have had their penises surgically rerouted—which, needless to say, causes persistent frustration.[9] Once cows in heat are detected, insemination specialists are hired to expertly designate and insert the sperm. First, they must grope around in the cow's rectum, shoulder deep, to clean the area out and to locate the uterus and cervix. Later, once the cow's vagina is spread, the specialist syringes sperm through the cervix with a straw-loaded inseminator gun.[10]

Embryo transfer similarly involves invasive techniques, which utilize high-quality eggs harvested from select females for implantation into numerous surrogates.

Hogs do it, turkeys do it

Hogs. Somewhat similar techniques are used with today's swine. To get a boar excited—apparently not an easy task when all you have is a small bench-like "stool" called a training dummy—the stock hand is advised to take it slow, become the animal's friend, and vocalize in encouraging tones. "Stimulate his sides, testes and prepuce [foreskin],"[11] one veterinary Web site instructs. But if that doesn't work, allow the boar to mount the stool while standing directly behind him. "Reach forward to massage the sheath and apply pressure with your legs to his rear. Allow the penis to [become] erect and continue massage."[12]

Turkeys. Because of intensive trait selection, the breasts of male turkeys have become so large that copulation can no longer physically take place. All commercial turkeys raised for meat today must therefore be the result of artificial insemination. On turkey breeding farms, "milking" the males in one barn and depositing the semen into hens in an adjacent one is not only cruel to the birds but also monotonous and degrading for the farm hands.[13]

Mean, obscene cruelty machine

From the producer's point of view, the efficiency of artificial insemination is, shall we say, exciting. In just a few decades, the technique has produced profitable, albeit freakish, genetic traits in farmed animals. Despite the inherent perversity, no one seems to be complaining. For the producer, the technique works far too well. For the animals, it's another story.

56 Chemical castration

MANURE DOWNSTREAM MENACE

"Once it [manure] comes out the tail end of a cow we haven't been interested. Now we need to reconsider our assumptions."—Louis Guillette, researcher studying fathead minnows downstream from a Nebraska feedlot[1]

The world is in the midst of a pharmaceutical revolution. Not only are we humans medicating *ourselves* with colossal amounts of drugs for every pain, condition, cosmetic flaw, or garden-variety angst under the sun, we're drugging up our livestock with no less reckless abandon. The phenomenon has ushered in an unanticipated environmental menace to our waters: drug pollution. There are the trace amounts of caffeine, aspirin, cholesterol-lowering medications, and birth control pills—the people drugs. And there are the growth-promoting steroids and antibiotics—the livestock drugs. Consequently, endocrine-disrupting substances are getting into our water via human and animal waste—this, after standing up to digestion and even treatment and filtration systems.

The pharmaceutical as pollutant

So far, few people have begun to grasp the idea of pharmaceuticals as water pollutants. Others dismiss the phenomenon because concentrations tend to be fantastically small—in parts per billion or even parts per trillion. The drugs' damaging effects, however, are far from insignificant. Research, though still a bit sketchy, is linking the presence of trace pharmaceuticals in the water to the partial or even full sexual reversal of some aquatic animals. In several documented cases females have been observed displaying male traits and males have been observed displaying female traits downstream from factory-farm operations.

There are hundreds of animal drugs and chemicals used today on farms. Each has its own chemical stability, meaning that each degrades to a benign state at its own rate. These vaccines, parasiticides, hormones, insecticides, feed medications, and antimicrobials are making their way into our creeks, rivers, and lakes, it happens, via the feces and urine excreted by the animals.[2] This becomes quite an important piece of information when one considers that livestock in America, according to a 1997 U.S. Senate report, produce 130 times the waste that the people do.[3] And water samples show that a significant amount of the chemical-infused effluent ends up in our water.

Loss of species, the cost of feces

In a groundbreaking University of Florida, Gainesville, study, conducted downstream from a Nebraska feedlot, male fathead minnows were found to have abnormally small testes and significantly less testosterone than normal fathead minnows.[4] Females of this species exhibited decreased egg production,[5] but, more surprisingly, they grew bumps, or tubercles, on their heads, the outward sign males normally display when reproductively active.[6] The ramifications of the study, which some see as just the tip of the iceberg, are frightening, given that the vast majority of the nation's 35 million beef cattle are routinely pumped up with the suspected causal agent: growth-enhancing hormones. The hormones enhance growth in the beef cattle by spurring feed conversion. But apparently, when allowed to get into the environment, they can play havoc with the reproductive abilities of non-target species downstream.

In another groundbreaking study conducted in 2004, researchers from Colorado State University found three kinds of antibiotics identified specifically as livestock drugs in the Cache la Poudre River, which flows within the confines of the western state. Of the three drugs, one that is normally administered to cattle, Monensin, was found in the river's sediment at levels 1,000 times greater than in the water.[7]

The more scientists look, the more they find. A study of the Chesapeake Bay watershed has detected hormones in its streams, undoubtedly originating with area livestock operations.[8] European and Canadian studies have similarly found animal agriculture suspect for drugs in local waterways.[9] Antibiotics, pesticides, and fungicides used in aquaculture operations are even more easily passed along in fluid environments, eventually lodging in mounds of sediment.[10]

Just say no

The human-health ramifications of hormones in beef have been the overriding concern of a trade dispute between the United States and the European Union for well over a decade. One could argue that the environmental issues surrounding these drugs are more troubling. In the meantime, people might consider "just saying no" to the foods that cause drugs to infuse our water supplies.

57 Industrial-size farm

BIG AND INFLEXIBLE

"Specialization produces efficiencies, but carries risks."—Ron Plain, agricultural economist, University of Missouri.[1]

There has been one all-consuming trend in agriculture for the last century: higher volumes of output by fewer producers with more specialized operations. In 1920, most farms diversified with a variety of operations, breeds, and species. There were 44 times as many hog operations that year as in 2000.[2] Now, 70 percent of the hogs are produced by 7 percent of hog producers. Similarly, 60 percent of the nation's cows are milked by seven percent of dairy producers. Most dramatically, 85 percent of feedlot cattle are fattened on just 2 percent of feedlot operations.[3] Today's farms often produce only one commodity.

In the late 1980s there were 2,500 egg producers. By 2002, only 300 were left.[4] Between 1980 and 2000, 300,000 farmers of all kinds exited the business.[5]

These numbers illustrate how concentrated farm production is today. Call it a mental block, but most people who have little difficulty understanding what this means for other industries cannot seem to visualize how industry consolidation applies to their food. (Can we blame the children's picture books—the ones with the cow and the pig and the chicken?)

The fact is, farm consolidation over recent years has been especially harsh and abrupt. It seems that when no one was looking—perhaps when people thought all our community problems were urban ones—a Robert Moses-esque highway of sorts cut a swath across our land. There was nothing to stop it: no laws, no ethic, no useful political analysis, and almost no populist mobilization.

Indeed, consolidation ran amok, while public policy seemed clueless. Subsidies figured in prominently—they still do—bestowing advantages to the largest operators. A quarter of the subsidy payments today go to farms with sales of $500,000 or more.[6] Always touted as a safety net for small family farmers, the multibillion-dollar handouts actually work to put them out of business. Giant monocultural grain growers are some of the biggest winners. But their windfalls only get passed on again to the livestock producers in the form of low grain prices. In the end, it all works to place vast supplies of animal-based foods into the marketplace at bargain prices shoppers have long learned to expect.

For the individual farmer, the specialization that makes for efficiency leads to inflexibility in response to market conditions. Modern confinement systems are designed with only one species in mind. A barn for pigs cannot easily be converted to one for chickens, for instance. In eras past such a change would have been a viable option.

Pork glut '98–'99

A particularly cataclysmic consolidation took place in the hog world in 1998 and 1999. A freakish glut was brought about by a perfect storm of economic factors. Efficient factory-farm production greatly augmented supply; severe financial woes in Russia and Asia lessened demand.[7] Add in curtailed slaughterhouse capacity, and prices dipped to numbers not seen since the Great Depression. Hog operations were abandoned, leaving animals to starve. Farmers advertised hog hunts and charity pork giveaways—anything to unload the massive stores. Ultimately, 20,000 U.S. hog farms, or about 20 percent, were pushed out of the business within this short time frame.[8]

The big got bigger

The slaughter industries, whether in beef, pork, or chicken, are also highly concentrated. In the 1980s, smaller meatpackers were swallowed up, one by one, by bigger ones.[9] The few mammoth-size firms still around today were those able to monopolize butchering by acquiring expensive, automated machinery and hiring cheap labor. Cuts of meat in consumer-ready portions are now shipped directly to supermarkets in refrigerated trucks. Moreover, vertical integration defines the pork and poultry industries, and the beef industry to a somewhat lesser extent. The control allows the processors to dictate wages, specifications, schedules, and prices from their employees and suppliers in order to shave fractions of a penny off selling prices.

In the end, when it comes to food, local is fresher, smaller is safer, and vegetarian is kinder. With monolithic meat companies, you get none of these. All you get is efficiency at the expense of absolutely everything.

58 Moo!

MODERN DAIRY COW LIFE

"A cow's a piece of machinery. If it's broke, we try to fix it, and if we can't it gets replaced. Today, every cow has a number and a page on the computer."—Gene Koopman, dairy farmer, quoted in *The New York Times*[1]

Cold, hard cost analysis will show you that it is more profitable to maintain one cow than four, if the one cow gives as much milk as four. Indeed, after just several generations of selective breeding, exactly this kind of efficiency now exists. In 1940, a cow in the United States produced an average of 2.3 tons of milk per year.[2] Today's cow yields a staggering 9.1 tons per year, with some regions specializing in cows yielding an inconceivable 13 tons per year.[3] Daily milk output of the most fecund of these super-producers comes to 70 pounds per day. A cow's udder can weigh as much as a full-grown man,[4] causing leg problems to be widespread.

The stress on cows is tremendous. Five hundred gallons of blood have to circulate through a cow's udder to provide the nutrients for a single gallon of milk.[5] It takes 350 squirts to accumulate a gallon.[6] Cows may be lying around most of the day, but their bodies are working overtime—in fact, for the peak performers, the equivalent of a man jogging six hours per day.[7] Though cows formerly lived 20 years, today's superlactator is usually "spent" after a 4–year life that imposes three rapid-fire milking periods,[8] preceded by three requisite pregnancies. Furthermore, mastitis, a painful udder disease that infects 40 to 50 percent of U.S. cows,[9] is essentially man-made. Cows get infected by a combination of factors, including over-milking, improperly functioning milking machines, growth hormones, and injuries. To treat the malady, farmers usually administer antibiotics, aggravating that much more the public threats of drug resistance and end-product residues.

Kindness for profit's sake

Conditions for cows vary widely across the United States and among producers. With consolidation in the industry taking hold, larger modern dairies have been influenced by new scientific findings that discourage rough handling in favor of comfort for the animals—for profit's sake. Comfort perhaps, but the necessary evils of dairy production haven't gone away: the serial pregnancies, young taken away from their mothers within 24 hours of birth, mutilations such as tail docking, the preponderance of "downed" animals (those incapacitated by injury and disease), and involuntary inseminations (artificial and otherwise). And finally, no matter if a farmer raises his animals traditionally in pastures or intensively tethered at the neck, virtually no cow gets a retirement package after her heroic term of service. Fast-food burgers are such a bargain because of plentiful supplies of the ground remains of under-producing dairy cows.

Conditions sorely wanting

The cows people see from the road are the lucky ones. The vast majority of cows in the United States live much if not all of their lives in barns or, if outdoors, in barren dirt pens devoid of grass. Especially abusive are the Midwest and Northeast dairies. Cows in much smaller, mostly outmoded operations are chained at the neck to stanchions. They are forced to endure confinement that prevents them from grooming and socializing.[10] These cows often live in filthy conditions, doing their best to avoid being tangled in their tethers or slipping on mattresses befouled with waste. Cows need to stand up and lie down numerous times during the day. If nothing but concrete is below them, hocks and rumps will become swollen, abraded, abscessed, and bruised. Early confinement systems for cows were designed with the laborer, not the cow, in mind. Some systems make it difficult for cows to lunge properly to get to a standing position.

The U.S. government subsidizes the dairy industry to an extent bordering on the absurd. Yet, with the slightest research, one can easily learn of milk's less-than-wholesome aspects. On your next trip to the store, reach for the oat, almond, rice, or soy beverage. Many brands come fortified with vitamin B12, vitamin D, calcium, and omega-3 fatty acids. They also come in a dazzling array of flavors.

59 Biotech and cloning

THE CRUEL FRONTIER

"Deaths and deformities in cloned animals are the norm, not the exception."—Wayne Pacelle, CEO, Humane Society of the United States[1]

Genetic manipulation of livestock has long been an effective instrument in bringing down the cost of meat. It's a tool, however, that has made, and continues to make, farmed animals into freaks.

High-tech gene splicing, with its pinpoint accuracy, now holds even more potential for the meat industry. It gives modern agricultural geneticists the precision they need to readily design animals to even greater ideals of farm-output perfection than are already available. Taking genes garnered from across the kingdom of life, they cobble like digital artists with pixels. Later, in theory, cloning holds promise to lock in the results. Final outcome: more trait monoculture, more animal suffering, and more alienation from the natural world.

Biotech: A technology for the producers

Scientists have amassed hundreds of transgenic and cloned animals. The genes of some have the farm of the future as their destiny. Experiments all, these creatures reside in living laboratories across the United States and the world. They include the super-producers, of course, but also such amalgams as the "enviropig," a farmed animal designed to excrete less-noxious waste to lower pollution.[2] A chicken born resistant to disease is also on the horizon.[3] Other species have been engineered with "reduced sentience" to allow them to withstand the stresses of intensive confinement.[4] Outside of a few cases, the marvels of the biotech toolbox speak to the concerns of producers, not consumers. It remains unknown whether the meat from these creations will foster allergic reactions (due to spliced-in genes),[5] antibiotic resistance, or yet-unknown health risks for those who consume it.

GE out of the bottle

Transgenic farmed fish that grow to market weight five times faster than regular fish could be the first government-approved, genetically engineered (GE) animals designated for commercial production. So far, approval has been stalled, thanks, undoubtedly, to a National Academies of Sciences report warning that mobile GE creatures, such as farmed fish, pose a grave threat to the environment if they escape their pens and displace species in the wild.[6] Indeed, escapees could prey upon, interbreed with, and spread disease to their wild cousins.[7] They could compete with indigenous fish for food and mates.[8] A USDA-funded study of transgenic fish determined that such an ecological assault could bring certain native species to extinction.[9]

A Pew Initiative on Food and Biotechnology study determined that escaped GE organisms, such as fish, could theoretically wreak permanent ecological damage[10] and that the FDA lacked the appropriate authority to deflect lawsuits brought by biotech firms pushing their products.[11] Meanwhile, GE fish proponents say their creations are engineered to be sterile. Others say it only takes two.

Send out the clones

The approval of GE fish could eventually open the door to a menagerie of GE species that, once perfected, stand to be duplicated out, en masse, via cloning. At first, clones might function as breeding stock. But eventually, entire herds could be made up of the most highly productive.[12] So far, however, miscarriages, stillbirths, birth defects, and premature aging have slowed the establishment of cloning technologies.[13] A study in 2002 found cloned mice with hundreds of abnormal genes.[14] And not only does cloning research inflict cruelty on its test subjects, but the flesh of these experimental animals is predicted to become part of the food supply. Already, the Food and Drug Administration (FDA) has determined that cloned animals are safe to eat, eliminating any reason for labeling the resultant meat at the supermarket.[15] "Cloning can help livestock producers deliver what consumers want: nutritious, wholesome food products in a repeatable and reliable manner and at an affordable price," crowed one industry spokesperson after the FDA determination.[16]

A science of defiance

Gene splicing is considered an additive or ingredient, so biotech comes under the purview of the FDA, an agency many believe to be ill prepared to handle such high-tech science. Moreover, standard FDA procedure nudges aside the public during product-approval periods in order to protect companies' trade secrets—a dangerous restriction, considering this technology is so riddled with societal risk.

For that matter, the United States probably needs to consult with the rest of the world before introducing technologies we may be unable to control. In the meantime, when consumers purchase cheap and uniform meat, they just encourage these modern-day Frankensteins.

60 Death by algae

SHAFTING FISH AND GRASSES

"Now it is clear. The size and duration of the hypoxic zone is very clearly driven by the nutrient load in the Mississippi River."—Donald Scavia, Senior scientist, NOAA[1]

In 2004, the executive director of the UN Environment Program (UNEP), Klaus Töpfer, warned that "humankind is engaged in a gigantic, global experiment as a result of inefficient and often overuse of fertilizers." Along with other pollutants that are generated by cities, the fertilizers are contributing to vast areas in coastal waters that are devoid of life.[2] Sadly, the experiment is on track to continue. The UNEP has warned that by 2025, the release of nitrogen fertilizer into the environment will double worldwide from year-2000 levels.[3] A UNEP report has in fact declared that so-called "dead zones" are the greatest emerging environmental challenge.[4]

The number of "dead zones" in the world has doubled to 150 since 1990.[5] This trend is largely the result of explosive growth in livestock production—from excessive cultivation of feed grains to the continued growth of factory farming. Suffocating algae results when fertilizers and manure run off of farm operations into the world's bays, estuaries, lakes, gulfs, and seas. One-celled phytoplankton eventually die and fall to the water's floor, where oxygen becomes depleted by the decay.[6] The hypoxia, or oxygen deficit, that occurs is what causes thousands of square miles to become devoid of life. When you're in the midst of one of these vast aquatic graveyards all you see are rotting fish and wilting plant life. Tragically, the world's dead zones develop in coastal waters, the critical areas where fish spawn and in fact spend most of their lives.[7]

Midwestern nutrients feed Gulf dead zone

The Gulf of Mexico contains the third largest dead zone in the world, spanning in 2001 an area the size of Massachusetts. Billions of creatures are suffocated by it every midsummer.[8] (Imagine the same size area on land as devoid of life.) It is estimated that 70 percent of the runoff that causes this phenomenon comes from agriculture,[9] which, up the Mississippi River in America, means animal agriculture. About 6.3 million tons of nitrogen and 2.7 million tons of manure wash down the river every year.[10] All told, the amount of these nutrients has tripled since 1960.[11]

Underwater grasses take a hit

Nutrient pollution is the cause of over half the degradation of U.S. estuaries, according to the National Oceanic and Atmospheric Association (NOAA).[12] Sea grasses, which provide shelter and spawning grounds for fish, are a primary casualty of the runoff, as the resultant algae growth blocks the sunlight they require. In parts of the Gulf of Mexico, sea grasses have diminished by 20 to 100 percent (depending on the location) over the last 50 years.[13] Grasses in the Chesapeake Bay, in general, are down to a tenth of the area they once covered, largely due to chicken and dairy operations upstream and on nearby land.[14] During most summers a third of the Chesapeake Bay is essentially empty of life.[15]

Scientists have compared sea grasses to rainforests. According to the *Baltimore Sun:*

> "Underwater vegetation not only provides critical habitats for sea life but also regulates the marine environment. It slows the flow of water, settling out sediment, and absorbs nutrients, making water clearer and cleaner. It also dampens wave energy, reducing shoreline erosion, and helps offset global warming by absorbing surprisingly large amounts of carbon from the atmosphere."[16]

These submerged jungles are vital signs to the health of waterways as well as a critical restorative for keeping them healthy. When habitats and nurseries for fish and crabs are lost, entire ecosystems collapse. Studies have shown that even small amounts of nitrogen can severely impact underwater grasses. Fish can be threatened directly by nutrient runoff even before the grasses disappear.

A world transformed to vegetarianism would go a long way toward transforming dead zones back to live zones.

61 Mining the aquifers

THIRSTING FOR MEAT

"Groundwater is part of a system of powerful hydrological interactions—between earth, surface water, sky, and sea—that we ignore at our peril."
—Payal Sampat, Worldwatch Institute, 2000[1]

Demand for fresh water has soared in recent generations, thanks in large part to unprecedented increases in world meat production that have taken place.[2] Agriculture consumes most of these vital reserves; two-thirds of the world's fresh water is used for irrigation. This use by farms would not have to be so great if not for the 37 percent of the world's grain (70 percent in the United States) that is cycled through animals. This grain represents a massive amount of crop cultivation and therefore water usage.

In many ways, our great supplies of fresh water actually preceded the demand for them. The powerful pumping technologies that are now in use all across the globe became available only in the middle of last century.[3] Once they were adopted, it wasn't long afterward that people became accustomed to the bounteous supplies of water they delivered. The new availability of water allowed grain supplies to explode, bringing a seismic shift in the human diet. Now, the practice of eating meat is considered a birthright for huge pockets of the human population.

The wellspring of underground water today, though vast, should of course never have been considered a bottomless pit. The dire consequences of overpumping have already been felt in some areas of the world. Although water crises tend to be local affairs, increasingly they are becoming more widespread.

Scientists warn that overpumping has set the stage for famine. India, perhaps more than anywhere else, faces this threat. Aquifers there are predicted to run dry from the country's 21 million tube wells stuck hundreds of yards below the surface of the earth.[4] As water tables become progressively lower, there is no turning back to the hand-dug wells of old; they no longer extend deep enough. India is not alone. Just about everyone is tapping unsustainably into their groundwater. For example, China is predicted to be dependent on grain imports in the near future, since some of its most important underground water stores are running dry. Grain, now, is seen as "virtual water." To produce a ton requires a thousand tons of water.[5]

According to Lester R. Brown, this increase in international demand could suddenly price some countries out of grain markets altogether, bringing famine to the least fortunate of the world. A corollary to this, according to Jacques Leslie, a journalist who observes water issues: "Agricultural prices are now at their lowest point in two decades and have forced some American farmers out of work, but if overpumping were to cease, grain prices probably would rise significantly."[6]

That sinking feeling: Aquifer mechanics

Aquifers can be thought of as colossal sponges, with sediment the medium that allows them to hold their shape. Indeed, 97 percent of the planet's fresh-water supplies are below ground.[7] This represents vast amounts indeed. However, people can manage to deplete them. And in doing so, they disrupt several physical mechanisms that aquifers provide.

Far from inert masses, aquifers are in constant flux, interacting with earth's other freshwater reserves: clouds, lakes, and rivers. Aquifers accept overflows in times of flood and release supplies in times of drought.[8] When aquifers have their water pumped from them, rivers above flow in to fill the void and eventually run dry. Moreover, the earth above can literally sink when an aquifer collapses from overpumping. Once this takes place, the utility of an aquifer may be transformed from that of a sponge into that of a brick. At this point, the aquifer's role as a vital storage tank in times of surface-water imbalance is lost forever—or at least until the next geological age. Furthermore, overpumping can create voids into which polluted or salt-contaminated sea water may flow.[9] Aquifers have no natural cleansing mechanisms.

Aquifers that have had their supplies diminished are often not readily replenished by other water systems, such as rainfall or even monsoons. Taxing them in this way essentially mines the earth of an indispensable resource, but with graver consequence than just depletion. As people make withdrawals, they literally destroy the physical foundation upon which they must live.

Ogallala nourishing feedlots and slaughterhouses

Close to home, America has its own story of water squandering—the extraction of vast reserves from the Ogallala Aquifer, which lies under parts of eight High Plains states. Except for a rare wettish decade from time to time, the climate above this underground lake is essentially bone dry. But ever since the mid-twentieth century, the land has been blanketed with thirsty feed grains—thanks to titanic amounts of water pumped up from below. Farmers have for decades been depleting the Ogallala by the million-acre foot to irrigate their land. Since the 1950s the aquifer has diminished in volume by a third, a quantity equivalent to half of Lake Erie.[10] The water was used to nourish an infrastructure of feedlots and industrial slaughterhouses.[11] The experts predict that a mere 60 years of supply remain.[12]

The United States has actually entertained thoughts of grandiose replenishment schemes for the Ogallala. Some people even envision siphoning water from the Great Lakes[13] or from Canada,[14] allowing America, we suppose, for a time to hold on to its penchant for water-guzzling burgers—12 billion per year.[15] Don't hold your breath on that one, though. Meanwhile, do hold the meat.

62 Predator control

OPERATION EXTERMINATION

"But killing [prairie dogs] was time-consuming and sometimes costly. Therefore, as usual, stock men turned to the taxpayer."—Lynn Jacobs, *Waste of the West*[1]

Eradicating wildlife for the benefit of cattle ranching is an American tradition, one that began with the near extermination of the buffalo in the late 1800s. No matter that cattle don't even belong in most parts of North America because the environment is not conducive to them (nor they to the environment), the killing ethic on their behalf goes on—though recently with a little more consciousness about it. Predators of cattle and sheep, in particular, continue to be rifled down, poisoned, or trapped, as a matter of public policy and expense. Official federal government indulgence toward the predator-control needs of cattlemen has been America's public policy since 1931 and by now is undoubtedly seen by its recipients as a right. Few ranchers understand that their enterprises are operating in a wild setting that should command their respect, not be the victim of their destruction. Just the same, the nation's taxpayers fork over $14 million annually so this destructive policy can continue.[2]

Interestingly, the threat of predators to cattle is often nonexistent or exaggerated. What may look like a predator eating the carcass of a cow is often just an opportunistic scavenger.[3] The cattle die easily on the range, since they are essentially ill-equipped to physically withstand the Western environment. Wild animals naturally take advantage of the situation.

Animal Damage Control—euphemistically renamed Wildlife Services—is the official U.S. program charged with exterminating primarily badgers, bears, mountain lions, bobcats, foxes, and coyotes. Throughout the 1990s, nearly 100,000 animals were killed per year. Death instruments of choice include leg hold traps, neck snares (strangulation), sodium cyanide, helicopters for aerial gunning, and shovels used to pry coyote pups out of their dens.[4] Not only are non-target wildlife easily victimized by predator elimination campaigns, but the efforts themselves can backfire.[5] For instance, targeted species may become adept at avoiding the lethal measures that are used against them. They may even "learn" to populate themselves more efficiently as a result of being hunted down.

Though non-lethal solutions are more effective, ranchers don't usually adopt them.[6] Indeed, employing noise-making devices, keeping a guard dog, corralling livestock at night, and quickly disposing of deadstock can eliminate most predator problems.[7]

Not for predators only

Predators are not the only perceived enemies of ranching. Wildlife in general seems to pose a threat or, at best, is unnecessary to the rancher. If a species does not kill cattle, it is readily thought to compete with them—or it may simply have some characteristic that ranchers do not like.[8] Unfortunately, the wholesale extermination of wildlife causes surrounding ecosystems to suffer.

This last statement could not be more true than in the case of the prairie dog. The range of this burrowing ground squirrel, whose habitat once stretched across the North American continent covering an estimated 100 million acres, has been reduced by 99 percent. The near-extermination took place despite the fact that at least 150 other animal species either benefit from or are wholly dependent on the creature.

It is believed that prairie dogs compete with cattle for forage, and that their burrows cause cattle to stumble. Neither notion holds up under scientific scrutiny. In fact, the activities of prairie dogs actually engender rangeland health—a necessity for the lush vegetation that cows need to thrive.[9]

Not for cattle only

Depredation has recently been permitted against double-crested cormorants. The proliferation of open-air catfish pens in the South—each able to hold up to 60,000 fish per acre—has given the birds what appears to them to be a ready-made banquet, and their populations have exploded as a result.[10] Ironically, in years past the greenish-black water birds have more than once actually needed government protection from extinction.

63 Animal transport

ACCIDENTAL TRAVELERS' BYWAY TO HELL

"Even with a zero death rate that might be associated with providing more space on the truck, the hogs that we save would not be enough to pay for the increased transportation costs of hauling fewer hogs on a load."—Kenneth B. Kephart, swine specialist[1]

The majority of farmed animals in the United States are transported at least once in their lives when they are sent to slaughter. Many, however, experience their first ride when, only days old, they are trucked out of hatcheries, ranches, or farrowing operations. Every year, millions of chicks are in fact sent through the U.S. mail.[2]

Creature discomforts

Intensive crowding is standard for animals in transit. Chickens, for example, are loaded in stacked cages, four birds per cubic foot.[3] Larger animals may be packed in tiers. Floors quickly become besmirched with urine and feces, making conditions conducive to slips and falls. The hapless may be trampled upon or suffocated. At any time mechanical breakdowns or accidents may occur. Wide, swift turns can cause injuries to animals simply standing without restraint—although tight packing is considered the working answer for the absence of seat belts.

All in all, no niceties are provided for doomed animals. Aside from the standard lack of food and water, livestock in transit must go without heat in the winter and cooling in the summer. Transported animals may freeze to the sides of trucks or become frozen in the urine and feces that build up on vehicle floors; they will be pried away with chains.[4]

Negotiating truck on- and off-ramps remains a cruel challenge for large mammals not bred or raised for dexterity. Rough goading by stock men—even genital hot shotting (hand-held electric prodding)—is not an uncommon motivator of stubborn or immobile animals.[5] And assume "broken bones on board" when "spent" egg-laying hens—

weakened by a life of intense egg production with no exercise—are transported. Industry research in 1994 found one in four so afflicted.[6] The laborers who gather up the birds into transport cages are paid scantily by the job, not by the hour, and so typically are swift and brutal on the fragile birds.

Transit fundamentals

Because prices for cattle and feed are prone to fluctuation, beef animals tend to be shipped around frequently—five times, on average, in a short lifetime, so owners can take advantage of the best commodity prices.[7] Pigs and chickens, in their more monopolistic markets, tend to stay put throughout their lives, which makes their final trip to the slaughterhouse all the more foreign and wildly disconcerting. Some truck trips across country will drag on for as long as 60 hours.[8]

U.S. hog imports and exports amount to about 6 million live animals.[9] Though most U.S. trade in livestock takes place within North America, some of the nation's animal exports, such as hogs, actually go to other parts of the world, particularly Asia. By ship, such excursions can take months. Live animals, rather than prepackaged meat, are transported, because refrigeration is not universally available in every part of the world.[10] In the case of the Middle East, animals are shipped as meat "on the hoof" rather than "on the hook" to fit with on-site halal slaughter requirements.

Mortalities: The cost of doing business

Novel situations without assurances from a human or fellow creature will cause intense stress for nearly all animals. Indeed, transport is something most animals simply cannot comprehend. Stress can be so intense as to be lethal. Over 250 hogs show up dead at U.S. slaughterhouses every day, most because of porcine stress syndrome,[11] a recessive trait that was inadvertently bred into their bodies along with the genes that make their flesh super-meaty. As for spent layer hens, millions die of heart failure in transit because of stress.[12] Losses, as per usual, are figured into the cost of doing business.

64 Illegal fishing

THAT FINAL NIHILISTIC GRAB

"Soon some oysters may be as rare and costly as pearls."—Peter Benchley, author, *Jaws*[1]

In 1994, *The Economist* ventured a guess as to the extent of worldwide illegal fishing: as many as one in every three landed fish, it surmised, was illegally caught.[2] About a decade later, the experts were guessing that the proportion of illegal catches had jumped to one in every two landed fish.[3] Of course, these estimated levels are just averages for all fish. In one extraordinary year, 1998, the haul for Patagonian toothfish (better known as Chilean sea bass in restaurants) was estimated at 10 times the legal catch.[4] This species continues to be a prized cargo for the world's fish-pilfering pirates.[5]

So, how can one tell if the fish on the menu at the local Red Lobster was caught by upstanding people who harvested their catch in the right waters, within the right seasonal time frame, within the right weight parameters, from the right species, at the right stage of the fish's life, and with the right gear—in other words, according to the law? While you're pondering on the answer, consider the fact that 80 percent of the seafood Americans eat comes from other countries.[6] And most fisheries around the world are rarely monitored.[7]

Plummeting wild fish stocks around the world have prompted governments to regulate fish catches. But invariably, black markets have arisen, spurring collapse all the faster. Even when governments show the will and can afford to go after poachers and smugglers, enforcement systems can easily become tainted by corrupt surveillance officials and bribe-taking inspectors. Some markets, as with Russian caviar[8] and South African abalone,[9] have acquired all the brutish characteristics of illicit narcotics trafficking. A corollary to this is that two-thirds of all the cocaine destined for the United States (275 tons or so) is transported via ocean-going vessels—often, it is believed, in the holds of tuna boats—according to a 1997 U.S. government report.[10]

No region untouched

Illegal fishing is rampant and may occur with the tacit approval of world governments.[11] The following provides but a tiny glimpse at the various scenarios playing themselves out across the globe.

- A siege is taking place along the coast of West Africa.[12] Weak or corrupt local governments have succumbed to fishing pirates—who are sometimes armed—hailing from richer nations. The offshore trawling disrupts coastal fisheries, leaving native inhabitants with harbors nearly bereft of fish.[13]
- Small-scale fishers that operate using illegal gear in Cambodia have devastated the Mekong River, the largest inland fishery in the world.[14] Corrupt regulatory agents, as well as the country's own military, have been complicit in the habitat's demise.[15]
- The crisis of overfishing has even reached the remote environs of the Amazon. Local fishermen's patrols regularly go after poachers there who see great rewards, despite armed threats, in landing the area's mighty pirarucu, a type of striped peacock bass that can grow to 200 pounds.[16]
- Nine hundred angry fishers staged a violent demonstration in the Galapagos Islands in 2000, making death threats, blocking roads, ransacking the Charles Darwin Foundation research station, and even taking a giant tortoise hostage, as they demanded absolute liberty to fish with any method they choose, no matter how destructive.[17] This protest continues to erupt from time to time.
- After a decade of industrial trawling, Mexico's Gulf of California fishing grounds have nearly collapsed. Meanwhile, small-scale fishing boats, unlicensed and ungoverned, finish up the destruction in a final grab for what's left.[18]
- According to one California-based Fish and Game official, there aren't enough cops in Los Angeles to track down all the small operators illicitly taking ground fish off the coast.[19]

Convenient loophole

Probably the worst illegal fishing today is practiced by so-called flag-of-convenience (FOC) vessels.[20] While every nation is responsible for the ships that sail under its flag, a few small, seemingly inconsequential countries are turning a blind eye to violations of international fishing laws. At the same time, they are allowing general use of their flags in exchange for hefty fees. The pirates not only fly the FOC flags but also bring their catches to market via "ports of convenience" after "laundering" trawler-fulls of fish via illicit at-sea transshipments. Some 1,300 industrial-scale fishing vessels are estimated to be cloaked by this system.[21] They are not only well financed but also well equipped with destructive fishing gear. Only dogged paper-trail sleuthing and even drawn-out sea chases bring any of the rogues to justice.

It may be that only draconian measures can truly put an end to illegal fishing. Iran, albeit a case unto itself, has been known to enforce a zero-tolerance policy for poaching when it comes to caviar, which is derived from the endangered sturgeon. If you poach you could be put to death or, more likely, have your hands chopped off.[22]

65 Boosting output

THIS IS YOUR COW ON HORMONES

"As every awkward adolescent or expectant mother knows, sex hormones can have profound effects on the body."—The Economist[1]

About 35 percent[2] of the approximately nine million dairy cows in the United States are regularly subjected to the effects of Recombinant Bovine Growth Hormone (rBGH), a drug that synthetically duplicates the animals' own hormones and boosts milk output by 10 to 25 percent.[3]

Consumers should assume that essentially every carton of commercially purchased milk contains some portion produced from cows administered this genetically engineered drug. Since milk is normally pooled from many dairies, a processor wishing to guarantee for his customers an rBGH-free product must impose herculean levels of control. Proponents of rBGH contend that since trace amounts in the final product are indistinguishable from those produced by the cows themselves, labeling is not necessary. Opponents sorely disagree.

Milking dubiously

The United States is the only major country that allows the use of rBGH. Even the Canadians, who have legalized hormone use in beef,[4] eschew the drug because they believe it causes health problems in the cows.[5] In 1999, Canada called into question the original FDA research used to prove that the drug was safe for human consumption,[6] charging that one study showed that rBGH caused cysts in a significant number of male laboratory rats.[7]

Activist groups, such as the Humane Farming Association and the Consumers Union, have charged that the FDA worked with the creators of rBGH to suppress information that would put the hormone in a negative light. A key researcher, Richard Burroughs, was fired because he was slowing down the approval process by raising questions about the drug's health effects on both cows and humans.[8]

Opponents of rBGH point to the fact that milk from cows administered with the drug contains high levels of insulin-like growth factor (IGF-1),[9] a substance that most scientists believe survives the digestive process and raises risk for disease.[10] IGF-1 is naturally found in the human bloodstream, and excessive amounts of it are linked to breast, prostate, and colon cancer.

The animals' sacrifice

The European Union (EU) says rBGH causes fertility problems and lameness in cows.[11] Even product directions for rBGH concede that use of the drug could result in more cases of bloat, diarrhea, and mastitis.[12] Moreover, a significant amount of pus and bacteria tend to be found in rBGH-treated herds, and therefore in the milk, according to data gathered by the manufacturer itself.[13] Furthermore, rBGH increases the level of immune-system-compromising stress in the animals. A cow may even go into a kind of shock if her body is not metabolizing food fast enough for the demands of the drug.[14]

Due to decades of intense selective breeding, today's cows already produce milk to excess. So why would anyone develop such a drug? The manufacturer guessed, and correctly, that larger farms able to ride out prolonged periods of low prices resulting from gluts would be willing to use it. Of course, the government is always there to maintain price floors and to buy up the surpluses.

Beef pumped

Hormones in beef cattle constitute a separate issue that seems to be more about U.S./EU trade rancor than anything else. These drugs are used to stimulate faster growth and bigger muscles in the animals. The EU contends that at least one of the six hormones that are used on 95 percent of U.S. beef cattle is carcinogenic.[15] It also points to the ever-present potential for abuse—multiple implants, miscalculated dosage intervals, and black-market brands—as further vindication of its stance. Besides, the EU asserts, its consumers just don't want them.

The FDA requires no pre-slaughter withdrawal periods for the six beef hormones, which it says mimic those that occur naturally inside the animals.[16] As long as the drugs are administered properly, the FDA sees no reason for concern. The World Trade Organization has, in fact, ruled that EU alarm over the synthetic hormones is simply a cover for protectionism and has allowed the U.S. to impose nearly $120 million in yearly retaliatory tariffs. The EU adamantly continues to prefer to be free of hormone beef nonetheless.

In the end, the world is left with a lot of drugged-up cows and more unnecessary tension between nations.

66 Exotic meat

HERALDING EXTINCTION, DISEASE

"New research has identified other SIVs [simian immunodeficiency viruses], raising the possibility of more catastrophic epidemics with the increased consumption of bushmeat."—Kerry Bowman, bioethicist, founder of the Canadian Great Ape Alliance[1]

Notwithstanding the people who eat squirrel brains in Kentucky or attend the annual Rocky Mountain Oyster (bull testicle) Festival in Montana every year, Americans tend to avoid "exotic" meats. When U.S. entrepreneurs try their hands at raising ostriches, emus, turtles, elk, bison, goats, frogs, yaks, and alligators, their products usually get a chilly reception from the locals.

The rest of the world is, on the other hand, less finicky. Indeed, people readily eat horses in Europe, dogs in Korea and Taiwan, cats in China, kangaroos in Australia, moth larvae in Thailand, insects just about everywhere, bat blood in Vietnam, and guinea pigs in Ecuador—just to name a few. Some of the same negatives associated with factory farming of more familiar species (at least to Americans) also apply to these more unusual food animals—although cruelty tends to stand out, with no laws against abuse.

Human see, monkey eat

For some uncommon meat animals—rare breeds of domesticated cattle and sheep in particular—the only chance of avoiding extinction is in becoming a deli item. For others, simply being considered meat at all courts demise.

The UN has amply warned the world to rein in the growing African bushmeat trade. According to leading primate expert Jane Goodall, more than a million metric tons of meat from elephants, antelopes, gorillas, chimpanzees and other threatened species are taken from the forests of the Congo Basin each year,[2] increasingly to be sold in European restaurants.[3] Without prompt intervention, African apes, in particular, are likely to be wiped out within a matter of years.

Meanwhile, the Chinese are vacuuming up their wildlife to extinction, not only for aphrodisiacs and medicinal cures, but for a "taste of the wild."[4] In any case, once the desire for these meats is established, outlawing their lucrative markets invites all the perils of prohibition.[5]

Tradition: A formidable foe

The world has tried to shame the Japanese into giving up their practice of eating the flesh of whales. But the taste of it for some has long been fully acquired. Whale meat was sold by street vendors during the lean years after World War II and now invokes memories of a glorified collective past.[6] Today, especially older Japanese sorely resent outsiders telling them that whales need to be protected.[7]

Though not as endearing as whales or primates, sharks claim a critical place in the ocean's ecology. Yet fate has given them dorsal, pectoral and lower tail fins that, when dried, provide a key ingredient in an Asian soup that is considered a delicacy. Fishers slice the appendages off living sharks, later tossing the mutilated animals back into the water to die slowly of hunger or be killed by predators or scavengers against whom they have no defense.

Exotic and deadly

The quest for exotic and often endangered animal cuisine increasingly threatens to become a conduit for disease. In fact, every emerging human disease that has been introduced into the world in the last twenty years has originated in animals, whereas only 60 percent of human disease in general is so derived.[8] Based on recent history, the Royal Society, the independent scientific academy of the United Kingdom, predicted in 2004 that the world would see the emergence of 30 new diseases in as many years.[9] SARS, for example, which in 2003 infected 8,500 and killed 800 people in 30 countries,[10] is linked to at least seven wild animals considered culinary delicacies in southern China. Such animals are typically kept on display in filthy, stress-inducing Asian "wet" markets. The practice will be slow to die.

In addition, it is believed by some that humans first contracted HIV/AIDS in Africa after exposure to blood from SIV-infected chimpanzees who were killed for their meat.[11] Similarly, the Ebola virus is believed to be transmitted to humans through the consumption of wild boar[12] and gorilla[13] meat.

67 Protein, iron, zinc

YES, WE HAVE NO DEFICIENCIES

"We were all brainwashed to believe that the only source of protein was meat and cheese."—Suzanne Havala, RD, charter fellow of the American Dietetic Association[1]

Despite everything, don't we still need meat for protein, iron and zinc? No, no, and no. In fact, vegetarian foods are healthier sources for these nutrients.

Established guidelines suggest a healthy diet includes a mere 10 to 15 percent of calories as protein.[2] Few plant foods (aside from fruits) provide less than 10 percent, and many give much more. It would be difficult not to obtain adequate protein on a whole-food vegetarian diet that includes a variety of foods. Protein deficiencies are usually reserved for situations resulting from famine or calorie deprivation.[3] On the other hand, people in Western countries—meat eaters in particular—tend to get far too much protein in their diets.[4] Indeed, the Cornell-Oxford-China Study linked the consumption of animal protein, but not plant protein, to chronic disease.[5]

In 2001, the National Institutes of Health found that women who get most of their protein from animal sources have three times the rate of bone loss and hip fractures as women who get most of their protein from vegetable sources.[6]

Furthermore, too much protein can damage the kidneys, which are constantly stressed through the filtering and removal of waste from the body.[7] The American Dietetic Association listed lower levels of protein as an advantage of the vegetarian diet.[8] And single-meal food combining of essential amino acids (protein building blocks)—once thought mandatory for vegetarians—is not necessary.[9]

The Atkins scourge

What of that nemesis of the vegetarians, the Atkins Diet, which has thoroughly permeated our culture? Condemned as dangerous by the American Heart Association,[10] the high-protein/low carbohydrate weight-loss plan not only allows its adherents *carte blanche* to gorge on buckets of animal protein and tubs of saturated fat but discourages them from eating foods with essential nutritional merit.[11] According to vegan nutrition educator George Eisman, excess fat metabolism causes the production of ketones, which are difficult to flush out of the body. In excess, they cause a person to experience a simulated starvation.

High amounts of protein stress the liver and kidneys with excess ammonia and urea. Calcium ends up being leached from the bones.[12]

A high-fat, low-carbohydrate diet causes nitrogen buildups in the blood and dehydration without signals of thirst.[13] The Atkins Diet is not only dangerous to the body, but it causes the brain to alter its metabolism, a condition that is not normalized when the dieter drinks more water.[14]

The Partnership for Essential Nutrition, a consortium of 11 health organizations led by former U.S. Surgeon General C. Everett Koop's group Shape-Up America!, has cautioned potential adherents to the diet. It has pointed to studies that show that the low-carb approach can, to quote the *Washington Post*, "starve the brain of carbohydrates, produce constipation and other gastrointestinal problems, reduce energy levels, and cause difficulty concentrating."[15] In the long run, the diet can "increase the risk of liver disorders, gout, coronary heart disease, diabetes, stroke, and several types of cancer."[16] And sadly, evidence shows that these diets don't even keep the weight off.[17]

The Atkins Diet *has* been shown to lower LDL (bad) cholesterol. But any type of weight loss will do this. The diet has also been shown to raise HDL (good) cholesterol. But as Dean Ornish, M.D., explains, HDL cholesterol can be equated with garbage trucks. Their appearance is welcome but also signals that you've got refuse to cart away—refuse you didn't need in the first place.[18]

Paleolithic peculiarities

It is not possible to compare, as some have, today's Atkins-style diets with those eked out by some of our Paleolithic ancestors 10,000 to 40,000 years ago—some of which consisted of as much as 60 percent protein by calorie.[19] Compared with today's commercial meat, the game our ancestors ate contained a small fraction of the fat—about one-sixth—and plenty of omega-3 fatty acids. Our precursors expended vastly more energy than today's couch potatoes and, most telling of all, most of them ate huge and diverse amounts of plant-based foods still in their natural state. The veggies gave them 5 to 10 times the fiber that today's *Homo sapiens* ingest.

Scrapping the metal woes

As for iron, vegetarians do not experience anemia at any greater rate than meat eaters.[20] Non-heme iron, which comes from non-meat sources, has been found to be less absorbable than heme iron—the kind found in meat, fish, and poultry. But vegetarians make up for the shorfall with typical eating patterns.[21] First, vegetarian foods are—contrary to popular belief—abundant in iron. Second, vegetarians tend to consume more vitamin C, which enhances the absorption of iron. Moreover, it is now known that people can, in fact, accumulate too much iron in their bodies.[22] Men and postmenopausal women who consume a diet particularly rich in heme iron are at a greater risk of fatal heart attack.[23] Cancer and diabetes are likewise associated with too much iron.[24]

As for zinc, again, vegetarians can easily attain requirements here, particularly if a variety of beans and nuts, as well as pumpkin seeds and sunflower seeds, are part of the diet—foods that tend to be staples for the meat-free. On the other hand, here again, too much of this nutrient is tied to disease. Prostate cancer, in this case, is linked to overdoing it with zinc supplements.[25]

68 Marine refuges

THE VIRTUES OF ABSTINENCE

"It's no longer a question of whether to set aside fully protected areas in the oceans, but where to establish them."—Jane Lubchenco, Professor of Zoology, Oregon State University[1]

In the span of just a half a century, industrial-scale fishing has robbed the oceans of 90 percent of its large predatory fish—from the "Porsches of the sea," such as shark, marlin, sailfish, swordfish, and bluefin tuna, to the somewhat less stunning cod, flounder, and hake. A 10–year study, financed by the Pew Charitable Trusts and published in the journal *Nature* in 2003, found that decades of increasingly efficient fishing methods have brought marine stocks to ruin. The study, which involved sifting through dusty records amassed by fishing fleets and research boats, was unprecedented in its detail and scope.

No matter where the researchers looked, the findings were the same: only a small fraction of former fish numbers remained. Moreover, the study revealed that, in general, it took only about 10 to 15 years for each species to crash.[2] Researchers also discovered that industrial fishing has spread to nearly every corner of the globe.[3] There are, in fact, precious few places left for fish to hide anymore.

Refuge for the weary

We can now say that fisheries management around the world has been a dismal failure—generally little better than controlled plunder. Now, marine biologists are sounding what may be a last-chance red alert to convince the rest of us to do the right thing to save the oceans and the animals in them. We must, they say, ban fishing from a *third* of the ocean in a system of marine reserves, policed by naval patrols and guided by satellites.[4] Currently, less than one percent of the world's waters is off limits.[5] The pronouncement in 2003 was the logical conclusion of a group of British researchers, led by internationally known marine conservation biologist Callum Roberts, who had analyzed 300 studies of 60 small marine reserves. Their conclusions rested on the simple observation they found over and over: stocks rebound when protected from human designs—and usually in spectacular ways.

The virtues of designating so-called "no-take zones" first became known in 1999 when a study of the Cape Canaveral marine reserve was released. The reserve was designated in 1962 to protect people from rocket-launch failures, but it inadvertently became a sanctuary superabundant with fish. During a lull in shuttle activity after the 1986 Challenger disaster, scientists began gathering data in protected areas. After chronicling over 20,000 specimens representing 50 species over a four–year period, they found densities of spotted sea trout, red drum, black drum, common snook, and striped mullet to be significantly richer than in nearby areas where fishing was allowed.[6] The fishing-free zones were found to contain 2 to 12 times as many fish as adjacent waters, depending upon the species.[7] The overall mix of fish was more diverse, and individual fish were generally larger. Similar findings were found in a 2001 California study that examined 102 reserves.[8]

Terrestrial come-back

As a consequence of the Missouri River floods of 1993, mounds of sand unfit for crop cultivation replaced some fields where corn and soybeans once grew. Left untouched for just six years, these areas reverted to a naturalist's wonderland of cottonwoods, willows, native grasses, insects, and birds.[9] One can only imagine what it would be like if all the oceans were similarly left alone to rebuild! Certainly, highly migratory pelagic species, such as bluefin tunas, marlin, and sailfish, would appreciate the reinstatement of vast areas of habitat.[10] Nature, we see, can often be more than forgiving when given half a chance—which a vegetarian world could automatically provide.

69 Gastroenteric emissions

BURPING COWS HEAT THE PLANET

"Methane is the second-most-important greenhouse gas in the atmosphere now. The population of beef cattle and dairy cattle has grown so much that methane from cows now is big. This is not a trivial issue."—Ralph Cicerone, atmospheric scientist, UC, Irvine[1]

There is no doubt among America's climate experts: Global warming is real.[2] The Food and Agriculture Organization of the UN has predicted that the earth's temperature will rise by 2.5°F to 10°F by 2100.[3]

Over the next century the world must face the prospect of melting polar ice caps, songbirds relegated to northern climes, once-temperate regions dried to dust bowls, and New England maples a figment of memory.[4] Fourteen laboratories around the globe concluded in 2004 that global warming will cause a quarter of the species they have studied to go extinct or nearly so by mid-century.[5] One hundred years from now Australia's Great Barrier Reef, the world's largest coral system, could very well be gone.[6]

A Swiss insurance company forecasts worldwide expenditures of $150 billion per year within the next ten years because of the heating of the atmosphere.[7] Even the Pentagon predicted in a 2004 worst-case-scenario report that abrupt climate change within the next 20 years could bring anarchy to the planet and cost millions of lives in wars between people vying for habitable real estate and scarce natural resources.[8]

The power of ruminant burps

Global warming is primarily caused by elevated carbon dioxide (CO_2) levels from human-generated fossil-fuel emissions in the atmosphere. Levels of CO_2 are up 31 percent from pre-industrial times.[9] Trace gases, however, such as methane, also contribute to the thermal trend.

It is believed that 13.2 percent of planetary warming is caused by anthropogenic methane, that is, emissions caused by human activities.[10] The world's belching ruminants, which emit 80 million metric tons of methane every year,[11] contribute 20.5 percent of this proportion.[12] Cow-generated methane is created by billions of bacteria breaking down grass and hay in the rumens of the animals—a process known as enteric fermentation. Manure from all livestock contributes an additional 5.6 percent of anthropogenic methane.[13]

Each dairy cow can fill 200 two–liter soda bottles with methane each day.[14] Every pound of meat represents half a pound of methane floating into the atmosphere.[15] Meanwhile, humans have doubled the world's cattle population over the last 30 years to 1.3 billion animals, bringing the total number of ruminants (the chief livestock emitters of methane[16]), including sheep and goats, to 2.4 billion animals. Collectively, livestock have been transformed by sheer numbers into instruments of climate change.

A little bit goes a long way

Methane is an especially potent greenhouse gas. It is 21 times more effective at trapping heat in the atmosphere than carbon dioxide over 100 years.[17] So any reduction in the causes of methane emissions is particularly valuable for reducing global warming.[18] Furthermore, methane has a relatively short lifetime—12 years, versus 120 years for carbon dioxide—making it, again, a good candidate for mitigation.[19] So the present is as good time as any to start trimming those ruminant hordes!

Animal agriculture must take the heat for other contributions it makes to global warming. This is a human activity that is highly dependent on CO_2-creating fossil energy, from temperature-controlled indoor housing for the animals to extensive refrigeration systems, to motorized vehicular transport. All in all, animal agriculture is a great, yet unnecessary, contributor to the whole of human-generated global warming.

Forest demise

On a related subject, the Amazon rainforests, considered the oxygen-producing "lungs of the world," are rapidly being cleared, primarily for two reasons: first, for ranching,[20] and, second, to grow 20 million metric tons of soybeans annually[21] for export to China, primarily for use as animal feed.[22] World demand is robust thanks to the fact that Brazil's meat is considered BSE (mad cow)-free and its soybeans are known to be GMO (genetically modified organism)-free.[23] Destroying the Amazon, as well as forests elsewhere, contributes significantly to the forces of global warming. The Amazon, in particular, functions as an important planetary "carbon sink."

All over the world wholesale obliteration of carbon dioxide-absorbing forest and grassland is taking place to create farmland, much of it to produce animal-based foods. Meanwhile, the fires that are set to clear rainforest land create smoke that effaces clouds and disrupts vital systems of precipitation.[24] The burning of the Amazon accounts for 75 percent of Brazil's greenhouse gas emissions, ranking Brazil as one of the world's top ten polluters.[25] In 2004, annual Amazon deforestation showed no sign of slowing after a Brazilian government report claimed that nearly 10,000 square miles (an area about the size of Massachusetts) of rainforest was destroyed over the previous year.[26] At this rate, the forests are projected to be gone in this century.[27]

70 Pick your *poisson*

DIOXIN, MERCURY, OR PCBS

"The funny thing is, people got better when they stopped eating it."—Jane Hightower, M.D., researcher, referring to fish that gave people mercury poisoning[1]

Seventy-five thousand chemicals are registered with the Environmental Protection Agency (EPA), yet only a fraction of them have been studied to any adequate degree. Billions of tons of them have entered the environment. A few, such as dioxin, mercury, and polychlorinated biphenyls (PCBs), are very toxic and virtually non-biodegradable. They not only linger in the environment, but their cloud of toxicity can drift halfway around the world. Studies of sperm whales[2] and remote Arctic peoples—the Inuit, most dramatically[3]—attest to this.

Even minute amounts of these types of poisons are a cause for concern. Some of the deadliest of them tend to settle in the fat or the flesh of animals, including humans. A person who eats a fish, who ate a fish who ate a fish, and so on, assimilates the cumulative and collective toxicity of the whole lot of them. Even an animal that takes in only grain is the toxic product of a lifetime of eating. For this reason, meat, eggs, dairy, and farmed fish are always more contaminated than those from plants. Indeed, random-sample tests, conducted periodically by consumer groups, reveal dangerous levels of mercury, dioxin, and PCB contamination in store-bought, animal-based foods.[4]

According to the EPA, about 102,000 lakes and about 846,000 river miles were under fishing advisories in the United States in 2003 due to toxic chemicals found in the fish.[5] This amounts to over a third of the total lake acres and nearly a quarter of the river miles in the nation that people are being warned about because of mercury, dioxin, DDT, and three dozen other chemicals. Advisories, which are issued by the states, range from specific restrictions regarding certain fish to outright bans on all fishing.

Dioxin debacle

Scientists say that traces of dioxin are to be found inside the bodies of every person on the planet. But people who eat excessive amounts of fatty animal-based foods have been found to have significantly higher levels of dioxin than the general population.[6] According to the EPA, 95 percent of dioxin exposure comes through dietary intake of animal fats.[7]

The World Health Organization and the EPA have declared dioxin to be a known carcinogen.[8] According to some calculations, 1 in 14 cancer deaths in the United States, or 100 per day, are attributable to it.[9] Dioxin is also linked to birth defects, learning disabilities, and developmental problems in babies, as well as immune-system deterioration.[10] Breast milk can be a point of exit for the toxin in women nursing their babies.[11] Safe levels, if there are any, are unknown.[12] "It's the Darth Vader of toxic chemicals, because it affects so many systems [of the body]," according to Richard Clapp, a cancer epidemiologist.[13]

The EPA has assured citizens that dioxin emission levels have fallen dramatically in recent decades, thanks in large part to its regulatory actions against municipal incinerators, paper mills, and those who manufacture certain herbicides.[14] Critics complain, however, that while the agency has focused on these successes, it has neglected to push for other necessary controls.[15] Meanwhile, the agency tells people to change their diets to reduce the amount of animal fat they consume.[16]

White wine with your mercury?

Another pollutant also makes its way into food animals: mercury. A heavy metal, it is converted by bacteria into the organic neurotoxin methylmercury. Fish are the primary conduits for its entry into the human body. Coal and oil-fired power plants are the primary sources of the poison in our environment, although a significant amount of mercury lingers from various mining processes used during the California Gold Rush in the mid-nineteenth century.

Today, women put their babies at risk for irreparable brain damage when they eat seafood high in mercury while pregnant, and even beforehand.[17] According to the EPA, about 630,000 newborns in the United States every year—roughly 15 percent of all—may be exposed to dangerous levels of mercury in the womb.[18] When the Mount Sinai Center for Children's Health and the Environment (New York City) looked a number of studies, it found that lower IQ levels are linked to mercury exposure in the womb and cost the United States $8.7 billion a year in lost earnings potential.[19]

Heavy fish eaters in general can fall victim to low-level mercury poisoning, which can result in headaches, hair loss, fatigue, depression, and memory loss.[20] And doctors tend to misdiagnose the source of these symptoms. When victims quit eating fish, however, their suffering ends within a couple of months.

Mercury is the source of most freshwater fish advisories. The government recently added some ocean species to its list of mercury-contaminated fish (swordfish, shark, king mackerel, and tilefish). These types of fish were so designated because of their particularly long life spans, which allow ample time for large amounts of mercury to accumulate in their bodies. The government, however, has failed to adequately warn people, primarily those at highest risk (pregnant women, and those wishing to become pregnant), about the most popularly consumed fish species in America of all: tuna. A 2004 University of North Carolina at Asheville questionnaire found that a person who eats four or more 6-ounce servings of canned tuna per month (tuna type was not distinguished) has a 33 percent chance of having dangerous levels of mercury (as defined by the EPA) in his or her body.[21] The FDA has warned that canned albacore, in particular, has three times the mercury as chunk light. "They [the FDA] have completely failed in their obligation to protect the public," says Richard Wiles of the Environmental Working Group.[22]

Sedimental journey: Dredging up the past

In 1979, the manufacture of PCBs was banned in the United States, 50 years after they were first introduced. A majority of Western countries have also banned their manufacture. Nonetheless, millions of tons of them still fester in river sediment due to past dumping—and industries in many developing countries in particular still release them into the environment. Being fat-soluble, these persistent poisons continue to contaminate the food chain, notably via fish. Aquatic organisms have been known to contain 2,000 to more than a million times the PCB concentrations of surrounding waters.[23] A study released in 2004 showed farmed salmon to contain ten times more PCBs and other contaminants than wild salmon.[24] Ninety percent of fresh salmon eaten in the United States is farmed.[25]

In the mid-sixties, fish placed in an Alabama creek that was contaminated with concentrated amounts of PCBs were observed to die within seconds. They spurted blood and shed their skins as if dropped into boiling water.[26] Companies that have been indicted for dumping PCBs have defended themselves from cleanup costs by arguing that to dredge the chemicals would only stir up their poisonous effects. But sand under waterways is hardly an inert substance. On the contrary, sediment is alive with tiny organisms assimilating the toxin. Consequently, the pollutants filter up the food chain into the bodies of surrounding fish, eventually into the bodies of fish eaters, human and otherwise.

71 Links, lost and found

ECOSYSTEMS IN TURMOIL

"The message is that overfishing and massive extraction can lead to food web impacts that are unexpected and unintended."—Alan Springer, oceanographer[1]

What goes on down there, where we cannot see, when humans remove a species from nature's aquatic web of life, or add one? Following are two tales of tampering that show that it's not nice to disrupt the food chain.

Introducing invasive species, deliberately

As European settlers made their way across the American continent in the nineteenth and twentieth centuries, they seeded the lakes they found with alien, predatory fish species[9]—those best suited, as far as they were concerned, for the frying pan. The native fish, which the frontiersmen saw as inedible, were labeled "trash."

Before their arrival, however, only five percent of the 16,000 high-elevation lakes had contained any fish at all.[10] Mountain lakes were inhabited primarily with frogs and amphibians. To this day, most of these lakes continue to be regularly stocked with various species of non-native hatchery trout to indulge "sport" fishers, and the practice has invariably led to the loss of indigenous species.[11] The introduced fish have devoured the native wildlife,[12] upending food chains.[13] One study involving several lakes showed that frogs do flourish again once trout are removed—a painstaking process to say the least.[14]

Stocking is, however, far from confined to mountain areas. In the case of salmon, the practice has disguised the long-term problem of dwindling wild species[15] and, in fact, has become a leading factor for the overall decline of native fish.[16] And, incredibly, Lake Michigan is stocked with baby salmon to grow up for anglers to catch, though, of course, this environment is utterly alien to salmon, which are strictly suited for ocean and river environments.[17] Stocking of fish even takes place in our national parks, where the ethic of preserving native species is otherwise esteemed. Indeed, where park visitors are urged in no uncertain terms to not remove any other wildlife, angling is allowed.[18]

Finally, stocking fish in itself can be cruel. One study showed that half of the trout fingerlings dropped from one Fish and Game airplane died upon impact with the water.[19]

Be careful what you fish for

In recent decades the Aleutian Islands of Alaska have been the scene for environmental mayhem. New relationships between predator and prey and explosions and implosions of species populations at all levels have brought this ecosystem to ruin and disarray. Steller sea lions and sea otters have nearly vanished from the environment—and these are just the obvious signs of more than a half-century of ecological upheaval.

After years of meticulous study, scientists believe they have deciphered the riddle of the ecosystem's collapse. They've concluded that cascading predation—originally put in motion by the commercial slaughter of baleen, bowhead, humpback, and sperm whales, which began over half a century ago—lies at the source of the disruption.[2] With the removal of this colossal-sized food source, killer whales were forced to move down the food chain to disastrous consequences. Populations of harbor seals, fur seals, and Steller sea lions were, one by one, brought to collapse, as none of these species was able to stand up to the killer whales' food needs.[3] Meanwhile, industrial-scale trawlers, with their coastal catches of herring and ocean perch, imposed "nutritional stress" on the sea lions and speeded their demise.[4] Finally, killer whales went after a most unlikely target, sea otters, whose swift depletion caused perhaps the greatest ecological disruption of all. With the sea otters nearly gone,[5] sea urchins—the food source of the otters—proliferated out of control.[6] The overpopulated sea urchins at this point began overgrazing their own home, the kelp forests, which serve as a refuge, feeding locale, and spawning ground for countless other creatures who have since been unable to survive the habitat rout.[7] Whaling ended in the 1970s, but the otter population has yet to rebuild, and kelp beds remain barren.[8]

72 Dirty dining

CONTAMINANTS BY THE POUND

*"You couldn't find (a cow carcass) that wasn't too rotten, cancerous, or putrid they wouldn't grind up and turn into feed."**—Howard Lyman, former cattle rancher[1]

You have to wonder about an industry that when left to its own devices degenerates into a ready conduit for disease, bacteria, and filth. By mistake, conscious deception, or even common practice, a bit of that extra weight that came with your meat—and which you paid for—could have easily been from adulterants.

Spittle, rats, and dung

The famous author Upton Sinclair wrote in *The Jungle* in 1906 that in his day tubercular cattle were welcomed by cattlemen, because the disease made the animals fatten more quickly.[2] Then there was the spittle, the rats, the dung, the sawdust, the nails, and even the odd human finger that the early twentieth-century muckraker revealed tainted slaughterhouse meat. One corroborated story of Sinclair's time told of the flesh and blood of a man's entire body that became part of a vat of offal rendered into lard—his bones fished out by coworkers.[3]

A century later, the scandals continue. Periodically, we hear about condemned meat entering the human food supply.[4] Broken hypodermic needles—from veterinary care—sometimes find their way into salable muscle tissue.[5] In 2003, European poultry processors were caught adding pork protein filler to their chicken, to the consternation of those with allergies and those who keep kosher or choose to eat halal meat.[6] In 2004, suspicions surrounded a Vancouver pig-farmer-turned-serial-killer, who may have spiked his ground pork with human remains.[7]

The above cases are unusual—we hope. On the other hand, the contamination of meat via machinery or specific production processes probably warrants a lot more concern.[8] Take for instance the communal chilling bath into which just-degutted birds in processing plants are dunked for cooling. This "fecal soup," is where cross-contamination is allowed to take place as a matter of course.[9]

Advanced meat recovery (AMR) is another. This slaughterhouse process is performed on large mammals with a motorized device that

* Nearly all aspects of feeding ruminant remains back to cattle have since been banned in the United States.

retrieves every last bit of flesh from bones, including the craggy areas around the spinal column. The resultant trim adds about 45 million pounds per year of salable product in the United States.[10] The extracted material would not consist of anything particularly dangerous, except that the industry can't always be bothered to first remove spinal cords from carcasses. Central nervous system tissue, such as spinal cord, is where mad cow's infectious agent, the prion, tends to lodge. In 2002, the USDA conducted a survey of 34 meat plants that produce beef products from various meat-removing systems. Thirty-five percent of samples tested came back positive for the prohibited material.[11]

Guess what's coming to dinner

In 1998 the USDA reclassified a number of animal diseases as part of a pilot project, allowing them in meat as long as lesions are cut away. The diseases, such as cancer, airsacculitis (poultry pneumonia), lymphomas, sores, infectious arthritis, and illness caused by intestinal worms rarely, if ever, present a public health risk, the agency explained.[12] In any case, it is common practice for a spent or diseased animal to be rushed to slaughter in order for a rancher to optimize his returns.[13]

In 1999, an in-depth survey of several hundred USDA inspectors conducted by Public Citizen found that 41 percent saw fecal material, 56 percent saw vomit, and 61 percent saw hair or feathers on meat products on a daily basis.

So it's hard to feel assured that meat is adulterant-free. Then again, it would not be unwise to first consider the fact that every hamburger is, in fact, comprised of the flesh of dead cows!

73 Aghast from the past

VENOMOUS COASTAL CELL

"I think pfiesteria has probably been around for millions of years. It's just that right now we're making conditions a lot more comfortable for it."
—JoAnn Burkholder, Ph.D., pioneering pfiesteria researcher[1]

It could have been just one more sediment-dwelling microorganism lying dormant, unknown and harmless in estuarine waters for a million years. But nutrient overload generated by chicken and hog farms on the Delmarva Peninsula and Eastern North Carolina—as well as a number of other un-ecological human activities—changed all that. Harmless became harmful. Soon this one-celled critter, drunk with spilled or runoff manure and fertilizer, might have been heard to stutter: "It's time to party!" But while this venomous "cell from hell" was getting what it needed, fish up and down the Atlantic shoreline were dying, rather, being killed—at least a billion of them off the shores of North Carolina alone in the early 1990s.[2]

Depending upon your perspective, *Pfiesteria piscicida*—the second word is Latin for "fish killer"—is either a triumph of evolution or the advent of environmental Armageddon. In stealth and deadliness, it puts both James Bond and the Terminator to shame. Douse it with bleach or sulfuric acid—as has been done in the laboratory—and it still has a 20 percent survival rate after an hour.[3] You can't kill it without also killing everything around it. All you can hope for in the field is to return the little monster to dormancy and harmlessness. To do that, you must take away the things that it needs: sewage and waters rich in nutrients—particularly phosphorus and nitrogen from factory farms.

Demise in disguise

Pfiesteria is phenomenally—no, freakishly—versatile, manifesting itself in 24 known forms. So novel are its abilities that pfiesteria has been classified as a whole new family of life, not just a new species.[4] Few fish can survive its attack methods. First, it masquerades as harmless algae, tricking fish to come close. Upon detecting fish, it transforms itself into a predator, enveloping its victims in toxic secretions, which are emitted in doses a thousand times more concentrated than cyanide.[5] The fish are disoriented, defenseless, and finally devoured. Sometimes a hole is eaten straight through a fish's body.[6] By this time, the pfiesteria cell has transformed itself yet again into a hungry amoeba, sucking away flesh through a straw-like arm. Simultaneously, the microscopic predator commences to reproduce itself. Finally, organic matter that is released into the water by the bloody kill attracts yet more hungry pfiesteria—and so the process continues. A 20-pound fish will be dispatched in four hours and a guppy in 10 minutes[7]—this by creatures so small that a thousand could fit on the head of a pin.[8]

Human exposure to pfiesteria by direct contact or through inhalation of vapors is also horrible, causing acute memory loss, disorientation, and bizarre behavior.[9] Divers and fishers have reported festering sores on their bodies, similar to the ones found on exposed fish.[10]

Blooms of doom

Pfiesteria was discovered in 1988—just one of many newfound toxic microorganisms thriving in polluted waters today. So-called harmful algal blooms (HABs) are on the rise all over the world and are a fixture all along American's ocean coasts.[11] Eruptions cause the water to turn yellow, red, or brown, and can harm fish. When the algae are lodged in the food chain, fish become poisonous to consume. HABs deplete the water of oxygen and can displace indigenous species. Only three kinds were known until recently. Today we have some 50 HAB species to contend with.[12] Perhaps we're just looking harder. Or, more likely, modern animal agriculture and aquaculture have tilted earth's ecological balance way out of kilter.

74 Living laboratories

TO BE OR NOT TO BE VEGETARIAN

"Both Chinese and non-Chinese should think about drinking more green tea, eating more vegetables, and eating less meat and dairy products."—Dr. Kam Woo, researcher of Pan Yu (China) diet[1]

One really needs to consult epidemiological evidence to truly establish what the optimal diet is for the human species. An epidemiological study, which compares various aspects of diet and lifestyle over large population samples, is far superior to any that might simply single out individual nutrients or foods for examination. To paraphrase *New York Times* food writer Marian Burros, Americans tend to cherry-pick. They may hear "olive oil," for instance, and add it to their meals, while missing the point about the virtues of the Mediterranean Diet as a whole.[2] Remember oat bran, beta-carotene, and vitamin C? These foods are only as good as the diets they're part of. The following cases should make this clear.

Mediterranean connection

The tiny, mostly impoverished nation of Albania became the setting for an epidemiological study in the late 1990s that compared the diets of two ethnically similar segments of its population, isolated from each other by geographic barriers. The mountain dwellers subsist on foods that are mostly of animal origin; the coastal group enjoys what is today termed the Mediterranean Diet, consisting mainly of fresh fruits and vegetables, cereals, some fish, and olive oil. Death rates were found to be significantly higher for those on the high-meat diet,[3] while the low-meat diet kept cholesterol levels in check and cardiovascular disease at bay.[4] (Vegetarians wishing to follow the Mediterranean Diet can eat ground flax seeds daily as a substitute for fish.)

Okinawa: Land of the centenarian

Researchers who studied the traditional Okinawan diet over a recent 25–year period found that the people of this island are the healthiest and longest-lived in the world, boasting the highest percentage of people on earth who make it to 100 years of age. And longevity is only part of the story. The country's super-seniors tend to retain their mental keenness into their twilight years, and few need to live in nursing homes.[5] Not surprisingly, the Okinawans were found to eat very little food of animal origin and consume easily 10 servings of fruits and vegetables per day.[6]

Sadly, the era of superlative longevity in Okinawa is coming to a close. Over a half-century of American military presence on the island has enticed the younger generation to fast-food hamburgers and chicken nuggets. In the coming years we are likely to see older Okinawans outliving their children. "It's not only a health problem, it's also about protecting our culture," lamented one Okinawan old-timer quoted in *The New York Times*.[7]

And they smoke, too

Japanese men live on average five years longer than American men. Exceedingly low incidence of prostate cancer is one reason, as is low incidence of heart disease. Their secret? Perhaps it's soy and green tea. But, more importantly, Japanese men eat very little meat.[8] Similarly in Pan Yu, China (about 100 miles from Hong Kong), people eat lots of vegetables, very little meat, and almost no dairy.[9] Indeed, they have one of the lowest rates of heart disease in the world to show for it, even though the villagers have high rates of smoking.

In peace

In Poland in the early 1990s, a 25 percent decline in heart disease coincided with the country's switch to a market economy that ended government subsidies to meat. The general replacement of animal fats with vegetable fats and the increased importation of fruit were seen as factors in the decline, according to a report made by a team of multinational researchers.[10] The authors of the report noted that the decline was "apparently without precedent in peacetime."

And in war

During World War I, Denmark was confronted with life-threatening shortages by the Allied blockade. It had no choice but to institute a rationing program that prohibited feeding grain to its livestock. The people were forced to subsist on scarce stores of grain without cycling it through animals first. Inadvertently, the country's three million people were forced to take part in a bit of state vegetarianism. Despite the hardships of war, the mortality rate from disease dropped 34 percent during this period.[11]

75 Carnivore conflicts

MEAT MILITATES AGAINST PEACE

"If the EU does not lift this [hormone] ban, we will retaliate this summer."
—Peter Scher, U.S. trade negotiator on agricultural matters, 1999[1]

The more people choose to put animal-based foods in their diets, the more the world risks being embroiled in the "carnivore conflicts" they provoke. From trade disputes to disagreements over animal drugs and diseases, to battles over fishing grounds, to the endless wrangling over country-to-country equivalency in processing-plant sanitation, it is not an exaggeration to say that meat consumption contributes greatly to international tensions. And the discord often escalates to the point of requiring officials from the highest levels of world governments to intervene.

Russia, which buys more chicken than anything else from the United States, has periodically halted millions of dollars in poultry imports, citing worries over salmonella and feed contaminants, including antibiotics.[2] Over the years, vice presidents Gore and Cheney have both been called into service to bring back the business.

In 2002, Mexico cried foul as barriers to free trade were disintegrating and heavily subsidized, low-priced U.S. poultry, beef, and pork were flooding its markets. A precipitous drop in Mexican poultry tariffs was scheduled to go into effect in 2003, and several thousand Mexican farmers threatened by the changes erected roadblocks.[3] The impasse became a challenge to the North American Free Trade Agreement itself.

Disease, drugs, and contaminants halt trade

The discovery of a single cow with bovine spongiform encephalopathy (BSE) in Canada in May 2003 caused at least 30 countries, overnight, to refuse imports of Canadian beef.[4] The yearly export of 1.7 million Canadian cattle into the United States stopped on a dime. Needless to say, the United States got a comparable dish of trade-ban pudding seven months later, only worse, when confronted with its own BSE-infected cow. Import bans by 50 nations, representing 90 percent of a significantly larger U.S. export market, immediately went into effect.[5] It was soon found that the Washington state "mad" cow originated in Canada. The situation continues to foster ill will between the two North American neighbors.

Throughout the 1990s, thousands of similarly afflicted animals in Great Britain prompted the same kind of draconian trade bans. Likewise, in 2001, a massive outbreak of foot and mouth disease resulted in countries all over the world closing their borders to EU meat, although the disease was primarily confined to the United Kingdom. London fielded the wrath of much of the European continent at that time, as did Belgium in 1999 when dioxin-contaminated feed originating in that country was found to have been widely exported.[6]

Meanwhile, the EU has remained steadfast, on grounds of human health, against purchasing U.S. beef from animals treated with growth hormones. It has chosen instead to accept WTO-imposed multimillion-dollar punitive tariffs on an array of unrelated export items.

Fish fights threaten fragile relations

A bitter trade dispute between the United States and Vietnam continues to simmer. It concerns low-cost Vietnamese catfish entering American markets. In 2001, House members from southern U.S. catfish-producing states became proponents of a labeling law to require the imported fish to indicate "product of Vietnam" and buttressed their cause by noting, apparently without irony, that Vietnamese catfish may be contaminated with high levels of Agent Orange, the defoliant used by American forces during the Vietnam War.[7] The law was passed. In addition, these imported fish are no longer allowed to go by the name "catfish," because technically they are a different species from the U.S. fish. In any case, duties have effectively forced any remaining imports out of the United States. All together, the rulings have sent many dirt-poor fish farmers in the Mekong Delta to ruin.

In 1997 the United Nations reported that over 100 countries were involved in fishing disputes.[8] A particularly volatile one today is taking place at the border between North Korea and South Korea. Flouting the UN boundary designated in 1953, fishermen from the north stray southward to catch blue crabs in May and June. Their incursions have prompted exchanges with the South Korean navy patrol—encounters the North Koreans say are intended to incite a larger fight.[9] Numerous skirmishes have ended in casualties and even sunken ships. And now, as the United States accuses the North Koreans of harboring a clandestine nuclear weapons program, the slightest increase in tensions could escalate into a resumption of the Korean War, or worse.

76 Slaughterhouse sludge

HAPPY ENTRAILS TO YOU

"[The record-breaking penalty accused] Smithfield of committing a host of environmental violations, submitting false reports to regulators, and destroying evidence."—Bloomberg, Oct. 2, 2000[1]

It was a "bust" to remember when in 1999 the *Washington Post* caught Tyson Foods trucking plethoric amounts of decomposing chicken heads, entrails, and feathers to a 105-acre field in Berlin, Maryland. Memorable indeed, because the crime was so blatant, so visible, and until then so unstoppable. Citizens had apparently pressed for two years to get the poultry giant to end its dumping. State soil tests determined that the nutrients that were present on the field could have fertilized the land for anywhere between 13 and 45 years into the future.[2] Regulators who had served notice to the plant two months prior to the *Post* exposé had been stymied. Even in the shadow of the nation's capital, across the Chesapeake Bay, it wasn't until the *Post* published its damning front-page report, with photos, that Tyson finally ended its dumping spree.

Legal sludge fest

Legal loopholes provide the key to this case. Tyson chose Maryland as its "toilet" for a reason. Here, nitrogen (in the form of slaughterhouse waste) was legally regarded as fertilizer, and not a pollutant, no matter the quantity. For the same reason, Perdue Farms, another poultry conglomerate, had also been trucking millions of gallons per year of slaughterhouse sludge into the state, the *Post* later found.[3]

The Delmarva Peninsula, where Berlin, Maryland, is located, teems with poultry processors in addition to its many farms. Twelve slaughterhouses in the region use over 12 million gallons of water to butcher two million birds every day.[4] Slaughterhouses, as with other "point-source" polluters, are allowed through permits to discharge treated waste water into local waterways. Treated though the water may be, the EPA has determined that nutrients from poultry productions have fouled the Chesapeake Bay, sending more than four times as much nitrogen into the water as the number-one non-agricultural source—leaky septic tanks and runoff from developed areas.[5]

Dumpers get dumped on

It's the EPA that is responsible at the federal level for limiting slaughterhouse pollution under the Clean Water Act. However, this top agency typically delegates its authority to the states, where regulators tend to be cozier with local polluters. Each state has a unique regulatory culture, but, by and large, oversight is found wanting.[6] In a number of high-profile cases, however, dumpers have had the book thrown at them. Following are a few examples.

Central Industries, a Jackson, Mississippi renderer, earned itself a $14 million penalty in the fall of 2000 for dumping carcass material into the Shockaloo Creek nearby.[7] The company kept taking in raw input beyond its capacity. Apparently, it didn't know how to say no.

Darling International, a California-based renderer with 30 plants across the country, received a $4 million fine for similar infractions in the early 1990s.[8] The company argued that it wouldn't make sense for it to discharge the very material that was its bread and butter—tallow, bone meal, yellow grease, and feed additives. The company fired four employees associated with the "uncrime," just the same.

When Darling's Boyle Heights, California operation was given a notice of violation from the local air-quality agency complaining of foul odors, it quite unceremoniously shut down—not, however, because of the violation, according to the company. Soon afterward, nearly 300 dead cows accumulated at nearby dump sites in a sweltering rigor-mortis salute.[9] A vomit-inducing stench—not to mention the lack of any viable rendering facility nearby—soon put the Darling plant in a very good bargaining position to negotiate the terms of its restitution.

Smithfield Foods, slaughterer of 12 million hogs per year, was fined $12.6 million in 1997 for committing nearly 7,000 violations of the Clean Water Act over six years.[10] Specifically, infractions included habitual dumping of thousands of gallons of intestinal waste into Virginia's Pagan River. According to Smithfield's defense, the discharges were deemed legal, per an agreement with Virginia's state regulators. A plant manager served a 30-month prison sentence for actions he claims Smithfield officers told him to carry out.[11]

Buckeye Egg Farm, at one time the fourth largest egg producer in the country with 15 million hens, was eventually driven out of business by environmental lawsuits. According to the "The Rap Sheet on Animal Factories," which was compiled by the Sierra Club, the Ohio company disposed of dead chickens by dumping them in a nearby field and violated its clean water permits over 800 times.[12]

77 Health claims

THE CATCH ABOUT FISH

"The crowding out of nutritious omega-3s has serious implication for health and chronic disease...the imbalance in an all-plant diet may be even more pronounced."—Brenda Davis, R.D. and Vesanto Melina, M.S., R.D., co-authors, *Becoming Vegan*[1]

Vegetarians have an Achilles heel—that is, in obtaining a couple of nutrients abundant in fish but otherwise not always easy to come by. And certain aspects of modern diets tend to further aggravate the deficiencies. The nutrients, eicosapentaenoic acid (EPA) and docosahexaenoic acid (DHA), or the omega-3 fatty acids, help the body form cell membranes and regulate important processes.[2] The body can manufacture them as long as certain foods are consumed. However, many vegetarians neglect these foods, often because they simply do not know of their importance. Unfortunately, without EPAs and DHAs, a vegetarian can end up canceling out his or her natural survival advantages against heart disease, stroke, and certain cancers.[3] And, worse, the oils used in processed foods (the omega-6 fatty acids) tend to cancel out the generally limited omega-3s that vegetarians take into their bodies in the first place. Processed food manufacturers tend to replace omega-3s with omega-6s in their products for the sake of extended shelf life.

Why not eat fish?

The flesh of certain fish is, without question, an incomparable source of DHAs and EPAs, allowing fish eaters to achieve their requirements for these very important and essential nutrients from small and infrequent portions of species rich in omega-3s. However, no benefits accrue from increased amounts, and indeed, after taking into consideration all aspects of fish as a food, after the DHAs and EPAs, it's basically downhill from there. Neal Barnard, M.D., gets right to the point in this regard: "Fish and shellfish contain too much protein, fat, and cholesterol to be healthy."[4]

Otherwise, fish, like any animal flesh, lacks fiber, is devoid of complex carbohydrates, is deficient in life-giving phytochemicals and vitamin C, and is high in kidney-straining animal protein. Oily fish—the food source which many people choose for their omega-3 fatty acids—is, by calorie, about 20 percent heart-unhealthy saturated fat.[5] In fact, the cholesterol content of fish may be as high as or higher than that of beef or chicken.[6]

Furthermore, fish oil supplements can cause nausea, diarrhea, halitosis, nosebleeds, and easy bruising.[7] The increased risk of uncontrolled bleeding that can result from fish oil supplementation or excessive fish consumption is problematic when a person experiences an injury or laceration.[8] Also, fish have even been found to contain prions, those mutant proteins considered to be agents of so-called transmissible spongiform encephalopathies (TSEs), among which you can count mad cow disease. Now, apparently, we have the prospect of "mad fish disease.[9]" Finally, even the FDA and American Heart Association are at odds as to whether the omega-3 fatty acids in fish can really reduce the risk of coronary heart disease—the former says this has yet to be proved.[10]

Fish dilemma

So where is a vegetarian to get his or her EPA's and DHAs? We still need to know. Fortunately, there are direct plant sources for these essential nutrients: microalgae. Fish in fact, have EPAs and DHAs in their bodies because they eat microalgae in the wild, or eat fish who ate microalgae. (Incidentally, this is why grain-fed, farmed fish have essentially no omega-3s.) A person can eat these microscopic organisms directly. However, they're only available in supplement form, which can, over time, strain the pocketbook.

A better choice may be indirect sources for DHAs and EPAs. A person *can* eat foods that contain the building blocks the human body needs to manufacture the omega-3s on its own. These foods include flax seeds and oil, hemp seeds and oil, walnuts, and soy oil.[11] Eating copious amounts of green vegetables also promotes a good omega-6-to-omega-3 balance. (Again, omega-6s can cancel out one's omega-3s.) One Toronto researcher, Dr. David Jenkins, points to several studies suggesting that omega-3 fatty acids found in plants—in particular, walnuts—are as beneficial to the heart as eating fatty, cold-water fish.[12] Michael Greger, M.D., who closely follows issues of vegan nutrition, urges vegetarians to consume two tablespoons of ground flax seeds every day as the best way to derive the equivalent of the American Heart Association-recommended one or two servings of fatty fish per week.[13] Greger also suggests that vegetarians avoid corn, safflower, sunflower, and cottonseed oils, which are rich in omega-6 fatty acids. Minimizing one's omega-6's in general is as important to optimal vegetarian health as getting enough omega-3s, he says.

In conclusion, it is nutritionally quite safe (see reason #100) to exclude fish from one's diet and still retain one's natural vegetarian advantages against a host of life-threatening diseases. Adopting a few simple practices is all that it takes. And just think how the fish and the oceans will benefit from your efforts.

78 Mutilating animals

A VERY BAD HABIT

"Sloppy castration means lower profits."—Matt Claeys, Purdue Cooperative Extension Service, beef-cattle specialist[1]

Debeaking, branding, castration, ear notching, wing and comb removal, dehorning, teeth clipping, and tail- and toe-docking—these standard procedures of the ranch and farm add yet one more layer of barbarism to the business of animal agriculture. Flipping through the hundreds of illustrations in the comprehensive *Handbook of Livestock Management Techniques*, the uninitiated may think that those who handle livestock do nothing but surgical procedures all day—operations that invariably are performed on the animals without anesthesia.

Animal welfare advocates have observed that sometimes the mutilations don't even bring any practical benefit to the animals' owners. The procedures continue just the same, apparently out of habit or tradition. Indeed, more humane management techniques often exist. The alternatives are not used, however, because they usually require a more sophisticated, read expensive, work force. The trend has been toward highly mechanized systems that are custom-made for cheaper, uneducated labor. Moreover, as long as any procedure is considered "common and accepted practice" in the United States, it remains perfectly legal. The mutilations exist as part of a general ethic that favors convenience over proper care and profit over mercy. Not one of them would be necessary in a vegetarian world.

Castration without representation

America's ranchers don't have to castrate their cattle. The Europeans raise bulls just fine. The procedure is even somewhat illogical from the industry's own set of criteria. Bulls naturally grow faster with their own hormones provided by intact testicles.[2] In the United States, hormones are routinely, and often imprecisely, administered to steers after their castration, usually in the form of an ear implant. Moreover, bull meat is naturally lean—what today's market demands.

American ranchers castrate, however, because it makes the animals fatten more quickly, and it usually makes them more docile. A castrated animal can be mixed with females of his own species, minimizing management problems in feedlots.

There are three castration methods, two of which shut off the blood supply so that the testicles either are reabsorbed into the animal's body or simply fall away after a couple of weeks. In a third method, the scrotum is cut so that the testicles can be pulled out.[3] Castration is a surgical procedure that can easily be bungled. Yet it is commonly performed by people who learn on the job without formal veterinary training. Again, anesthesia is rarely given—the argument being that such niceties would take too long and cost too much.[4] Still, some argue that anesthetics would reduce the number of botch jobs.

Dehorning: Extreme solution

Cattle with horns require too much space, the industry says, and horns damage valuable hides, or worse. For these sins the horns must go. Caustic chemicals do the job, particularly on calves. For older animals, stock men use clippers and saws, which soon becomes a bloody mess. The fact that older animals lose two weeks of growth immediately after the procedure is a testament to the extreme pain and stress that dehorning causes.[5]

Branding: The third degree

Cattle branding for some may evoke a certain romance about the Wild West. Yet this traditional identification tool for ranchers sears a third-degree burn into flesh. Some animals may have to endure the torturous procedure more than once as they are passed from owner to owner. There are branding technologies that generate less or even no pain. Still, none has offered a mark that is as completely fool-proof, visible from a distance, and, most importantly, inexpensive as the burned-on variety—so the practice continues. Just the same, and despite the ubiquity of the brand, today's rustler increasingly slaughters stolen animals so quickly that any physical evidence the brand may have provided is simply butchered away.[6]

Piglet assaults

Piglets have their teeth clipped to prevent laceration of sow udders, their tails docked to prevent the tail biting that occurs because of the intensely crowded conditions in which they are raised, and their ears notched, often with numerous clips, to aid in identification. Males are castrated to remove foul odors, or "boar taint," from their meat. Finally, vaccination rounds out the battery of invasive procedures endured by piglets before they are even ten days old.[7]

The last de-tail

Dairy cattle often have their tails docked. Farmers say the procedure reduces the incidence of mastitis. But the painful amputation is probably more a cause of the udder disease than not, since it can cause infection, lower immune response, and produce extreme stress in cows. Essentially, only those dairy farms that cannot keep conditions clean and sanitary for their cows would see the procedure as necessary.[8]

Burning beaks

Battery hens are squeezed into cages like sardines in tin cans—sometimes nine at a time. Their natural response is to fight and peck. Such behavior as feather pulling, as well as toe-, head-, and vent-picking, is referred to disparagingly by industry people as "cannibalism" and is seen as shortcomings in the birds. To reduce economic losses, the industry removes part of the animals' beaks. It is a haphazard procedure, accomplished with a hot (1,500°F) knife. When performed, the chicks will chirp shrilly, defecate in panic, and flap their wings in desperate attempts, to avoid being wounded.[9] Many bleed from botched attempts, and some may never be able to eat. The mutilation may have to be repeated. The birds are initially debeaked sometime between 10 days and three weeks of age, although some chicks may endure the procedure soon after hatching. Debeaking can cause lifelong chronic pain or even death.

Chickens raised for their meat are usually spared the debeaking process. However, intensively confined male turkeys will endure the procedure in order to reduce aggression.[10] Ducks raised in crowded conditions may have only the top portion of their beaks removed.[11]

Other industry mutilations inflicted on poultry include dubbing (removing combs) to preempt frostbite, toe-cutting to reduce bird-on-bird injury, and de-winging to keep the animals grounded. Caponization or poultry castration—easily a deadly procedure—promotes rapid growth and tender meat.

79 Recalling meat

OVERDUE AND INCOMPLETE

"The ConAgra recall is not an aberration. It is another example of a food safety system that is teetering on the brink of collapse."—Wenonah Hauter, director, Public Citizen[1]

In 2002, the United States saw a record number of federally ordered meat recalls, 113 in all.[2] At first glance, a person may assume that the government must be doing something right. On the other hand, one may wonder, why the need for so many recalls? And what effect are they having ultimately? An Ohio State University review of government records found that only half of the meat that is ordered recalled ever gets returned.[3]

When you get down to it, this is an industry that essentially lives not by government directives but by an honor system, at best. At worst, food safety programs are a smoke screen to shield the meatpacking industry from liability.[4] Tens of billions of pounds of meat are sold to consumers every year, yet the USDA conducts only one salmonella test per day per plant.[5] And these are for facilities the size of airplane hangars. If tests repeatedly come back positive, it is assumed that other bacteria may also be lurking. In theory, such a system makes sense. In practice, we have a different story.

Far from total recall

In 2002 19 *million* pounds of contaminated ground beef were ordered recalled from a ConAgra plant on account of the deadly pathogen E. coli

O157:H7. According to an inspector-general investigation into the case, federal inspectors had done nothing, despite being aware that the plant had failed 63 tests for the deadly pathogen over the course of a year. Blurred lines of authority were cited. According to the report, the inspectors actually believed they were not empowered to rectify the situation. The recall was deemed "ineffective and inefficient" simply because too many weeks had passed before necessary action was taken.[6] Ultimately, only about 16 percent of the designated tons of meat were recovered.[7] With a mixture of bravado and wishful thinking, the American Meat Institute declared at the time that it was "likely" that most of the product had "already been safely consumed."[8]

Paper tiger

According to a Government Accounting Office (GAO) investigation into meat-inspection oversight in 2002, the USDA had not followed through on threats to shut down 60 meat plants for food safety infractions, despite repeated violations.[9] The USDA's timorous stance has everything to do with a government food safety force rendered powerless by legislation, lawsuits (or threats of them), and budget shortfalls. Specifically, the GAO declared that America's food safety systems do not train inspectors properly, are deficient in their record keeping, and seem incapable of enforcing their own "zero-tolerance standard" for fecal contamination.[10] "No matter how much fecal contamination they find, it never seems to trigger shutdowns," one consumer advocate exclaimed at the time.[11]

Just prior to the ConAgra recall an investigation by two watchdog groups showed that USDA microbial testing was essentially rigged by selective examinations and strategic delays. The maneuvering by the agency not only allowed the USDA to report that the testing process was "working" but permitted plants to stay open despite numerous violations.[12] It was discovered in 2003 that though U.S. producers bring the carcasses of 300 million turkeys, representing 5.6 billion pounds of meat, to market per year,[13] the USDA had reduced the number of turkey processing facilities it tested for salmonella to a single plant[14]—no doubt a particularly clean one. This was down from 38 the year before.

Resistance not futile: Comply if you want

ConAgra complied with the USDA's 2002 recall request but was not legally compelled to do so.[15] Incredibly, the USDA has no authority to recall meat, nor can it issue fines. It cannot shut down a plant, though it can, at the risk of a lawsuit, remove its inspectors—thus having the same effect since no plant can operate without inspectors assigned to it. Furthermore, the government cannot compel a company under a recall to reveal its proprietary list of wholesale customers, leaving consumers in the dark as to whether they may have been exposed to contamination.[16]

Now, how would you like your mystery meat today?

80 Storm stories

TORRENTS OF TRAGEDY

"When producers lock up huge numbers of animals, there's the potential for huge numbers of victims."—Karen Davis, Ph.D., United Poultry Concerns[1]

Weather calamities are murder on farmed and ranched animals. In no time at all, a facility or an entire region of farms or ranches can become a scene out of hell involving thousands—or even millions—of terrified creatures, trapped, crushed, drowned, hurled, pinned, baked, frozen, impaled, or washed downriver.

Any person witnessing such a tragedy must begin to question the wisdom of confining huge numbers of animals in concentrated areas. The waste of life is horrendous, and the environmental fallout of inadequate disposal methods for the casualties is always disastrous.

Hoofnotes to history

Droughts, floods, blizzards, tornadoes, hurricanes, heat waves, and snow storms happen, and they affect animal operations more often than people realize. Perhaps the first livestock weather calamity to hit America was the one that took place between 1885 and 1887. Eighty percent of America's Plains cattle died after two dry summers were followed by two harsh winters. Today, weather disasters affecting legions of animals are a regular part of the agricultural landscape.

For example, there was the stifling heat wave of 1998 that baked seven million chickens to death in factory sheds across America's southern states over a four-week period. Were television stations called to the scene? Hardly. A small Reuters piece actually emphasized how inconsequential the bird deaths were to markets. It predicted that the drop in supply would have little effect on retail prices for chicken, noting that the seven-million-bird shortfall, large as it was, paled in comparison with the 600 million birds that would be slaughtered anyway within the same period.[2]

More people, no doubt, took notice of the January 2000 winter storms that ruined approximately 535 poultry houses across several southern U.S states—if only because the event involved millions of dollars in property damage beyond the loss of the birds. It killed perhaps eight million chickens under the weight of collapsed ice- and snow-laden roofs.[3]

Of course, it would have been difficult to ignore 50,000 head of cattle being swept downriver, as they were in 1998, when rain pelted 60 southern counties in Texas.[4] While some of the cows survived to walk the streets in towns down the way, others drowned after being chewed up by floating fire ants or gnawed on by snakes. Similarly, in 1999, Hurricane Floyd tore through eastern North Carolina, leaving an estimated 100,000 hogs and three million poultry birds drowned. Across hundreds of square miles, the flood waters became a multimillion-gallon witches' brew of decomposing carcasses and excrement from 225 washed-out cesspools of hog waste.[5]

Perhaps more widely known is the tornado that demolished 12 barns holding, all told, a million egg-laying hens in Licking County, Ohio, in 2000. Birds that weren't gassed and rendered, or rescued by animal protection groups, were bulldozed away with the wreckage two weeks later, some still trapped and alive during the process.

Death by bankruptcy

Imprisoned factory animals are also killed in great numbers by fires and electrical failure. The energy crunch that hit California in 2001 produced rolling blackouts across the state and put millions of chickens at risk. Without electricity to power giant ventilating fans, hundreds of thousands of birds can die almost immediately.[6]

Lack of electricity is equally deadly for aquaculture and swine operations. In 2003, three million farmed Atlantic salmon in Maine suffocated when a fire destroyed an oxygen-pumping system that funneled fresh water to their 100 circular holding tanks.[7] Two years earlier, a malfunctioning feed motor ignited a fire that caused approximately 12,000 sows and piglets to be burned to death at the Circle Four Farms in Utah. Decomposing carcasses soon became a serious health risk. Eventually, the bodies were buried on the spot, but groundwater was threatened with contamination.[8]

Ultimately, perhaps, bankruptcy is the most grisly cause of death for farmed animals of all. Stories of producers simply walking away from their operations because they can no longer pay the bills are reported periodically. Animals are simply left to starve to death. In one case in 2003—a ten-thousand-head pig farm in Ontario, Canada—animals were found in piles of decomposing carcasses, some still barely living among them reduced to cannibalism.[9]

81 Endocrine pump

HORMONAL CANCERS AND MEAT

"Fat is a remarkably active substance."—George Bray, obesity scientist[1]

The link between excess body fat and heart disease is well established. But excess body fat also provides the stimulus for the development of so-called hormonal cancers—those of the breast, prostate, ovary, endometrium, and testes. Studies suggest that too much fat acts like an endocrine pump, exuding hormones and growth factors in excess into the bloodstream, later causing robust cell division and raising the risk for mutation.[2] Specifically, a diet rich in animal fat is now associated with both prostate cancer[3] and breast cancer.[4]

Of fiber, menarche, and breast cancer

An English study published in the *International Journal of Cancer* found "strong inverse trends" between consumption of vegetables and breast cancer.[5] Dietary fiber was found to facilitate healthful mechanisms, due to its ability to soak up estrogen in the intestines and send it on its way. Without dietary bulk, which is derived only from plant foods, the intestines tend to recycle estrogen right back to the bloodstream, raising risk for the disease.[6]

Historically, as the amount of fat on our plates has gone up, the average age in which girls begin menstruating has gone down.[7] The average fat content of the meat-centered American diet is a whopping 37 percent of calories, and U.S. girls have the early menarche to show for it. Aside from the obvious drawbacks, early menarche is a risk factor for breast cancer as women advance in age.[8] In contrast, Asian girls, who eat only one-half to one-third as much fat as Americans, begin menstruating three to six years later than American girls and only rarely get breast cancer.[9]

Arachidonic acid, phytosterols, and prostate cancer

According to the Cancer Project, a program of the Physicians Committee for Responsible Medicine, "We know that daily meat consumption triples risk of benign prostate disease, regular consumption of cows' milk doubles it, and failure to regularly consume vegetables almost quadruples it."[10] Such poor eating habits must be on the rise, since the incidence of prostate cancer went up 23 percent between 1983 and 1998.[11]

Research has revealed that arachidonic acid—a fat primarily derived from foods of animal origin—is converted by cancer cells into a substance prostate cancer needs for its progression.[12] Moreover, too much meat in the diet nudges out the foods that provide fiber, which acts to soak up excess testosterone, long linked to higher risk for prostate cancer. Finally, vegetarian foods produce plant-based fats called phytosterols, which are believed to reduce testosterone levels in the bloodstream.[13]

Prostate cancer now occurs ten times more frequently in the United States than in Japan. Diet seems to be the reason for the discrepancy.[14] According to the U.S. National Library of Medicine and the National Institutes of Health, "the lowest incidence [of prostate cancer] occurs in Japanese men and vegetarians....Adopting a vegetarian, low-fat diet, or one that mimics the traditional Japanese diet, may lower risk."[15]

Moreover, those Japanese men who do contract the disease find their illnesses progress more slowly than those of American men.[16] Nutrition experts suggest that the traditional Asian diet, which consists of rice, soy, and generous portions of vegetables, and which relegates meat to a side dish, is the distinguishing factor. Japanese men who migrate to America and take on the rich dietary lifestyle of the locals raise their risk for prostate cancer demonstrably.[17]

A study conducted by the Preventive Medicine Research Institute, which began in 2002, put 84 prostate cancer patients into two groups. Those men who made lifestyle changes, including adopting a vegetarian diet, regular exercise, and stress management, saw their conditions improve, compared to those men who were simply monitored.[18]

82 Clinical consensus

FISH FEEL PAIN

"We found 58 receptors located on the face and head of the rainbow trout that responded to at least one of the stimuli."—Lynne Sneddon, lead researcher, trout study, "Do Fish Have Nociceptors?"[1]

It's just a tad too convenient. Anglers, in particular, but anyone, really, who catches, processes, or consumes fish, tends to, or pretends to, believe that fish do not feel pain. Fish do not yelp or whimper when you hurt them. This is true. But science now begs to differ with the apologists for fishing. Fish feel pain, and the evidence is now irrefutable.

Pain systems are present

A study conducted in 2003 at Edinburgh University and the Roslin Institute in Scotland concluded that fish react adversely to painful stimuli. Electrophysiological measurements detected not only immediate responses to applications of physical pressure, heat, and chemical irritants (bee venom and vinegar) but profound and prolonged behavioral and physiological distress over extended periods afterwards—similar to normal reactions expected in mammals.[2] In particular, after trout lips were subjected to chemical stimuli, the fish were seen to rock and to rub their mouths across the tank's gravel in apparent attempts to find relief.[3] Furthermore, the fish required extended recovery periods before resuming feeding activity.[4]

Other studies have revealed that fish adrenal systems function in similar ways to those of mammals, indicating that fish experience sensations that humans would describe as panic, fear, or stress.[5] Indeed, Donald Broom, an animal welfare adviser to the British government, says, "The scientific literature is quite clear. Anatomically, physiologically, and biologically the pain system in fish is virtually the same as in birds and mammals."[6] According to S.C. Kestin of Bristol University, "All the fundamental structures and modulation processes necessary to achieve a perception of pain are present in fish."[7] And fish release opiate-like substances in response to stress, which implies our piscine friends have the capacity to feel pain.[8]

University of Oxford zoologist Dr. John Baker concluded from his studies that the "powerful struggling movements" that lobsters display when boiled alive in preparation for a meal indicate efforts to escape pain. It takes up to two minutes for a lobster to die in this manner. Lobsters' sensory organs are highly developed, and they possess highly complex nervous systems.[9]

Hooks hurt

Fishing inflicts pain with gill nets, drag nets, purse seine nets, driftnets, longlines, and hooks. And these are just the conventional tools of the trade. Let's not forget that fish are "harvested" with bows and arrows, spears, guns, dynamite, and cyanide as well. Gear can strangle, puncture or tear flesh. Side-piercing hooks are routinely used to sort fish on deck into catch and discards, snaring anything—a torso, a fin, or an eyeball.

So-called sport fishing amounts to a sick game in which one plays a sentient creature to exhaustion for the fun of it. "Catch and release" may impact fish stocks less severely than catch and consume, but what's the cost in terms of suffering, when studies have found that some fish may be caught as many as ten times a year?[10] A report published in the journal *Science* in 2004 estimated that 20 percent of those fish caught via methods of catch and release ending up dying from the stress.[11] Similarly, on fish farms, crowding, handling, and transporting are highly disruptive to the fish. Oxygen deficiencies, high ammonia or nitrate levels, and pH shock are also great stressors.[12] All of these things can cause farmed fish to stop eating, get sick, or die.

Good vibrations

Fish possess intricate nervous systems and are capable of learning complicated tasks.[13] They can express vibratory sounds to form various "calls" that have been identified by researchers as communicating alarm and aggravation.[14] Some fish have been found to recognize individuals in their group.[15] Fish also have been seen to perform amazing navigational feats.[16] As animal activist Dawn Carr once put it: Fish are not merely vegetables that can swim.[17]

83 Apocalypse then

FOOT AND MOUTH DISEASE

"This disease doesn't kill the animals. It doesn't have to. The human fear of contagion kills them."—Verlyn Klinkenborg, editorial observer, *The New York Times*[1]

Foot and mouth disease (FMD) is wildly contagious. The infectious bacteria that cause it can remain airborne for up to 40 miles.[2] Indeed, clothing, shoes, the breath of a pig, or the dust on a car-radio antennae may harbor the disease, which can live up to three weeks.[3] Blisters on lips, teats, muzzles, and hooves are the first signs that an animal is sick. Loss of appetite sets in. Feed conversion and milk production soon begin to falter. Though some people confuse it with that other livestock scourge, mad cow disease (which has a very different source of infection—the prion), FMD is nothing more than a really bad cold for animals.

A capital crime of under-performance

Foot and mouth disease is rarely fatal. However, to cloven-footed and split-hoofed livestock, it carries a death sentence. Livestock must perform up to precise commercial expectations at all times. It's nothing personal. It's just business. For some countries, the value of an export trade in meat and live animals free of the disease is worth more than the losses incurred by a mass cull. A country that is not FMD-free is prohibited by rules of international trade from exporting meat from diseased or even vaccinated animals.

Particularly devastating was the 2001 FMD epidemic in England that ended in six million cows, sheep, and pigs destroyed, 10,000 contiguous farms closed off from traffic at one time or another, and losses of $9 billion.[4] The actual number of animals afflicted came to just over 2,000; the rest underwent eradication as a buffer.

The carnage brought grown men to tears. When the slaughter man's gun was just around the bend, some livestock owners said they would place themselves between the executioner and their herds.[5] A number of rare breeds were threatened with extinction by the giant cull.[6]

"First they lock you up. Then they shoot your livestock, and then they force you to breathe in the smell of your burning livestock for the next week," fretted one rancher just after English authorities liquidated his sheep.[7] On some farms, contagious animals were simply left to starve to death.[8]

Dead animal disposal naturally became an environmental disaster. According to the Food and Agriculture Organization of the UN, total dioxin emissions from the burning carcasses amounted to 18 percent of the UK's annual dioxin output for the year.[9] People worried that water tables would become contaminated.[10] Others feared the infectious agent that causes mad cow disease—possibly lurking in some of the animals—would become airborne.[11]

Profits supersede all

Foot and mouth disease is generally endemic in poor countries and is simply allowed to run its course when it presents itself. Afflicted animals eventually recover, though later tend to be much less productive. The British solution played out in stark contrast. With its $1-billion-a-year export trade in meat and live animals, it felt compelled to extirpate its FMD epidemic completely. The use of vaccines—the more humane, farmer-friendly, and lower-cost alternative to eradication—was rejected, since antibodies produced in response to them are indistinguishable from those of infected animals. Vaccinated animals or their meat would have been unable to leave the European Union with FMD-free export status.

It is not an exaggeration to say that this disease could severely impact the U.S. economy if it were to come to American shores. But perhaps the ultimate disaster of a U.S outbreak would be if wildlife in this hemisphere were to become long-term or even permanent reservoirs for the disease.[12] Were this to happen, the meat industry would surely demand a government campaign to eradicate wild animals that threatened its livestock. Such a program would not be without precedent. The U.S. government maintains ongoing cull campaigns against wild deer and elk because of chronic wasting disease and bison because of brucellosis.

84 Ammonia rain

FUMES OF DESTRUCTION

"If you have a sensitive woodland...you should not allow it to be downwind from a major pig or chicken farm."—Dr. Phil Ineson, regarding his research into the destructiveness of livestock-generated ammonia[1]

Proponents of factory farming's so-called "lagoon system" sing its utilitarian praises, saying the giant pits of urine and feces not only function as holding tanks, they work as bacterial digesters. But before we sigh with relief, we need to consider the destructive gas that is the by-product of this digestive process. Much as coal dust and smokestack emissions cause acid rain, ammonia fallout (ammonia volatilization) from animal waste lagoons adversely affects environments many miles away.[2]

A hard rain for others

Gigantic open-air lagoons that are positioned next to factory farms are particularly potent exit portals for ammonia emissions into the environment. The urine and feces volatilize (change from a liquid to a gas) to later rain down their toxic particles on distant waterways, forests, and nitrogen-sensitive plants.

In rivers and estuaries, ammonia contributes to algae growth, which eventually chokes the water of oxygen. According to the Agriculture Research Service of the USDA, a total of 50 to 70 percent of organic nitrogen (animal waste) can be converted to ammonia.[3] Atmospheric deposition accounts for between 25 percent and 80 percent of the total nitrogen load entering the Chesapeake Bay.[4] Much of the acidic fallout is surely floating over from North Carolina's many swine operations.[5]

Ammonia volatilization also takes place over crops where excesses of fertilizer are used. Nitrogen levels in rain over Midwestern states—cultivated primarily with feed crops—are 5 to 30 times higher than in non-farmed areas.[6]

The ammonia rain is particularly harmful to plants that thrive on little nitrogen. Too much can become poisonous. Rare prairie plants in a remote Minnesota nature reserve, for instance, have disappeared from the effects of excess airborne ammonia.[7]

In the Netherlands, scientists discovered that 90 percent of its acid rain resulted from ammonia.[8] So open-air lagoons were outlawed. Farmers are required to inject manure into the soil rather than spray it over fields.[9]

A study in 1999 surprised at least one British scientist when he discovered that manure is as damaging to trees as industrial soot. On a relatively small farm of only a few hundred pigs, researcher Dr. Phil Ineson found plumes of ammonia emanating from what he described as colossal amounts of manure. A shaft of heat from the animals themselves drove the ammonia skyward to later descend on a nearby wood. Tree branches were found denuded and dying from a coating of ammonium sulfate.[10] "Farmers have been getting away with things that no factory owner would ever be allowed to," Ineson later exclaimed.

Atmospheric ammonia damages vital leaf absorption capacities. It also acidifies soil, further interfering with trees' nutrient absorption. The latter phenomenon tends to take place more readily in naturally nitrogen-poor ecosystems such as forests.[11] Ammonia pollution has, in fact, been blamed for some of the Black Forest dieback in the Netherlands.[12]

Grilling up the carcinogens

On a related subject, fine particulates from the cooking of meat are a significant source of smog.[13] The fatty fumes—the kind you smell when you walk past the local chophouse—are in the same class of pollutant as diesel emissions, cigarette smoke, and car exhaust. Los Angeles restaurants in 1994 were found to emit 33 tons of meat particles into the air every day, equivalent to the hydrocarbons that might be emitted by an oil refinery, or nine times more soot particles than all the region's buses.[14] Industrial chain-driven restaurant charbroilers were eventually regulated in Los Angeles and other cities. Yet emissions from this type of cooking device actually represent a small fraction of the total meat particles contaminating the air.[15]

85 Colorectal cancer

OPTING FOR PREVENTION

"Tomorrow on [the Today Show] I will give them the true 'inside story'—sharing exclusive video of my very own colon, shot during my first colonoscopy."—Katie Couric, NBC's *Today Show* host, who champions screening for colon cancer[1]

Colorectal cancer is a killer, and not just because you have to use the words enema, rectum, anus, and bowel movement when you're discussing it. It is the second most lethal cancer in America after cancer of the lung. About 57,000 people die from the disease in the United States every year,[2] even though there is a 92 percent survival rate for those whose cancer is detected and treated early.[3]

Holding the bag

How far the disease has progressed determines your treatment. You may only need a polypectomy, the surgical removal of cancerous growths. Or, in more advanced cases, your surgeon will carve out entire sections of your colon and reattach the ends. Sometimes the reattachment procedure cannot be performed immediately, or ever, forcing you to wear an external bag so your feces can collect for disposal.[4] Highly malignant cases may require the complete removal of the colon.

A University of Oxford study that followed 10,000 people for 17 years found vegetarians to be significantly less likely to develop colon cancer.[5] Apparently, excluding fruits and vegetables from the diet is an important a risk factor. Study subjects who ate five servings of fruit per day were 40 percent less likely to develop the disease.[6] Among other factors, the fat in red meat increases the excretion of bile acids in the body, which produce other substances that encourage tumor growth.

In 1990, the Harvard Nurses' Study of over 88,000 women found that those who ate beef, lamb, or pork on a daily basis ran two and a half times the risk of developing colorectal cancer as did those who ate these meats less than once a month.[7] The head researcher exclaimed at the time, "The optimum amount of red meat you eat should be zero."[8] So-called white meats were similarly indicted in 1998.[9]

Epic findings

The EPIC Study (European Prospective Investigation into Cancer and Nutrition), which involved over 400,000 subjects in nine countries, reported in 2001 that eating excessive amounts of red meat promotes the creation of N-Nitroso, a carcinogen, in the colon. The fecal material of people who eat a lot of red meat has been found to contain this suspect chemical in equivalent concentration levels found in tobacco smoke.[10] N-Nitroso is believed to be created when heme—the pigment that makes meat red—combines with bacteria in the colon. According to the study, preserved meats, such as bacon, cured ham, salami, corned beef, and pastrami, are particularly dangerous—a finding that confirmed numerous previous studies. The study further found that risk of colorectal cancer is reduced by 40 percent when one adopts a high-fiber diet.[11] The best way to obtain fiber, of course, is from whole vegetarian foods; those derived from animal-based foods are devoid of fiber.

Across the cultures

The incidence of colorectal cancer varies particularly widely between cultures. The evidence that the high-fat, meat-based diets of the United States, Canada, Western Europe, and Australia promote the disease is essentially airtight. The prevalence of colorectal cancer in developed countries is three to eight times higher than in countries such as China, Colombia, Greece, and India, where diets include far fewer animal-based foods.[12] Moreover, when people from countries with low cancer rates move to those with high ones, they take on the higher risk for the disease if they adopt local eating habits, proving no genetic advantages.

86 Concentrated and centralized

THE BIG-MEAT STEAMROLLER

"Federal case law, underfunded enforcement, and a reliance on unfounded efficiency claims have greatly diminished the competitive environment in the farm sector."—Sen. Charles Grassley (R-IA)[1]

Today the local farmer, butcher, fisher, and fishmonger are no longer a fixture in the neighborhood. Their ruddy images have long been lost among the plastic packages at the supermarket.

Producers operating coast to coast have adopted an industrial model for their businesses. Meat and dairy foods arrive via multi-sectored, fully integrated, non-stopping conveyor lines. Huge fishing vessels are controlled by global concerns.

Meanwhile, a monoculture has invaded our fields, our barns, and our refrigerators. Nearly all dairy cows in the nation are closely related Holsteins, and twelve million hogs slaughtered each year by Smithfield essentially share the same genes.[2] The system is bad for the environment as well as our health, and animal diseases more easily get a foothold under such conditions. Food safety is a loser as well.

Today, farms essentially confine, coerce, pollute, poison, and stink for miles, and the little guy has been all but nudged out, leaving ghost towns to dot the rural landscape. While production may have been made more efficient in the process, did the road to "enough" have to bring us so many ills?

Gatekeepers asleep

During his tenure as USDA secretary under President Clinton, Dan Glickman once said that he heard more complaints about industry concentration than anything else.[3] Even auditors from the USDA's own inspector general's office have sharply criticized the antitrust division of the agency. It argued in 1997 that the USDA's antitrust officers were so ill equipped to investigate price fixing and other anticompetitive practices by large meatpackers that the function should be transferred to the Justice Department or the Federal Trade Commission.[4] Earlier, a 1996 panel of mostly livestock producers and packers had come up with an extraordinary 86 recommendations to improve the USDA's antitrust oversight.[5] Later, in 2000, a Government Accounting Office report found that the Grain Inspection, Packers and Stockyards Administration of the USDA—though adept at performing general economic analyses for the industry—was sorely lacking in its ability to investigate anticompetitive practices of powerful interests.[6] All in all, of a mere 74 investigations that the USDA initiated over a two–year period in the late 1990s, only 57 were completed, with violations found in only five.[7]

By the 1990s, meat production had become concentrated to an extent previously unimaginable. Yet even greater mergers were to come. Multibillion-dollar corporations with huge shares in processing and feed-grain markets—IBP and Murphy, Continental Grain and Cargill, Smithfield and Tyson, and later Smithfield and IBP—began pairing up. This finally sent clarion calls to government antitrust departments. However, one after another, the mergers passed legal muster. Moreover, a consensus was building that giant conglomerates were in fact better able to capture international markets, which by this time was hailed as a trade necessity.

Today, there's only one nail left to pound into the coffin of small-rancher and small-farmer independence, and that is meatpacker ownership of livestock. A few states still ban the control of such classic vertical integration. But pressure from slaughter interests mounts. Already, meatpacking companies control 83 percent of the nation's hogs and 32 percent of the nation's cattle through outright ownership or favorable contract agreements.[8] Ultimately, as long as gigantic concerns can own their own livestock, they are able to take from their own herds when prices are high and buy from the independents only if prices are low—a scenario that spells the demise of the independents.

A more basic question faces all of us: Why buy into any of these power grabs in the first place? Isn't it time we all headed for the produce section at the green market?

87 Greed before mercy

AGRICULTURE'S WALKING WOUNDED

"From a welfare standpoint, euthanizing downers on the farm would be ideal."—Temple Grandin, farmed animal welfare specialist[1]

In terms of cruelty, it's hard to choose which aspect of the meat industry is most heartbreaking. Up there on the list must be how some ranchers, slaughterhouses, and stockyards in America treat downers—those animals who, after factory lives, have become too crippled or sick to walk to their own slaughter. Undercover activists have videotaped torturous scenes of non-ambulatory animals, writhing in pain and crashing to the ground after being dragged with chains off of trucks. They have documented living creatures suffering in agony on piles of dead ones. They have shot videotapes of mangled animals, lowing and bleating, being scooped up in forklifts as if they were garbage. For these sick and injured creatures, veterinary care is out of the question, since they are not seen as worth the expense. Many are left to die of neglect.[2]

It is estimated that a third of the nation's calves arrive at auction too young to walk, according to livestock researcher Temple Grandin. They end up being thrown or dragged. For older animals, milk fever (hypocalcemia) is the usual cause of debilitation. "It is likely that 10 percent of the bad dairies are responsible for 90 percent of the downers," Grandin asserts.[3]

Inhumane at any price

To move an incapacitated animal humanely usually requires anesthesia, an amenity virtually nonexistent in the livestock business. Downers are doomed anyway. As soon as they become immobilized, they should be put out of their misery and their bodies prohibited from the marketplace. Yet handlers are reluctant to humanely euthanize an incapacitated animal. Sheer economics rules over mercy. Living, an animal fetches several hundred dollars; dead, about twenty.[4] Consequently, many downers end up being forced to live just a little longer so that they can go through the slaughter process. But, worse, this usually means waiting for the ambulatory animals to be processed first, since the downers cannot be allowed to slow the line. Sometimes the incapacitated animals end up outdoors having to endure bitter cold or scorching heat for an entire day.

Mad cow turn of events

Two days before Christmas 2003, America officially experienced its first case of mad cow disease. As a result, a federal decree prohibited all non-ambulatory ruminant animals from the human food supply. (The new policies do not pertain to non-ruminants, such as pigs.) In theory, the government considers the subset of downer cows as the place where mad cow disease is likely to emerge. The USDA's prohibition is meant to minimize the risk for human exposure to the disease.

In one swift stroke, what animal protection groups had lobbied for for years was achieved by way of a single sick cow. Overnight, any price a rancher might receive on a bovine downer was slashed to the floor, at least according to law. Performing euthanasia on downer cows at the farm or ranch suddenly became, for the producer, a matter of cutting one's losses. By way of economic incentive, the new rule that was instituted to protect people now inadvertently protects bovine downers from the agonies of transport and the slaughterhouse. The United States generates an estimated 600,000 non-ambulatory cows each year.[5]

Moreover, as long as crippled and sick cattle do not bring an adequate payback at the slaughterhouse, ranchers might have an incentive to maintain better conditions for them. It remains to be seen if the new rule is implemented in earnest. Already, the beef industry is complaining that the government's prohibition should not apply to cattle that are not sick but simply lame.[6]

In any case, however things play out, as long as animal agriculture continues to exist, the downers will be out there.

88 Meat, the sequel

HEART FAILURE, STROKE, AND BYPASS

"In a way, the epidemic of congestive heart failure is a sign of progress, evidence of advances in saving the lives of heart attack victims."—Denise Grady, for *The New York Times*[1]

A diet high in animal products inevitably causes arterial walls to become inflamed and hardened with atherosclerotic plaque. The condition is a setup for a rupture that can create a clot that can kill you. Diet and exercise are a good defense against this scenario, and you can choose this route. Or you can risk putting your life in the hands of modern medicine. Two invasive and expensive medical procedures are always there to come to your rescue.

First, there's balloon angioplasty, which presses plaque back against arterial walls. Then, there are the stents, or wire-mesh architecture, that are installed to keep the plaque in place. The operations work in tandem to hold arteries open so blood can flow and chest pain can be reduced. Unfortunately, these procedures may not remove the risk for a heart attack or "coronary event."[2] When this occurs, it's likely that yet again technology can intervene—but it's safe to say your life will never be the same.

Living with a broken heart

In the case of congestive heart failure—a primary side effect of successful heart surgery—your damaged heart is unable to circulate blood to the rest of your body adequately. The heart blows up in size. Fluid collects in the abdomen and lungs. And other organs, particularly the kidneys, also tend to be damaged by the lack of coronary pumping power.[3]

Heart failure is the only form of cardiovascular disease still on the rise in the United States.[4] Five million people are living with the disease in this country at any given time, and about 550,000 new cases are diagnosed each year.[5] This disease is the leading cause of hospitalization among the elderly.[6]

A stroke of bad luck

Stroke is another cardiovascular scourge that is linked to a high-meat, low-fruit, low-vegetable, low-legume, low-whole-grain diet, according to a study of 71,000 nurses and designed by a team of researchers at the Harvard School of Public Health. The study was published in the journal *Stroke* in 2004.[7]

Stroke is the third leading cause of death in the United States.[8] Yet people tend to fear it most because it is the nation's leading cause of serious, long-term disability.[9] The effects of stroke vary considerably, depending on what part of the brain is deprived of blood.[10] A victim may become paralyzed or blind. He or she may experience loss of sensation, balance, or bladder control. There may be speech impediments or swallowing difficulties. Depression is common, as is the telltale inability to remember things. Often the entire household is affected when a family member falls victim to a stroke.

Don't have a coronary

Coronary bypass is the quintessential, affluent-society, meat-eater operation—the inescapable result of a lifetime of daily intakes of pastrami on rye, ham and cheese, and chicken nuggets. Smoking and sedentary habits also raise risk. About 516,000 of these surgeries are performed in the United States every year.[11] And each has a hefty price tag to go with it—about $25,000 per procedure.[12]

The operation itself is gravely traumatic to the body. Joseph Epstein, who gave a blow-by-blow description of his bypass in a *New Yorker* article some years ago, said that his body was so mangled by the operation he feared his whole being had become fundamentally altered. Though anesthetics had erased his conscious memory of any pain, he was sure that his body held on to the violation deep within.[13] Just imagine having your rib cage opened, your heart stopped so it can be operated on, and your body hooked up to an external pumping machine so an artery or vein, taken from some other part of your body, can be grafted as a replacement blood vessel to your heart.[14] Memory, language ability, and spatial orientation become diminished in up to half of bypass survivors. For some, these side effects never completely go away.[15] It's not surprising that depression is common.[16] And about 40 percent of bypass patients have blockages within ten years, requiring a second operation.[17]

As fitness guru Susan Powter used to say, "Stop the insanity!" Better yet, send in the vegetarians.

89 Mephitic emissions

THE AIR OF DECOMPOSING WASTE

"It's this progressive loss of brain."—Kaye Kilburn, environmental medicine expert, describing the long-term effects of hydrogen sulfide exposure[1]

You have to wonder about a gas that has the ability to corrode metal—especially if you live downwind from that which creates it: millions of gallons of manure. Bacterial decomposition of animal wastes produces scores of volatile compounds, most of which do nothing more than stink to high heaven.[2] But at least one of the gases, hydrogen sulfide (H_2S), when combined with the natural moisture in the air, converts to sulfuric acid, a compound that can corrode the metal confinement buildings where masses of defecating animals are kept.

Farmers are warned to keep metal surfaces free of dust, because sulfide "growth" can cause electrical shorts,[3] ending life support for feeding, watering, heating, and cooling systems for thousands of confined beings. Electrical failure is the primary reason for barn fires.[4] Moreover, H_2S is heavier than air, so it is able to lurk below the surface of a pool of effluent slurry. When lagoon contents are agitated, fumes can unexpectedly burst forth to overtake a person or an animal.

Toxicity aloft

Of the four primary gases in manure and other decomposing organic wastes—ammonia, carbon dioxide, methane, and hydrogen sulfide—all can asphyxiate, methane and hydrogen sulfide are explosive in very high concentrations, and hydrogen sulfide can cause neurological damage.[5]

In 2003, a *New York Times* story featured an Ohio schoolteacher who said that a "swirling poison" invaded his home from a nearby hog farm and "robbed him of his memory, his balance, and his ability to work. It left him with mood swings, a stutter, and fistfuls of pills."[6] His diagnosis: irreversible brain injuries from hydrogen sulfide gas. He was lucky to even learn the cause of his symptoms. In general, the neighbors of industrial hog farms experience diarrhea, nosebleeds, earaches, and lung burns, yet these incidental victims don't always know the reason for their distress.[7]

In Iowa, the largest hog-producing state in the nation, a recalcitrant state legislature finally set limits in 2004 on air pollution from livestock operations, but there are no penalties for operators who exceed ceilings on gases such as hydrogen sulfide.[8]

Brain-eating gas

Hydrogen sulfide is also emitted by slaughterhouses and rendering plants. Downwind, it inflicts a cumulative assault on human respiratory systems and upends any semblance of quality of life. The gas, which smells like rotten eggs or a sewer, can cause eye irritation, sore throat, cough, and nausea. When taken into the body, it converts oxygen-carrying, iron-containing enzymes to ferrous sulfide, which works surreptitiously to impair a person's ability to breathe, eventually eating the brain. In 2000, *USA Today* documented the trials and tribulations of a Nebraska town that was host to a hydrogen-sulfide-emitting meat-packing plant.[9] It told of elderly residents shuffling around the local Wal-Mart with oxygen tanks in tow. Noxious fumes were found pouring out of the slaughter plant at nearly 20 times the concentrations at which companies are required to notify the government.[10] For residents of these towns, life had become a living hell. Over time, the gas may cause chronic sinusitis, hyperactive airways disease, atopic asthma, acute organic dust toxic syndrome,[11] and hydrogen sulfide poisoning.[12] People with pre-existing respiratory conditions or reduced immune function are particularly at risk.

Emissions accomplished

Ammonia emissions from manure that waft scores of miles away from livestock operations are also dangerous to human respiratory systems when combined with soot from vehicular traffic and dust from farms.[13] The result is a caustic vapor of ammonium nitrate particles, small enough to get past the natural defenses of the human nose and lung. The smoggiest place in the nation is just east of Los Angeles where ammonia and other pollutants from 300,000 dairy cows mix with the city's notorious smokestack and tailpipe emissions.[14] A number of published studies now exist that link such air pollution with birth defects, premature births, low birth weight, and even respiratory ailments that can kill a newborn.[15] More than sixteen percent of children in Fresno County—one of the areas worst-hit—suffer from asthma.[16] The dirty air in this region is blamed for 275 deaths per year.[17]

90 Nutrition Brownie points

OFFICIAL DICTA

"PCRM won significant victories in this case: soy milk is now part of the 'dairy group,' and the committee declared the foundation of a healthy diet is plant-based food."—Mindy S. Kursban, Esq., PCRM[1]

So, what do officials of major health organizations and government agencies have to say about vegetarianism? About eating meat? Surely some of them must see a conflict in designating meat as imperative to human health. The scientific literature certainly points to labeling meat as nothing more important than a food to be eaten sparingly if at all. Still, nearly all recommend meat as part of a "balanced diet."

Are all these food advisors merely indulging a public they're afraid will ignore more honest advice? Do the organizations they represent enjoy dubious ties to commercial food interests? Or are these people simply washed in the baptism of the prevailing meat culture? Perhaps a little of each. Just the same, the mainstream health organizations do at times tip their institutional hats to vegetarianism, albeit parenthetically. Following are a few examples:

"Appropriately planned vegetarian diets are healthful, nutritionally adequate, and provide health benefits in the prevention and treatment of certain diseases."[2]—**American Dietetic Association and the Dietitians of Canada**

Two-thirds of cancer deaths in the nation are linked to diet, and half of the fatalities could have been prevented by a diet rich in fruits and vegetables.[3]—**U.S. Surgeon General's Office**

"Choose foods low in saturated fat, trans fat, and cholesterol."[4] —**American Heart Association**

"Choose most of the foods you eat from plant sources....Limit your intake of high-fat foods, particularly from animal sources....Eating at least five servings of fruits and vegetables a day reduces the risk of cancer, especially colon and lung cancer....High-fat diets have been associated with an increased risk of cancers of the colon, rectum, prostate, and endometrium."[5]—**American Cancer Society**

The ACS also suggests eating beans as a substitute for red meat.[6]

Government pronouncements

Every five years, under the unlikely auspices of the USDA—the agency whose mission it is to promote American agricultural products—the government tells us what to eat. With its "Dietary Guide for Americans," the public purportedly gets an update on current nutrition science. The guide, which influences how billions of dollars are spent on federal food assistance programs, including the school lunch program, has also long promoted meat, poultry, fish, and milk in the diet. The Food Pyramid, the iconic distillation of the guide, is what the public knows best. Even more than the guide, it has endorsed the consumption of meat and milk.[7]

Some have rightly branded the dietary guide as "advertising from powerful food interests," although this characterization may not be quite as true as it once was, especially after 1999. That year, a successful lawsuit charged the USDA with illegally establishing and operating the advisory committee that writes the guidelines,[8] bringing to light the inner workings of industry influence.[9] "At least six members of the conflicted federal advisory panel have had financial ties to animal agriculture interests," accused the lead plaintiff, Physicians Committee for Responsible Medicine (PCRM).[10]

Promoting veggies, in spite of themselves

Nonetheless, if examined closely, the various incarnations of the guide have actually accommodated vegetarian and even vegan concerns. They have even told people to "eat less meat." They don't use those exact words—not since 1979 when the meat industry raised a hue and cry about it.[11] Still, the dietary guide does state: "Choose foods that are low in saturated fat and cholesterol." Unfortunately, this pro-vegetarian advice means very little to most people.[12]

The 1995 version of the USDA dietary guide acknowledged vegetarianism by name for the first time, adding, however, in telling detail all of the diet's supposed drawbacks compared to one with meat. The 2000 guide only alluded to vegetarianism, bunching it in with other "healthful eating patterns." This version, however, liberally endorsed fruits, vegetables, and beans as healthful foods. Tofu was mentioned three times, and the phrase "use plant foods as the foundation of your meals" was included. The 2000 version warned against saturated fats and also stated, "Foods that are high in cholesterol also tend to raise blood cholesterol."[13]

The 2005 guide was actually quite a breakthrough in that it substantially increased the amount of fruits and vegetables a person should eat every day to 4–1/2 cups, up from 2–1/2 cups. It also called for people to make half the grain foods they eat whole grains—no doubt an answer to the "carbophobia" that had swept the nation in preceding years.

The 2005 guide stayed the course in continuing to advise people to eat no more than 300 milligrams of cholesterol per day.[14] Of course, the human body needs exactly zero dietary cholesterol. The numeric limit no doubt exists simply so that people can continue to eat foods of animal origin, the only foods that actually contain cholesterol. Plants, as has been mentioned (reason #33), are free of cholesterol.

Interestingly, 300 milligrams do not go very far. A person handily uses up his or her entire USDA-designated daily quota for cholesterol after consuming two small eggs. How many would believe that the government actually advises people to completely curtail meat and dairy intake after that limit has been reached?

91 Listeria

THE PATHOGEN THAT CAME IN FROM THE COLD

"Pregnant women and immunosuppressed persons may choose to avoid foods associated with deli counters or thoroughly reheat cold cuts before eating."—fact sheet, Centers for Disease Control[1]

A relatively rare but particularly deadly pathogen has gained a foothold in ready-to-eat foods almost exclusively of animal origin. Soft cheeses, smoked seafood, meat pâtés, and cold cuts are the foods that are typically contaminated by it.

Despite amounting to only one percent of all foodborne outbreaks, the bacterium *Listeria monocytogenes* is the cause of 30 percent of all foodborne fatalities.[2] Listeriosis sickens 2,500 Americans every year. A fifth of them die from its effects.[3] These are the official statistics. Tracing deaths to the bug is difficult because of the two-week incubation period following an infection.[4]

L. monocytogenes is common in nature and is normally harmless to most people. When it comes to food, however, it is considered to be an adulterant. No amount of it is acceptable in any edible end product.[5] Yet when tests at meat processing plants are found positive for it, federal inspectors have tended to give plant personnel numerous chances to rectify the situation, to disastrous ends. In recent years, several recalls of tens of millions of pounds of meat were ordered because of *L. monocytogenes*. In each case, fatalities occurred.

Modern processing and preservation methods have provided the perfect conditions for *L. monocytogenes* to grow. Drains, air-conditioning units, and unreachable grooves in equipment are the places this bug tends to colonize. Once a processing plant is infected, eradicating it becomes nearly impossible. Hot dog producers have had to adopt the sterile, air-filtered conditions of the computer chip plant.[6] If the pathogen infects the meat, it tends to survive in-plant antibacterial saline and acid treatments as well as refrigeration—conditions that not only wipe out the bug's bacterial competitors[7] but also allow surviving bacteria to become more virulent.[8] "If you don't kill it, you make it stronger," explains Randall Phebus, a Kansas State University microbiologist.[9] In the future, more powerful strains could start affecting people with normal immune systems. In the meantime, when *L. monocytogenes* does emerge and survive, it eventually gets put away with its host—possibly for a long shelf life—in impermeable packaging, a mini-womb of safety where it can continue to multiply until purchased by the consumer.

A failure to communicate

In 2003, nearly five years after two particularly ugly outbreaks and recalls involving a total of 65 million pounds of hot dogs and luncheon meats (Thorn Apple, Arkansas, and Bil Mar, Michigan),[10] the USDA was still struggling to institute meaningful in-plant testing for *L. monocytogenes*.[11] In glaring detail, this pathogen has laid bare the entrenched dissemblance of American food safety. USDA's lack of regulatory muscle, the gray areas of accountability, and the furtive disingenuousness that permeates the process of meat-plant microbial testing are now seen as nothing short of scandalous.[12]

Heat your cold cuts

L. monocytogenes is particularly dangerous to pregnant women and their fetuses. Infection passed on to a fetus can result in premature delivery, miscarriage, stillbirth, or serious health problems for the child later in life.[13] The very young and the very old, as well as those with compromised immune systems, are susceptible to meningitis and encephalitis. Those in jeopardy are advised to heat the risky foods to 170 degrees, something that is surely counterintuitive in the case of soft cheeses and cold cuts. Warning labels on packages could add vital reinforcement to this precautionary advice, but the government does not require them.[14]

An overhaul of the U.S. inspection system (HACCP), which began in 1998, has inadvertently served to widen the chasm between pathogen and pathogen control at processing plants. While most meat plants do a superior, or at least a good, job at keeping their products free of contàmination, according to food-safety expert David M. Theno of Jack in the Box, about 20 percent can still be characterized as not clean at all.[15]

This is all getting to sound like a whole lot like Russian roulette.

92 Cyanide and dynamite

REEFS ON THE EDGE

"When times are really bad, when we can't even afford to buy rice, we use cyanide."—coral reef fisherman, the Philippines[1]

Coral reefs are resplendent concentrations of biological diversity that occupy but one quarter of one percent of the ocean, yet provide habitat for more than 25 percent of the world's known marine species.[2] Their richness is both their virtue and their vulnerability. According to Reef Check, a monumental five–year survey completed in 2002, these rainforests of the sea have been damaged more in the twenty years leading up to that year than in the prior one thousand years.[3] Ninety-five percent of the thousand-plus coral reefs researchers examined had been adversely affected by humans, primarily because of overfishing. Only one reef studied was still considered pristine.

A two–year British study of reefs near 13 Fijian islands found that even subsistence fishing, using traditional implements such as spears, hooks, and lines, could have a significant impact on coral reefs.[4] Twenty-five percent had been destroyed.[5] Reefs in the Caribbean[6] and Indonesia,[7] in particular, have been so ravaged that it is doubtful they can be restored.

Coral reefs predominate in underdeveloped regions of the world where burgeoning populations of the poorest people live. The reefs provide food for a billion people in Asia alone and, all told, are the source of about one-quarter of the world's harvested fish.[8] But coral-reef fish are increasingly being sold all over the world. Foreign markets for specific kinds have grown dramatically in recent years—and local people are more than willing to take in the quick cash to supply them. Indeed, when a certain species becomes popular in some far-flung region of the world, even extremely remote reefs can be adversely affected. Clams and sea urchins in the Philippines have been victims of this scenario, as have some large predator reef fish such as grouper.[9]

Reef-fish madness

In Asia, weddings and certain business occasions demand nothing short of an ostentatious show of wealth. As has become the custom, the menu includes reef fish, ceremoniously displayed live in a tank before being served. The restaurateur may receive $200 a plate for such an affair and, as can be imagined, will do what it takes to orchestrate a seamless production. If the fish are endangered or harvested illegally, it's a detail sure to be overlooked. Indeed, down the line, out of sight, and many miles away, a poor fisherman will be cashing in too. He is likely to use cyanide to capture his prize, even though the technique is illegal in the Indo-Pacific country where he probably lives.

Cyanide fishing is highly destructive. First the diver stuns his target with a squirt bottle filled with a sea-water-and-poison solution. Immobilization of the fish, however, does not take place until after the fish has had a chance to burrow back into the reef. The diver must extract the fish with a destructive tool. The cyanide itself also destroys the corals. Eventually, the cumulative effect of many divers destroys the reefs. Meanwhile, many people look the other way from these little crimes. For that matter, the customer himself, a big Hong Kong trader perhaps, might even have illicitly supplied the cyanide to the diver.[10]

Other fishing methods also harm the reefs—dynamite most notably. After a concussive blast in this case, the dead will float to the surface to be scooped up.[11]

Anywhere between one and nine million species inhabit the world's coral reefs. Yet no more than about 4,000 of them, as well as 800 species of reef-building corals, have been catalogued.[12] Some experts tell us that if the decimation continues, a million species could eventually be gone forever.[13]

93 Seafood surprise

PLATTER OF POISONS

"I would not call a [seafood] inspection system with little inspection and virtually no enforcement an inspection system. I'd call it an outbreak waiting to happen."—Sen. Tom Harkin (D-IA), commenting after a major Government Accounting Office (GAO) report, 2001[1]

It's been said you could drink the water from a polluted lake over a lifetime and not absorb the chemical contamination you get from just one fish meal.[2] And this does not take into account the viruses, parasites, tiny worms, flu-begetting bacteria, and biotoxins that also attack fish as our waters increasingly become polluted. Take sushi, for example. It may carry illness-promoting wormy parasites that are in fact visible to the naked eye. About 2,000 severe, sometimes coma-inducing cases of sushi food poisoning are reported in Japan every year—the tip of the iceberg, the experts say.[3] Indeed, according to the Food and Agriculture Organization of the UN, 40 million people worldwide—mostly in eastern and southern Asia—are infected with parasitic trematode worms, thanks to the widespread practice in this region of eating raw fish.[4] The parasite causes victims to suffer abdominal pain, fever, diarrhea, loss of appetite, swollen joints, skin rashes, and chronically enlarged livers that are sore to the touch.[5]

Pollution on the half shell

Eating raw or insufficiently steamed clams and oysters landed from sewage-contaminated waters is surely risky behavior. One oyster will filter 1,500 times its body volume in water per hour. It should not be surprising that approximately 100,000 annual cases of food poisoning in the United States can be linked to filter-feeding bivalves.[6] According to the FAO/UN, consumption of toxin-infused shellfish can cause diarrhea, vomiting, memory loss, paralysis, and death.[7]

Vibrio, another bug linked to shellfish, causes an estimated 8,000 illnesses and 60 U.S. deaths per year, according to the Centers for Disease Control.[8] Nearly all deaths associated with these bacteria, however, occur because of *Vibrio vulnificus*. This pathogen, which is in the same family as those that cause cholera, kills half that it infects. Immunocompromised victims, in particular, are susceptible to blood poisoning, blistering skin lesions, and septic shock.[9] Amputations may be necessary to save a person's life.[10]

All over the world, pollutants from human activities on land are running off into coastal waters and causing a historic rise in so-called harmful algae blooms (HABs). It is during these events that phytoplankton produce biotoxins that, once eaten by other aquatic organisms, find their way into the marine food web. Several of the illnesses that get passed along to humans in this way via seafood include amnesiac shellfish poisoning (domoic acid), diarrhetic shellfish poisoning, ciguatera fish poisoning, neurotoxic shellfish poisoning, and paralytic shellfish poisoning, the last derived from a toxin considered a thousand times more toxic than cyanide.[11] Flu-like symptoms are the typical result of exposure. However, neurological disorders such as memory loss, numbness, paralysis, disorientation, and brain damage can also occur. Some poisonings will cause death.

Doom, we presume

Scombroid poisoning, caused by histamine toxin associated with rotting tuna, mackerel, marlin, and mahimahi, causes victims to be suddenly overcome with abdominal pain, swollen throat and tongue, and disorientation—even a sense of impending doom.[12] Cooking and freezing have zero effect on this food toxin.[13]

Finally, no discussion of seafood would be complete without mention of fugu, the puffer fish that must be prepared by a trained, licensed chef. A slip of the knife can unleash bilious poisons onto edible parts, killing a diner within minutes. People actually eat it for the thrill of cheating death.

Oversight next to nil

Seafood is responsible for 15 percent of all the food-poisoning outbreaks in the United States—a lopsided proportion considering that Americans eat six times as much poultry and eight times as much meat.[14] The General Accounting Office reports that the nation's seafood companies are only in compliance with current food-safety rules 60 percent of the time.[15] Furthermore, the FDA does not force fishing vessels into compliance at all.[16] Fish processing plants are inspected by the government only once a year,[17] and half the time inspectors merely check a company's paperwork.[18] The United States imports 80 percent[19] of its seafood, yet in 1999 the FDA tested less than one percent of it.[20]

94 Veal calves

INCARCERATION OF THE INNOCENT

"On profit-driven factory farms, veal calves are confined to dark wooden crates so small that they are prevented from lying down or scratching themselves. These creatures feel; they know pain. They suffer pain just as we humans suffer pain."—Sen. Robert Byrd (D-WV), Senate floor, July 9, 2001

In every glass of cows' milk there lurks a shameful secret: the plight of the veal calf confined for life in a crate. A cow cannot give milk unless she regularly gives birth. But only those males who grow to serve as breeding bulls are of any use to the dairy industry. The excess male offspring have to go somewhere. The majority are siphoned off to the beef industry.[1] Many, however, become veal—either bob, red, or fancy. Most

U.S. veal is of the last sort, the fancy, "special-fed" type,[2] otherwise considered the end product of a horrendously cruel farming practice. A calf raised for this type of veal lives out a short life in a box just large enough for him to fit. In America, nearly a million calves annually are raised using these practices.[3] Because of their cruelty, such methods have been illegal in England since 1990.

Extreme cradle robbing

At only a day or two old, with umbilical cord still attached, the calf will be pried from his mother and presented at auction for "special-fed" veal production. In no time, he will be tethered at the neck and put in solitary in darkness in a stall. Though his body is full of energy and life, this vulnerable newborn will, against every inclination, be forced into inactivity, and worse, have no ability to groom, scratch, or even turn around until the day he is slaughtered, about 16 weeks later. No shifting in position will ever give him comfort.[4] As chattel, he won't even be able to touch or socialize with nearby calves who share his fate. If he had been allowed to live on pasture, he would have suckled his mother 16 times per day.[5] Pent up, he is presented with a witches' brew of milk replacer, antibiotics, and chemicals devoid of iron and roughage,[6] contained in a bucket set before him for two twenty-minute intervals per day.[7] Despite its strangeness, he will suffer to drink from it, since he is otherwise deprived of water. This concoction, combined with forced inactivity, transforms his flesh into a white, pasty, and anemic cut of misery.

Panoply of influences

By design, many of today's farmed animals are generally so unhealthy or sick by the time of slaughter that they may be ready to die anyway. By industry thinking, if an animal is healthy at the end of its life, it may mean the farmer spent too much money on him. In addition, most farmed animals are often very young when they die. If the geneticists have done their job, the animals grow to market size before they have had a chance to grow up. As far as the industry is concerned, fancy veal production fulfills these two criteria quite well.

Fancy veal, in fact, could only be a modern phenomenon—coming into being by way of a specific set of givens, each, it happens, now operating freely in the United States. You must have a sensitive market system at the ready to indulge the most perverse and bizarre culinary specifications of today's high-end chefs. You also need cheap inputs.

These arrive via a nationally subsidized dairy industry: male calves and by-product whey.[8] You need pharmaceuticals and a generally dispassionate inclination to make use of them.[9] Finally, you need a national policy that gives legal *carte blanche* to farmers, no matter how cruel their practices become.

95 Kandid kitchen

PATHOGENS WHERE WE EAT

"Are rubber gloves, forceps and sterilizing alcohol the kitchen implements of the future?"—Scott Williams, Farm Animal Reform Movement[1]

What does an environmental microbiologist find when he sleuths around your average household? Two hundred times the fecal bacteria on kitchen cutting boards as on toilet seats[2] and salmonella on 10 percent of hundreds of dishrags collected door to door.[3]

So how do these unsavory things get so near to the places we eat? Via mishandled raw meat and poultry, mostly, according to the sleuth himself, Dr. Charles Gerber, who says that the kitchen is the household portal for dangerous germs. Many people are ignorant of the hazards these foods pose. Moreover, the average homemaker tends to approach cleanup time in the kitchen with less rigor than in the bathroom.

Industry logic upended

The producers of meat, poultry, fish, and eggs claim that they don't have to provide pathogen-free food to their customers. They argue that bacteria are killed in the household when cooked.

Fair enough, perhaps. But what really happens down the line at the cooking end of things? How cautious is the average home cook? One researcher, Janet Anderson, from Utah State University, had a hunch that the industry's reliance on the good sense of home cooks would fall flat in the field. She set about designing an ingenious study, which gained funding from the USDA. Where similar investigations had relied on surveys of participants who tended to bend the truth about their own sanitary practices in the kitchen, Anderson's approach bared all with video-camera evidence obtained under strategically false pretenses.[4]

One hundred families from a middle class, well-educated Utah town became Anderson's willing subjects. They were given free ingredients to prepare meals they were later allowed to eat. Bonus checks of $50 per household were an added incentive. Each family had its choice of a salad and one of three entrées to prepare. The recipes were in fact designed to result in slip-ups. Participants were told that they were taking part in a market research study and nothing more. Food-safety was not mentioned. And, conveniently, the little white lie proved to be illustrative as each family prepared its meal without being self-conscious about cleanliness.

Ultimately, Anderson and her team were shocked by the results. They found 30 percent of the food preparers did not wash the lettuce, and many placed salad ingredients on raw-meat-contaminated counters. Thirty-five percent under-cooked the meat loaf, 42 percent under-cooked the chicken, and 17 percent under-cooked the fish.[5]

Menacing mamas

If these people represent prevailing practices in the kitchen, it seems that the babies of America are especially at risk. One woman dropped a bottle into a bowl of raw eggs and later rinsed it off with water, but no soap. Another woman, after handling raw chicken, readjusted her baby's bottle without first washing her hands.[6]

But the grownups were no less menacing to themselves. They neglected to wash their hands after handling potentially contaminated objects. They reused contaminated dishtowels. They stored leaky meat packages on upper refrigerator shelves.[7] And one subject took a taste of a marinade in which raw fish had been soaked.[8]

Twenty-five percent of reported outbreaks are the result of improper food handling in the home, according to a 2004 study published in the *Journal of the American Dietetic Association*.[9] An FDA telephone survey of nearly 4,500 adults across the nation found a significant number of the respondents admitting to lapses in proper sanitary practices in the kitchen. For instance, 15 percent did not indicate that they washed their hands after handling raw meat.[10]

The evidence seems clear. It's about time we start reexamining that industry assumption that allows contaminated meat to be sent to market. Or better yet, consumers should seriously consider taking foods of animal origin out of their kitchens altogether.

96 Necessarily soy

THE MOO-LESS WONDER

"In a face-off between a meat burger and an all-vegan soy burger, the soy version wins with only 8 percent of the fat, less than half the calories, and no cholesterol."—Keith Beaty, for the *Toronto Star*[1]

The soybean is poised to make cattle culture obsolete. Already, we have soy milk and soy burgers—not to mention every other soy-based mock meat under the sun. Soy even promises to nudge aside both slaughterhouse by-product and petroleum as industrial raw materials. The soybean is a key component in plastics, construction materials, glues (including epoxies), insulators, lubricants, inks, paints, solvents, disinfectants, cosmetics, crayons, candles, cement, rubbers, emulsifiers, and herbicides. As an antifoaming, dust-suppressing, wetting, dispersing, anti-static, and anti-spattering agent, soy is integral to many industrial processes as well. This legume is an astoundingly versatile, biodegradable, nontoxic, and renewable resource.

So who needs the cow?

At this point, if they weren't primarily grown from genetically engineered seeds and if human demand didn't force them into service as a feed for livestock (not their fault), soybeans would certainly be perfection incarnate.

A bean for the health of it

Calorie for calorie, soy is, of course, a powerhouse. Technically it is a complete protein—though low in methionine, an amino acid found in abundance in Brazil nuts. It provides vitamins such as folic acid, minerals, powerful antioxidants, and fiber—information not lost on the world's food producers. This amazing bean is now an ingredient in no less than 3,000 foods![2] In 2000, the American Heart Association (AHA) put soy protein on its list of foods most people should try to eat every day.[3] The best part about it, the AHA said, is its role as a substitute for cholesterol- and saturated fat-laden meat.[4]

Epidemiological studies have revealed that widespread soy consumption is associated with low rates of heart disease and certain cancers. Soy's phytoestrogens—its isoflavones—help reduce dysfunctional over-responsive signaling within human cells, thereby reducing cellular chaos that can lead to disease, according to government research.[5] Isoflavones are also believed to protect cells from the damage of oxidation.[6] Furthermore, clinical studies attest to the dramatic cholesterol- and blood pressure-lowering abilities of soy.[7] Canadian researchers found soy instrumental in lowering cholesterol, similar to the effects of cholesterol-lowering drugs.[8] There is some evidence that soy mitigates the symptoms of menopause, particularly hot flashes.[9] A study of post-menopausal women found soy protective against atherosclerosis (hardening of the arteries).[10] In addition, the bean is believed to boost bone density, lower the risk for prostate cancer, and brighten the skin.

Soy is a good food for diabetics, also. It has a very low glycemic index so is slow to set off an insulin response. Soy also reduces protein in the urine, forestalling kidney damage—a problem for diabetics.[11]

Soy prudence

In response to the burgeoning success of soy, industries that stand to lose to it have gone on the offensive. It's hardly a coincidence that studies have emerged linking soy to a host of health dangers. Much of the vitriol, however, has derived from dubious animal studies, hypothetical conditions, exaggerated claims, and plain hysteria.[12]

Of course even soy advocates concede that eating the bean in excess is unwise—something easy to do in Western cultures because of soy's current ubiquity as a processed-food filler and meat substitute. Others warn against taking isoflavones in supplement form.

Two-thirds of the world's population incorporates soy into their diets, and epidemiological observation suggests that this is a key to health.[13] But this chunk of humanity is generally eating soy in moderation and in "whole" form—that is as tofu, soy milk, edamame, tempeh, and miso[14]—not as soy energy bars, soy chips, soy cheeses, or soy sausages. Ultimately, the way to approach soy is the way one should approach aspirin—two tablets and it's a miracle cure, ten tablets and it can be a health hazard.

97 Contracts of betrayal

GROWER BE DAMNED

"It is difficult to get a man to understand something when his salary depends upon his not understanding it."—Upton Sinclair, author, *The Jungle*

Chicken meat is quite a bargain. But surely many wouldn't opt to purchase it if they knew that this dinnertime staple has placed a yoke of despair around America's poultry farmers. Indeed, today's poultry industry is a vertically integrated oligopoly, meaning that a few giant chicken companies control production from chick hatching to grocery store delivery. And those who raise the birds are on the low rungs of the pecking order.

For the 20 behemoths who control 85 percent of the nation's 36 billion pounds of chicken produced annually,[1] production costs are quite a bargain. The agreements they have forged with growers have allowed these poultry giants to reap extraordinary profits, especially as demand for poultry has grown feverishly over recent decades. The poultry-processor windfalls have been at the expense of the people who "grow out" the birds—those who are led to believe that contract growing can bring them the American Dream.

In exchange for literally hundreds of thousands of dollars in investment, today's contract grower just getting into the business will on average live on a paltry income in the neighborhood of $9,000 with no benefits until his or her debt is repaid. This can take 15 years.[2] And the debt burden can always be extended as nonnegotiable requirements to upgrade equipment are dictated to the farmer by the poultry titan.

Any talk of the endless debt, let alone hidden clauses that keep contract farmers from having any legal recourse, is missing from the rosy sales pitches when people get bilked into signing on the dotted line. As growers, these people find soon enough that the contract is really only there to serve the multibillion-dollar processor.

The bottom of the pecking order

Make no mistake. Today's growers are not independent business people—not the proud and self-sufficient individualists we picture living free on American's homesteads. For that matter, you can't call these people farmers. Serfs would be better, although even the lords of old had obligations to serfs.

The contract in this case is an agreement for grower subservience—by law, yes, but mostly by an implacable fiscal bondage. It dictates that the processor owns the birds and specifies the feed; the grower provides the farm hands and factory confinement hardware and is responsible for disposing of the mountains of resultant manure. With stricter federal rules about manure handling in the offing, this disposal factor is sure to become even more burdensome for the growers over the coming years. And though a grower never owns any animals when they are alive, the minute they die in his custody on the farm—which often amounts to piles of them at any one time—the carcasses become his responsibility.

Times are particularly tough on growers when chicken demand slows and the industry contracts. Processors are wont to inflict particularly onerous hardships on the growers to shake out the least efficient of them. At these times, growers are pitted against one another[3] with those on the bottom of the heap—like wounded gladiators—edged out. Suicides during these times are now legendary.

An offer not to be refused

True stories of betrayal are rife. Companies have been caught weight-cheating on carcasses and skimping on pay—even outright stealing from growers.[4] In one now-infamous case in 1995, ConAgra pulled out all the stops in crushing an Enterprise, Alabama "rebellion" made up of a band of 19 growers who refused to sign their contracts. The food giant not only punished the growers by sending them to the proverbial poor house, but it intimidated every sector of the society that might have come to the growers' aid—the state's agriculture department, the regulators, the local bankers and real estate agents, and the media.[5] ConAgra's ace in the hole was its heavy-handed threat to leave Enterprise, which would have reduced it pronto to a ghost town. The growers, each of them, were ruined.

98 Off the hook

FISHERS AS THEIR OWN REGULATORS

"As with virtually all species of marine fish, we had to nearly wipe them out before we managed them."—Ted Williams, columnist, *Fly Rod & Reel*[1]

People who eat wild fish might think that stocks are carefully guarded by world governments from unsustainable harvesting. As it stands, few fisheries are regulated at all.[2] And on the open seas, it's more or less a free-for-all.[3] Of the official oversight that does exist, it invariably tends to be tied to the industry itself—locked into a negligent state of denial, indulging fishers' short-term profit goals.[4]

A grand catastrophe

Arguably, the ultimate case of denial took place at the Grand Banks of Newfoundland, Canada, in the 1970s and 1980s. This fishery, which supported hundreds of small coastal communities for 400 years, was brought to collapse in just a couple of decades.[5] Destructive technologies, combined with irresponsible government policies, wiped away this rare Eden for marine life practically overnight. Canadian cod stocks collapsed, and now there is no hope in anyone's lifetime for their return.[6] But alas, not one lesson seems to have been learned. Even now, environmentalists are forced to use the courts to prohibit the very same types of boats that caused the damage—bottom trawlers in this case—from operating in Canadian waters.[7]

The name "Grand Banks" is invoked as the worst of all scenarios, yet New England and European cod likewise teeter on the brink. In the North Sea, which lies between the east coast of Great Britain and continental Europe, cod stocks have dwindled to one-tenth of 1970s levels.[8] Scientists warn that the entire North Atlantic basin could be reduced to nothing but jellyfish and plankton.[9] Nonetheless, spineless regulators dawdle and delay as they pander to fishing interests. In the meantime, scientists ratchet up their alarms and recommend a ban on fishing the hapless cod altogether.[10] The World Wide Fund for Nature (WWF) predicts that the world's cod stocks could be wiped out by 2020 because of overfishing, illegal catches, and oil exploration.[11]

Making quota and totaling the seabed

On the Pacific West Coast, U.S. regulators have, as per usual, also caved in to fishers' pleas, this time in the case of the rockfish. The result: nine species of the bottom dwellers are considered overfished, and these are just the ones that have been studied.[12] Some of the species will take half a century to rebuild, and this only if fishing is stopped altogether.[13]

These long-lived, slow-growing animals[14] have become the victims of the most misguided regulations anyone could dream up. Fishers have been restricted in the amount of any one species they can land, with no limits on incidental or collateral bycatch to obtain quotas.[15] Bycatch sea animals, with swim bladders already ruptured, are simply scraped overboard back into the water to avoid fines at port.[16] Twice as many of one species may become bycatch as fishers work to achieve a quota on another. Fishers explain that it isn't worth going out unless the quota is met.[17] A crisis intervention program, sponsored by the federal government, eventually decommissioned 260 rockfish trawlers in 2003 at $460,000 per boat.[18] It was a start, though an awfully expensive one for the taxpayers.

Forty-three percent of managed marine species in the United States are considered overfished[19]—a dismal assessment by any measure. In

2004, a federal commission on the oceans surprised environmentalists and others with a tough set of 250 recommendations to end further deterioration of coastal environments.[20] It described existing systems of fishing management as a "Byzantine patchwork" of agencies and councils incapable of reversing degradation. Furthermore, it recommended an end to America's 22–year-old refusal to join the UN Convention on the Law of the Sea, an international covenant of ocean stewardship.[21] Will the President and Congress heed its advice? An ocean of history says, "Probably not."

99 Foie gras

PÂTÉ WITHOUT PITY

"Tradition doesn't make something right."—John J. McEneny, assemblyman, New York, sponsor of legislation to outlaw foie gras production[1]

By some odd turn of history, humans saw fit to consider the diseased livers of ducks and geese a delicacy. But worse, they became hardened to the inherent cruelty required to produce this luxury food.

Fostering disease

Disease is normally something to be avoided on any farm. Yet with foie gras production, disease is itself the end product. Of course, illness does not end with the intended liver affliction, known as hepatic lipidosis. The birds are susceptible to infected feet, diarrhea, enteritis (bird plague), cardiac and renal failure, and liver hemorrhage.[2]

To make *pâté de foie gras,* which is French for "fatty liver spread," ducks and geese are systematically force-fed. Overfeeding causes the birds' livers to swell grotesquely to as much as twelve times their normal size.[3] To this end, captive birds are regularly dealt a pneumatic blast from an 8- to 10-inch steel pipe connected to a hydraulic machine[4] and loaded with a mix of grain, oil, salt, and water.[5] The instrument is rammed down the animals' throats two[6] to six[7] times per day. The mash is nutritionally deficient, by design—part of the formula that brings on the intended liver sickness.[8] Lack of calcium will result in multiple bone fractures for the birds at slaughter.[9]

Once a tiny niche market, today 20,000 tons of foie gras are produced worldwide.[10] One enterprising businessman in China is currently preparing to augment by a third the world's trade in foie gras made from goose livers.[11] All in all, prices have dropped for foie gras to the point where this cruel, fatty food has become just another ingredient in such commonplace dishes as pizza and quesadillas.[12]

Abuse by food

The daily torture goes like this: A worker grabs a bird—often lifting him off the ground by the neck—pulls on his head, and holds his feet in place. Once the tube is inserted, a lever is pressed. Four seconds of intense pressure later and the gorging "meal" is over.[13] Feed may bubble up, asphyxiating the bird. The traumatic feeding process injures birds' mouths, mangles their necks, damages their stomachs, and may rupture internal organs. If workers are not careful, they may cause birds' livers to burst.[14] Bloated, injured, or infirm from abuse, these animals—who are otherwise able to fly thousands of miles of migration routes—drag themselves along the ground in pathetic attempts to reach water spouts. When cage-bound, just before slaughter, they just sit still and pant. Barns are darkened to keep them calm.

Females are of no use in foie gras production, since they have less meaty livers than the males.[15] So they are disposed of, expediently. The animal advocacy organization People for the Ethical Treatment of Animals (PETA) has documented disposal techniques at a New York state foie gras farm. They observed sacks full of female ducklings being dunked in scalding water to extinguish them.[16]

Majestic birds imprisoned, denied, separated

In nature, these water fowl are able to fly at 60 miles per hour and dive 100 feet.[17] They take part in elaborate courtship rituals and engage in complex social behaviors. Imprisoned in pens or cages, the birds are denied exercise and freedom of flight. Moreover, they are separated from that which they take to most: water.

Foie gras producers defend their practices by saying that ducks and geese naturally gorge themselves before migratory flights. The truth is, at the time of slaughter, brutal factory conditions have brought each of these majestic creatures nearly to the point of death. None is able to eat on his own, due to mouth and esophageal damage. None is able to fly.

100 Longevity matters

TAKING OUR DIET FOR ALL IT'S WORTH

"We live in an unnatural world, which is compromising our health—compromising our vegetarian potential. But we can reclaim that potential with a few simple changes and live a long life in optimal health."—Michael Greger, M.D.[1]

This chapter is a synopsis of a lecture by Michael Greger, M.D., entitled "Optimum vegetarian nutrition: Surprising new research on omega-3's and vitamin B12." It can be viewed online at www.veganmd.org/talks.

The vegan diet—one comprised only of plants—is a healthier one. Of this we feel certain. Those of us who subscribe to this diet have an edge over those who do not because we consume more fruits and vegetables, more fiber and soy, and no animal protein. We are on the healthy side of things when it comes to most of the main risk factors for disease, such as high cholesterol, high blood pressure, and obesity. So we might find it surprising to have our diet challenged on the grounds of health, namely, to be asked whether vegans actually live longer than others, according to the clinical data. Common sense should tell anyone, yes!

Strangely, though, the little mortality data there is on vegans do not bear this out. According to Michael Greger, M.D., an expert in vegan nutrition, non-meat eaters can be subject to "counterbalancing forces" that work to cancel out some of their advantages, and vegans seem to be affected by these forces more than vegetarians. In any case, none of these drawbacks is intrinsic to the diet. They are a function of modern sanitation systems and today's food-processing methods. Thankfully, with simple remedies, vegans and vegetarians can easily regain all of their abundant advantages.

First with the bad news: In two modern studies[2] with Western subjects, it was found that the diet most conducive to human longevity is one with just a little bit of meat. What could that little bit of meat do for a person to provide longevity?

Vitamin B12, the homocysteine avenger

In his lecture on optimum vegetarian nutrition, Dr. Greger reminds us that we are all born with healthy arteries. But a cascading effect can cause them to harden. It is well established that meat eaters are highly vulnerable to these effects. But vegetarians and vegans are not always immune.

High levels of the neurotoxin homocysteine—a natural by-product of amino-acid metabolism—can lead to injured arteries as well as numerous other disorders. Those who eschew meat are generally protected from the ill effects of homocysteine because they tend to obtain plenty of vitamin B6 (pyridoxine), choline, and folate (vitamin B9) from their food. However, vegans in particular lack a fourth crucial homocysteine neutralizer, vitamin B12. This nutrient is readily found in animal-based foods, which vegans never eat. Otherwise, vitamin B12 is produced by bacteria, which people in modern societies tend to disinfect away. Consequently, homocysteine levels for vegans, which should be maintained around 10 µmol/l (micromoles per liter) or below, can clock in as high as 27 µmol/l. Vegetarians can reach levels as high as 17 µmol/l and meat eaters, 12 µmol/l.

Apparently, adequate intakes of vitamin B12 compensate for low folate levels for meat eaters.[3] However, folate still remains a problem for them, and barring adding copious amounts of oranges, beans, and dark leafy greens to their diets, or using supplements, meat eaters will tend to have some homocysteine problems.

Omega solution

Homocysteine-injured arteries are, unfortunately, prone to inflammation, which can lead to oxidized cholesterol, which in turn can lead to clotting, which can lead to cardiovascular disease and heart attack—the cascading effect. The meat diet is unalterably associated with oxidized cholesterol—the stage where, in fact, the vegan diet tends to naturally shine. There is no way around this degeneration outside of taking meat out of one's diet. Unfortunately, in the other stages, vegan and vegetarian diets can also fall short—but again, several dietary antidotes can easily rectify the problem.

An important factor for vegans and vegetarians at their problem stages, according to the Leon Diet Heart Trial, clearly seems to be imbalances between two polyunsaturated fats—the omega-6 and omega-3 fatty acids. (See reason #77.) Ratios of omega-6 to omega-3 should be no higher than about 4:1. Yet vegans average 15:1 and vegetarians average 10:1. Vegan kids, who tend to eat greater amounts of processed food, clocked in at a whopping 44:1, according to one study. Meat eaters average 7:1.

So meat eaters have the advantage when it comes to homocysteine levels and omega-6/omega-3 ratios. Thankfully, according to Dr. Greger, a few simple adjustments are all that are needed for non-meat-eaters—and vegans in particular—to get their numbers in line to "reclaim their advantages, and even surpass them beyond their highest expectations." And none involves eating animal foods—even fish.

First, vegans and vegetarians should eat two tablespoons of ground flax seeds every day to obtain a healthy omega-6/omega-3 balance. (Baking does not destroy the seeds' healthful effects; flax oil, on the other hand, should never be heated.)

In addition, to offset high homocysteine levels, vegans and vegetarians should take a total of 2,000 micrograms of vitamin B12 per week via supplementation or through fortified foods. The supplement, which in itself is vegan, is available as a chewable tablet or encased in veggie caps.

These simple habits can surely provide a healthier, less toxic, more environmentally sound, and humane alternative to diets that include animal-based foods. With these few measures, a modern-world plant eater, who eats a varied, whole-foods diet consisting of regular intakes of beans, greens, nuts, whole grains, calcium, water, and vitamin D (via supplementation or from sunshine), should have exceptional and abundant, long-lived health, better than any meat eater could ever hope for.

101 Planet lifeboat

THE EARTH'S INEXORABLE VERDICT

"According to a panel of experts, dwindling water, land, and oil, combined with population growth, will finally force Americans to adopt a healthy diet. Unfortunately, it will take another 50 years to happen.... Why wait until what is already clearly a problem reaches crisis proportions? Other than satisfying an addiction, meat has no benefits. Let's cut it out or cut it down."
—Henry Spira, letters, *The New York Times*, Feb. 25, 1995[1]

Have humans become the environmental victims of our own success? If so, the condition is nothing new. A look into history—and even the archeological record—shows us that human industry has gotten us into trouble before. For example, to fulfill a compulsion to erect iconic statues, the people of Easter Island perished 500 years ago after cutting down the last tree from the forests that sustained them.[2] Indeed, it seems that as long as technology allows it, people tend to deplete or pollute available stores of water, energy, land, forests, biodiversity, and marine and terrestrial wildlife until something forces them to stop. We humans have to work on this.

The so-called "ecological footprint" is venturing into unsustainable terrain—this time on a global scale. In the rich world, it's human greed; in the poor one, human privation. Whatever the motivator, earth's life supports are breaking down. If we want to buy ourselves some time—not to mention ensure our long-term survival—vegetarianism is a good place to begin. If we do not choose this path, earth's broken-down support systems will impose themselves on us whether we like it or not. Of this we can be certain.

Second to one

In 1999, researchers from the Union of Concerned Scientists examined various consumer activities and paired them off with their environmental repercussions. They concluded that the consumer choice to eat beef and poultry is the second most environmentally detrimental human activity after driving a car.[3] The researchers came to the conclusion after inserting mountains of government statistics into computer models they devised. They later commented that they were surprised that just two consumer items could have so much effect on the planet.

Spaceship vegetarian

Researchers at Cornell University were, in a way, also forced to "think plants" when they took on the task of developing menus for long-term space travel. Assuring prolonged and sustainable life support for the astronauts was the task at hand. Long-distance space travelers would not only have to prepare their own food; they would have to grow it first.[4] In such lifeboat conditions, meat and dairy would have to be off the menu. Indeed, it was clear to the scientists that unlike on earth, where people could run a natural-resource deficit with the planet for extended periods, astronauts would have to live in balance with limited on-board inputs right from the start. Spaceship earth could do with the same kind of reasoning.

Global warming's unsung sibling

In 2001, the journal *Science* published a study by a team of eight preeminent environmental scientists who compared the magnitude of agriculture's near-term environmental impacts with those prognosticated for climate change. The authors asserted that current trends presage agriculture becoming the overwhelming cause of damaging nitrogen runoff, species extinction, and loss of wild environments.[5] These, they said, will inevitably combine to vie with global warming as a distinct planetary threat. The scientists worried that the world's concern about global warming, although legitimate, seems to have overshadowed any discussion about the dire consequences of agricultural expansion.

In their report, the scientists projected that an additional 18 percent more farmland was going to have to be painfully eked out of the earth's crust by 2050 to supply food for an exploding world population bent on increasing its meat consumption.[6] This, they said, would dangerously encroach on the "ecosystem services" provided by areas of pristine wilderness. Beyond their intrinsic value, lead researcher David Tilman explained, untouched lands provide humans with purified water, soil fertility, insect pollination of crops, genetic diversity to supply medicine, timber, fiber, and actual physical barriers that meter the release of flood-controlling water into streams and rivers.[7] Forestalling our collective meat habits would go far to save wilderness areas, upon which we humans depend for our survival.

The reckoning

Six years earlier, another set of scientists made similar statements at a meeting of the American Association for the Advancement of Science. They predicted that while earth's resources dwindle and human population soars to twice its current numbers, a more plant-based diet is sure to work its way to America's dinner tables by mid-century. Oil wells, they argued, would be exhausted by 2015, 120 million acres of farmland would be taken out of production by 2055—due to erosion and urbanization—and using available water stores for irrigation would add to the eological stress.[8] Consequently, the percentage of animal-based foods in the American diet, they suggested, would shrink from 31 percent today to 15 percent in 2050.[9] The diet, which would be born of scarcity, would "actually be a healthier one," they acknowledged.

Surely the sooner we all start to enjoy this diet the better!

References

REASON #1

1. Testimony, USDA secretary Ann Veneman before the Senate Committee on Agriculture, Nutrition and Forestry, Sept. 26, 2001.
2. "Cattle ranches," *Modern Marvels*, The History Channel, May 8, 2002.
3. *Food and Agriculture Policy: Taking Stock for the New Century*, USDA, Washington DC, Sept. 2001, p. 16.
4. "Specialization shifting production into efficient but fewer operations," *Feedstuffs*, Mar. 6, 2000.
5. Joseph Weber, "Will agribusiness plow under the family farm?" *Business Week*, Oct. 10, 2000.

REASON #2

1. Brenda Davis and Vesanto Melina, *Becoming Vegan*, Book Publishing Company, Summertown, TN, 2000, p. 24.
2. Barbara Whitaker, "Medicare to run diet experiment for critically ill," *The New York Times*, Apr. 11, 2000, p. F7.
3. Quoted in Roberto Suro, "Hearts and minds," *The New York Times Magazine*, Dec. 29, 1991, p. 18.
4. *Heart Disease and Stroke Statistics—2004 Updates*, American Heart Assoc., Dallas, TX, 2003, p. 42.
5. Ibid, p. 3.
6. Ibid.
7. Lawrence K. Altman, "Heart disease can hit even the young, like Kile, at age 33," *The New York Times*, June 25, 2002.
8. Quoted in Neal D. Barnard, *The Power of Your Plate: A Plan for Better Living*, Book Publishing Company, Summertown, TN, 1995, p. 15.
9. Neal D. Barnard, "An interview with Colin Campbell, M.S., Ph.D.," *Good Medicine*, PCRM, Apr. 22, 1994, p. 11.
10. Geoffrey Cowley, "Healer of hearts," *Newsweek*, Mar. 16, 1998, p. 50.
11. Ibid, p. 53.

REASON #3

1. Peter S. Goodman, "An unsavory byproduct: Runoff and pollution," *Washington Post*, Aug. 1, 1999, p. A1.
2. "Pork Power," *60 Minutes*, CBS, Dec. 22, 1996.
3. *Animal Factories: Pollution and Health Threats to Rural Texas*, Consumers Union (Southwest Regional Office in Austin), May 2000, p. 9.
   Dale Dempsey and Laura A. Bischoff, "Megafarm has history of ignoring environmental laws," *Dayton Daily News*, Dec. 4, 2002.
4. "USDA, EPA, announce joint strategy for animal feeding operations," news release, EPA, Sept. 16, 1998.
5. "Animal waste pollution in America: An emerging national problem," report, Minority Staff of the U.S. Senate Committee on Agriculture, Nutrition and Forestry, Dec. 1997.
6. "The threat from behind: Manure happens," *The Economist*, Oct. 21. 2001, p. 35.
7. "Reducing water pollution from animal feeding operations," statement from the Office of Wastewater Management and the Office of Compliance (EPA) before the Subcommittee on Livestock, Dairy, and Poultry, and the Subcommittee on Forestry, Resource Conservation, and Research (Committee on Agriculture), U.S. House of Representatives, May 13, 1998.
8. Molly Ivins, "Home, home on the latrine," *Time* magazine, Aug. 6, 2001, p. 26.
9. Kevin O'Hanlon, "Massive manure fire burns into third month," AP, Jan. 28, 2005.
10. Robbin Marks and Rebecca Knuffke, "America's animal factories: How states fail to prevent pollution from livestock waste (Chapter 4: California)" NRDC, Dec. 1998.
11. Eric Whitney, "Can a hog farm bring home the bacon?" *High Country News*, Nov. 8, 1999.
12. Jackie Alan Giuliano, "Who's hogging the values," ENS, Jan. 17, 2000.
13. Judith Reitman, "Hog Heaven?" *Mother Jones*, Mar.–Apr. 2001.
14. Goodman, "An unsavory byproduct: Runoff and pollution."
15. Raf Casert, "Beer and manure," AP, Mar. 11, 2002.
16. Amy Lorientzen, "Environmentalists sue government over factory farm rules," AP, Mar. 11, 2003.
17. Emily Gersema, "Farmers need more land to spread manure, USDA study says," AP, July 10, 2003.
18. Katharine Q. Seelye, "U.S. report faults efforts to track water pollution," *The New York Times*, May 27, 2003.
19. Tim Molloy, "Pollution rules targeting manure could force dairies to relocate," AP, June 28, 2004.
20. Felicity Barringer, "A search for pearls of wisdom in the matter of swine," *The New York Times*, July 7, 2004.
21. Tom Horton and Heather Dewar, "Feeding

the world, poisoning the planet," *Baltimore Sun*, Sept. 24, 2000.

REASON #4

1. "The catch about fish," *The Economist*, Mar. 19–25, 1994, p. 13.
2. "Scientists sound alarm about ocean perils," AP, Jan. 6, 1998.
3. William J. Broad and Andrew C. Revkin, "Overfishing imposes a heavy toll," *The New York Times*, July 29, 2003, p. F2.
4. "Special: Biodiversity for food and agriculture, fish and aquatic life," *SD Dimensions*, FAO/UN, Feb. 1998.
5. Elaine Lies, "Japanese love fish too much for fragile stocks," Reuters, Feb. 20, 2004.
6. "Special: Biodiversity."
7. Erica Bulman, "UN and Nature Fund blame subsidies for global fisheries crisis," AP, June 2, 1997.
8. "Fewer fish in the sea," CBS, May 14, 2003.
9. "Factoids: World fisheries in crisis," ENN, July 10, 1998.
10. "Special: Biodiversity."
11. Juliet Eilperin, "Management blamed for depletion of fish," *Washington Post*, June 27, 2004, p. A3.
12. "Factoids."
13. Carl Safina, "The world's imperiled fish," special edition, the oceans, *Scientific American Presents*, Fall 1998, p. 61.
14. "The promise of a blue revolution," *The Economist*, Aug. 9, 2003, p. 21.
15. "Episode: In pursuit of the giant bluefin," *Living Wild*, National Geographic Channel, June 19, 2004.
16. Otto Pohl, "Challenge to fishing: Keep the wrong species out of its huge nets," *The New York Times*, July 29, 2003.

REASON #5

1. Kucinich for President, Web site, www.kucinich.us/issues/rightsanimal.php (viewed Aug. 2, 2004).
2. David J. Wolfson, "Farm animals and the law," *Satya*, May 1997.
3. David J. Wolfson, *Beyond the Law: Agribusiness and the Systemic Abuse of Animals Raised for Food or Food Production*, Farm Sanctuary, Watkins Glen, NY, 1999, pp. 13–14.
4. E-mail correspondence with David J. Wolfson, Mar. 29, 2004.
5. Wolfson, *Beyond the Law*, p. 10.
6. "Pig producer sent to jail," *Sanctuary News*, Farm Sanctuary, Fall 1995, p. 6.
7. "Changing the rules of the game," *Farm Sanctuary News*, Fall 1997.
8. Wolfson, *Beyond the Law*, p. 48.
9. Melinda Fulmer, "Eco-labels on food called into question," *Los Angeles Times*, Aug. 26, 2001.
10. "Home, home on the...small patch of dirt: Do free-range chickens taste better?" *Consumer Reports*, Mar. 1998, p. 14.
11. Patrick Condon, "Better Business Bureau nixes egg ads," AP, May 10, 2004.
12. Philip Brasher, "McDonald's pushes slaughterhouses to improve animal treatment," AP, Sept. 24, 2000.
13. Quoted in Jennifer M. Fitzenberger, "Senate report spells out concerns on 'factory farming'," *The Sacramento Bee*, Nov. 24, 2004.
14. "The cost of posh nosh," BBC News, May 30, 2000.
15. *WTO: The Greatest Threat Facing Animal Protection Today*, CIWF (UK), 2002.

REASON #6

1. Quoted in Doris Stanley, "Steaming out the salmonella risk," *Agricultural Research* magazine, ARS/USDA, Oct. 1997.
2. Jean C. Buzby and Tanya Roberts, "ERS estimates U.S. foodborne disease costs," *Food Review*, ERS/USDA, May 17, 1996, pp. 37–42.
3. Peggy M. Foegeding, et al., "Foodborne pathogens: Risks and consequences," Council for Agricultural Science and Technology (CAST), Sept. 1994.
4. "What are the most common foodborne diseases?" CDC, Sept. 3, 2003.
5. Stacey A. Zawel, "Is imported produce safe to eat?" letters, *Washington Post*, Aug. 5, 1997, p. Z4.
6. "Foodborne illnesses more common than previously estimated," Bloomberg, Sept. 17, 1999.
7. "CDC data provides the most complete estimate on foodborne disease in the United States," CDC, Sept. 16, 1999.
8. "Foodborne diseases are on the rise in Europe," news release, WHO, Feb. 25, 2002.
9. Patricia Reaney, "Study: Deaths from food poisoning underestimated," Reuters, Feb. 14, 2003.
10. Jane E. Brody, "A world of food choices, and a world of infectious organisms," *The New York Times*, Jan. 30, 2001, p. F5.
11. Marian Burros, "Health concerns mounting over bacteria in chicken," *The New York Times*, Oct. 20, 1997, p. A1.
12. "Bugged by disease," *The Economist*, Mar 19, 1998.
13. "Of birds and bacteria," *Consumer Reports*, Jan. 2003.
14. Sharon Durham, " 'Free-range' is not more free of salmonella," ARS/USDA, Sept. 20, 2004.
15. Emily Green, "The bug that ate the burger: E. coli's twisted tale of science in the courtroom and politics in the lab," *Los Angeles Times*, June 6, 2001.

16. Sarah Helm, "Americans play chicken with food hygiene rules," *The Independent*, Apr. 3, 1997.
17. "Is our food fit to eat?" *48 Hours*, CBS, Feb. 9, 1994.
18. Jane E. Brody, "A world of food choices, and a world of infectious organisms," *The New York Times*, Jan. 30, 2001, p. F5.

REASON #7

1. Matthew Scully, "Don't tolerate the cruelty on hog farms," *St. Petersburg Times*, Sept. 29, 2002.
2. "U.S. pig births decline 2.3 percent, signaling reduced pork supplies," Bloomberg, Nov. 27, 2002.
3. Bernard E. Rollin, *Farm Animal Welfare: Social, Bioethical, and Research Issues*, Iowa State University Press, 1995, p. 93.
4. "Pig births decline."
   "Pig in hell," *Viva!LIFE* (UK), Summer 2001, p. 2.
5. Gene Bauston, *Battered Birds, Crated Herds: How We Treat the Animals We Eat*, Farm Sanctuary, Watkins Glen, NY, 1996, p. 19.
6. "Pig in hell."
7. Richard A. Battaglia, *Handbook of Livestock Management Techniques*, 2nd ed., Prentice Hall, Upper Saddle River, NJ, 1998, p. 212.
8. Scully, "Don't tolerate the cruelty on hog farms."
9. Marc Kaufman, "In pig farming, growing concern," *Washington Post*, June 18, 2001, p. A7.
10. "Facts about hogs," Humane Farming Assoc., www.inmotionmagazine.com/pig.html, no date (viewed May 22, 2003).
11. Battaglia, *Handbook*, p. 217.
12. "Pig in hell."
13. "U.S. hog farms get bigger, but not better," *Farm Sanctuary News*, Spring 2002, p. 7.
14. Rollin, *Farm Animal Welfare*, p. 73.
15. Armelle Casau, "When pigs stress out," *The New York Times*, Oct. 7, 2003.
16. Quoted in Ibid.

REASON #8

1. Quoted in Ginger Otis, "A world without water," *The Village Voice*, Aug. 21–27, 2002, p. 62.
2. Otis, "A world without water," p. 63.
3. Danielle Nierenberg, "Factory farming in the developing world," *Worldwatch*, May–June 2003, p. 13.
4. "Institute warns of possible water shortage," AP, Apr. 20, 2004.
5. "The browning of America," *Newsweek*, Feb. 22, 1981, p.26.
6. "Institute warns of possible water shortage."
7. Jim Motavalli, "The case against meat," *E: The Environmental* magazine, Jan.–Feb. 2002, p. 29.
8. Mark W. Rosengrant, et al., "Global water outlook to 2025," IFPRI, 2001, p. 8.
9. Fen Montaigne, "Water pressure," *National Geographic*, Sept. 2002, p. 9.
10. "Growing water scarcity threatens global food and environmental security," news release, International Water Management Institute, Aug. 13, 2001.
11. Sandra Postel, "Troubled waters," *The Sciences*, Mar.–Apr. 2000, p. 19.
12. "Global water supply central issue at Stockholm conference," Reuters, Aug. 14, 2000.
13. "World meat demand to rise, animal disease fears—FAO," Reuters, Aug. 28, 2002.
14. Jim Suber, "Zinc man and iron woman save beef from vegetarian insults," *The Newton Kansan*, Mar. 6, 2003.
15. Alex Kirby, "Hungry world 'must eat less meat'," BBC News, Aug. 16, 2004.
16. "Shortage of fresh water predicted," AP, Aug. 27, 1998.
17. Mark Johnson, "Study urges water conservation on farms," AP, Jan. 10, 2005.
18. Michael Dorgan, "China: Running dry," Knight-Ridder/Tribune, July 11, 2000.
19. Cote D'Ivoire, "Expert warns of African water shortage crisis," Reuters, Feb. 9, 2000.
20. "Water shortages may make Africa more aid dependent," Reuters, Nov. 3, 2003.
21. Andrew Cawthorne, "Asian farmers are sucking the continent dry, says report," Reuters, Aug. 26, 2004.
22. Otis, "A world without water," p. 62.
23. Fred Pearce, "Thirsty meals that suck the world dry," *New Scientist*, Feb. 1, 1997.

REASON #9

1. Quoted in Neal D. Barnard, "An interview with Colin Campbell, M.S., Ph.D.," *Good Medicine*, PCRM, Apr. 22, 1994, p. 11.
2. E-mail correspondence with T. Colin Campbell, May 21, 2004.
3. Bob LeRoy, "China study indicts meat and fat," *Vegetarian Voice*, North American Vegetarian Society, Summer 1990, p. 3.
4. Jane E. Brody, "Huge study of diet indicts fat and meat," *The New York Times*, May 8, 1990, p. A1.
5. E-mail, Campbell.
6. Barnard, "An interview with Colin Campbell," p. 13.
7. Amy Norton, "Protein from red meat, dairy tied to heart risks," Reuters, Feb. 9, 2005.
8. Quoted in Ibid.
9. LeRoy, "China study indicts meat and fat," p. 4.
10. E-mail, Campbell.
11. T. Colin Campbell, "Chemical carcinogens: How safe are you?" *New Century Nutrition*, Dec. 1995.

12. Brody, "Huge study of diet indicts fat and meat."
13. Ibid.
14. Quoted in Ibid.
15. Brody, "Huge study of diet indicts fat and meat."
16. "China Study II: Switch to Western diet may bring Western-type diseases," *Cornell Chronicle*, June 28, 2001.
17. E-mail, Campbell.
18. Brody, "Huge study of diet indicts fat and meat."
19. Susan Lang, "CU—China study shows animal products aren't needed to improve growth," *Cornell Chronicle*, June 26, 1997.

REASON #10

1. Tony Horwitz, "These six growth jobs are dull, dead-end, sometimes dangerous," *The Wall Street Journal*, Dec. 1, 1994.
2. Eric Weddle, "Day job: Slaughterhouse human-resources director," *The New Yorker*, Apr. 24, 2000, p. 146.
3. Peter Coy, "Hiring illegals: The risks grow," *Business Week*, May 13, 2002, p. 94.
4. Laurie P. Cohen, "Free ride: With help from INS, U.S. meatpacker taps Mexican work force," *The Wall Street Journal*, Oct. 15, 1998, p. A1.
5. Bill Poovey, "Prosecutors: 'Corporate greed' behind conspiracy to smuggle illegal workers for Tyson plants," AP, Feb. 6, 2003.
6. Charlie LeDuff, "At the slaughterhouse, some things never die," *The New York Times*, June 16, 2000, p. A1.
7. Eric Schlosser, "The chain never stops," *Mother Jones*, July–Aug. 2001.
8. Eric Schlosser, "Meat and potatoes: Where the beef has been," *Rolling Stone*, Nov. 26, 1998, p. 79.
9. "Trouble on the line," *Consumer Reports*, Mar. 1998, p. 16.
10. Bureau of Labor Statistics, Dec. 2002.
11. Schlosser, "The chain never stops."
12. Bureau of Labor Statistics.
13. Brian Halweil, "The bioterror in your burger," Worldwatch Institute, Nov. 6, 2001.
14. Joby Warrick, "They die piece by piece," *Washington Post*, Apr. 10, 2001, p. A1.
15. "Livestock confinement dust and gases," National Agricultural Safety Database, Apr. 2002.
16. Rebecca Clarren, "Got guilt?" *Salon* magazine, Aug. 27, 2004.
17. Ibid.
18. Sheldon Rampton and John Stauber, *Mad Cow USA: Could the Nightmare Happen Here?*, Common Courage Press, Monroe, Maine, p. 70.
19. "Fishing at sea claims more than 70 lives a day, FAO says," FAO/UN, news release, Jan. 25, 2001.
20. "Fishing labeled 'most dangerous job'," BBC News, Jan. 25, 2001.
21. Peter Morris, "Vessel operations under 'flags of convenience' and national security implications," statement before the House Armed Services Committee, special oversight panel on the Merchant Marine, June 13, 2002.

REASON #11

1. *Living Planet Report: 2002*, WWF, www.panda.org.
2. United Nations projections, 2002.
3. Lester R. Brown, "Time for Plan B," *New York Press*, Sept. 10, 2003.
4. "The world's food: Feast or famine?" *The Economist*, Sept. 1, 2001, p. 40.
5. "Diverse diets, with meat and milk, endanger world food supply," Hearst, Mar. 8, 1997.
6. Glen Martin, "And baby makes 6 billion: As population hits milestone, scientists worry most about consumerism," *San Francisco Chronicle*, Oct. 11, 1999, p. A1.
7. Curt Anderson, "Study: World faces food shortfall," AP, Dec. 11, 1997.
8. "Undernourishment around the world," *The State of Food Insecurity in the World 2002*, FAO/UN, 2002.
9. Sue Leeman, "One-third of world's children [in the developing world] malnourished," AP, Mar. 13, 2002.
10. "U.S. could feed 800 million people with grain that livestock eat, Cornell ecologist advises animal scientists," *Science Daily*, Aug. 12, 1997.

REASON #12

1. Marc Bekoff, "Beastly passions," *New Scientist*, Apr. 2000, p. 32.
2. Rim Radford, "Do animals think?" *The Guardian*, Dec. 18, 2002.
3. Douglas Foster, "Open the labs and set them free," *Los Angeles Times*, June 2, 2002.
   Nicholas Wade, "A course in evolution, taught by chimps," *The New York Times*, Nov. 25, 2003.
4. Sharon Begley, "Clues to personality abound in sea life," *The Wall Street Journal*, Oct. 10, 2003.
5. Henry Fountain, "Snail-sustainable farming," *The New York Times*, Dec. 9, 2003.
6. David Attenborough, "The life of mammals," PBS, Nov. 27, 2003.
7. Sharon Begley, "Cultures of animals may provide insights into human behavior," *The Wall Street Journal*, May 7, 2004, p. B1.
8. Mary Carmichael, "Animal emotions," *Newsweek*, July 21, 2003.

9. Bekoff, "Beastly passions."
"Gorillas hold 'wake' for group's leader," CNN, Dec. 8, 2004.
10. Jeremy Rifkin, "Our fellow creatures have feeling—so we should give them rights too," *The Guardian*, Aug. 16, 2003.
11. Bekoff, "Beastly passions."
12. Carmichael, "Animal emotions."
13. Bekoff, "Beastly passions."
14. "Quoth the raven," *The Economist*, May 15, 2004, p. 77.
15. Quoted in Claudia Dreifus, "A conversation with Callum Roberts," *The New York Times*, Mar. 5, 2002.
16. Denise Flaim, "Keeping chickens without raising a squawk," *San Francisco Chronicle*, July 26, 2003, p. E9.
17. Alex Cukan, "Chickens more than just dumb clucks," UPI, Sept. 20, 2002.
18. Bernard E. Rollin, *Farm Animal Welfare: Social Bioethical, and Research Issues*, Iowa State University Press, 1995, p. 118.
19. Roger Highfield, "He's smarter than you think," *The Electronic Telegraph*, May 31, 1997.
20. Rifkin, "Our fellow creatures have feeling—so we should give them rights too."
21. Marcia Slackman, "How safe is the beef supply? The other secret—confinement practices," *San Francisco Chronicle*, Jan. 15, 2004.
22. Radford, "Do animals think?"
23. Helen Briggs, "Sweet music for milking," BBC News, May 26, 2003.
24. Keay Davidson, "Humans, animals share more DNA than previously thought: Santa Cruz study shows common 'junk' fragments," *San Francisco Chronicle*, May 8, 2004.
25. "Evolution," PBS, WGBH Educational Foundation and Clear Blue Sky Productions, 2001.

REASON #13

1. Quoted in Tom Horton and Heather Dewar, "Producing more nitrogen, not knowing where it goes," *Baltimore Sun*, Sept. 25, 2000.
2. Tom Horton and Heather Dewar, "Feeding the world, poisoning the planet," *Baltimore Sun*, Sept. 24, 2000.
3. Emma Ross and Joseph B. Verrengia, "Obesity becoming major global problem," AP, May 8, 2004.
4. Richard Manning, "The oil we eat," *Harper's Magazine*, Feb. 2004.
5. Horton, "Producing more nitrogen."
6. Heather Dewar and Tom Horton, "Seeds of solution to nitrogen glut," *Baltimore Sun*, Sept. 28, 2000.
7. Manning, "The oil we eat."
8. Frank Langfitt and Heather Dewar, "China's prosperity turns seas toxic in a generation," *Baltimore Sun*, Sept. 27, 2000.
9. "Environmental body studies U.S. coast," AP, Feb. 13, 1998.
10. "Massive red tide off China's eastern coast," AP, May 18, 2004.
11. Cecil Hammond, "Animal waste and the environment," U. of Georgia College of Agricultural and Environmental Sciences, Oct. 1994.
12. Dewar, "Seeds of solution to nitrogen glut."
13. "Flux and sources of nutrients in the Mississippi-Atchafalaya River Basin," NOAA Coastal Ocean Program, U.S. Dept. of Commerce, May 1999.
14. Richard Cooke, "Developments in agricultural drainage in Illinois," extension talk, Corn/Soybean Classics, Dept. of Crop Sciences, U. of Illinois, 2003.
15. Dewar, "Seeds of solution to nitrogen glut."

REASON #14

1. Quoted in "Loss of domestic animal breeds alarming," news release, FAO/UN, Mar. 31, 2004.
2. "Farm Animal Genetic Resources," *SD Dimensions*, FAO/UN, Sustainable Development Dept., FAO/UN, Feb. 1998.

REASON #15

1. Quoted in "Hong Kong's chicken killers haunted by guilt," CNN, Feb. 6, 1998.
2. Beth Gardiner, "Army kills sheep in Britain: Military joins fight on disease," AP, Mar. 29, 2001.
3. Peter Hetherington, "Farm crisis 'worse than war'," *The Guardian*, Mar. 23, 2002.
4. "USDA monitoring spread of cattle disease in Asia," Reuters, Apr. 7, 2000.
5. "A horrible end for Malaysia's porkers," *The Economist*, Mar 25, 1999
6. Andy Wong, "Malaysian farmers slaughter pigs to quash virus," AP, Mar. 22, 1999.
7. Rone Tempest, "New lethal flu may stem from 'chicken Ebola'," *Los Angeles Times*, Dec. 14, 1997.
8. Lawrence K. Altman, "UN agency to urge vaccinations to halt avian flu," *The New York Times*, July 30, 2004.
9. "Avian flu epidemic threatens PA poultry industry," Reuters, June 7, 1997.
10. Ralph Frammolino, "Avian virus surfaces in egg industry," *Los Angeles Times*, Dec. 28, 2002.
11. Andrew C. Revkin, "Virus is killing thousands of salmon," *The New York Times*, Sept. 7, 2001, p. A10.
12. Sam Howe Verhovek, "Virus imperils Texas shrimp farms," *The New York Times*, June 14, 1995, p. A16.

REASON #16

1. Quoted in Maggie Fox, "Eat veggies and avoid cancer, experts say," Reuters, Oct. 2, 1997.
2. "Cancer and diet," *Newsweek*, Nov. 30, 1998, p. 63.
3. Karen Collins, *Nutrition Wise*, AICR, Aug. 2, 2004.
4. " 'Plant-based' diets fight cancer," Reuters, Oct. 13, 1997.
5. David Brown, "Panel: Up to 40 percent of cancer cases are preventable," *Washington Post*, Oct. 1, 1997, p. A12.
6. Fox, "Eat veggies and avoid cancer, experts say."
7. "Eat your veg. It could be the next best thing to giving up smoking," *The Observer*, Oct. 10, 2004.
8. Neal D. Barnard, "A commentary: Redrawing battle lines on cancer," *Washington Times*, Jan. 4, 2000, p. A10.
9. "Eat your vegetables!" *Harvard Health Letter*, Nov. 1994, p. 8.
10. Jane E. Brody, "Chemicals in food? A panel of experts finds little danger," *The New York Times*, Feb. 16, 1996, p. A1.
11. Tara Meyer, "Experts: Food with pesticides safe," AP, Nov. 13, 1997.
12. "Charbroiled meat linked to breast cancer risk," Reuters, Apr. 5, 2000.
13. E.J. Mundell, "Meat preparation may cause cancer," Reuters, Oct. 17, 1997.
14. Seth Borenstein, "Cancer-causing list may expand," Knight-Ridder/Tribune, July 2001.
15. " 'Plant-based' diets fight cancer."
16. Patricia Reaney, "Why veggie diet may reduce heart disease, cancer," Reuters, June 27, 2001.

REASON #17

1. Richard A. Battaglia, *Handbook of Livestock Management Techniques*, 2nd ed., Prentice Hall, Upper Saddle River, NJ, 1998, p. 500.
2. "Use of animal drugs in livestock management," *NebGuide*, Cooperative Extension, Institute of Agriculture and Natural Resources, U. of Nebraska-Lincoln, June 1992.
3. Ibid.
4. "EU affirms ban on some beef imports," Bloomberg, Oct. 16, 2003.
5. "Use of animal drugs in livestock management."
6. "Tips on drug residue prevention in pork," fact sheet, Ministry of Agriculture and Food, Ontario, Canada, Oct. 1, 2001.
7. Janet Raloff, "Drugged waters," *Science News*, Mar. 21, 1998.
8. Beatrice Trum Hunter, "What is fed to our food animals?" *Consumers' Research* magazine, Dec. 1, 1996.
9. "Myths and realities about antibiotic resistance," fact sheet, Union of Concerned Scientists, www.ucsusa.org, no date (viewed Mar. 22, 2004).
10. Kevin L. Ropp, "Steroid substitutes: No-win situation for athletes," *FDA Consumer*, Dec. 1992.
11. "Livestock dealer pleads guilty," *FDA Consumer*, Dec. 1, 1994.
12. Beatrice Trum Hunter, "Reducing unwanted residues on food," *Consumers' Research*, Feb. 1, 1998.
13. Maria Hickey, "Small pork producers find ways to compete with big boys," Knight-Ridder/Tribune, June 27, 1997.

REASON #18

1. Quoted in Emma Ross, "Asia is the traditional cradle of influenza, although disease can originate anywhere," AP, Feb. 2, 2004.
2. Barry Gewen, " 'The Great Influenza' and 'Microbial Threats to Health': Virus alert," *The New York Times*, Mar. 14, 2004.
3. Lawrence K. Altman, "Spread of bird flu in Asia worries officials," *The New York Times*, Jan. 20, 2004.
4. "New clue why 1918 flu epidemic was deadliest," AP, Feb. 5, 2004.
5. Quoted in "WHO warns of dire flu pandemic," CNN, Nov. 25, 2004.
6. W. Graeme Laver, et al., "Disarming flu viruses," *Scientific American*, Jan. 1999, p. 79.
7. "Russian expert says flu epidemic may kill over one billion this year," MosNews, Oct. 28, 2004.
8. "Avian influenza: Wings across the world?" *The Economist*, Jan. 29, 2004.
9. Emma Ross, "Preliminary tests in Vietnam indicate pigs could be infected with bird flu," AP, Feb. 6, 2004.
10. Gretchen Reynolds, "The flu hunters," *The New York Times Magazine*, Nov. 7, 2004.
11. Vissuta Pothong, "Bird flu found in cats in Asia; Canada on alert," Reuters, Feb. 20, 2004.
12. "Mutation of bird flu virus into a new strain is possible, warn Japanese scientists," *Medical News Today* (East Sussex, UK), Apr. 18, 2004.
13. Michael Specter, "Nature's bioterrorist: Is there any way to prevent a deadly avian-flu pandemic," *The New Yorker*, Feb. 28, 2005, p. 52.
14. Lawrence K. Altman, "UN agency to urge vaccinations to halt avian flu," *The New York Times*, July 30, 2004.
15. Ibid.
16. Mai Tran, "Avian flu imperils livelihoods in Vietnam," *Los Angeles Times*, Feb. 7, 2004.

17. Merritt Clifton, "FAO/UN includes animal welfare considerations in plan to 'stamp out' deadly avian flu," *Animal People*, Apr. 2004, p. 1.
18. Maggie Fox, "Bird flu may be in Asia to stay, officials fear," Reuters, Aug. 26, 2004.
19. "Avian influenza: Wings across the world?"
20. Christina Toh Pantin, "Bird flu twice as deadly as last outbreak, doctor," Reuters, Feb. 8, 2004.
21. Michael Greger, "Bird flu: Meat eaters put the entire world at risk," www.veganMD .org, Feb. 26, 2004.
22. Debora MacKenzie, "Bird flu vaccination could lead to new strains," *New Scientist*, Mar. 24, 2004.
23. Gewen, " 'The Great Influenza' and 'Microbial Threats to Health .' "

REASON #19

1. Neal Barnard, *Food for Life: How the New Four Food Groups Can Save Your Life*, Three Rivers Press, New York, 1993, p. 130.
2. "Fiber helps diabetics control blood sugar, study says," Reuters, May 10, 2000.
3. Barnard, *Food for Life*, p. 129.
4. "High-fiber diet helps spare gallbladder," Reuters, Aug. 11, 2004.
5. Quoted in Neal D. Barnard, *The Power of Your Plate*, Book Publishing Company, Summertown, TN, 1995, p. 120.
6. "Fiber helps diabetics control blood sugar, study says."
7. "Fiber may reduce women's risk of heart disease," CNN, June 1, 1999.
8. "High fiber diet can cut cancer risk by 40 percent," Reuters, June 23, 2001.
9. "Studies revive fiber-colon cancer prevention link," AP, May 2, 2003.
10. T. Colin Campbell, "China report: Dietary fiber preventing cancer in China," *New Century Nutrition*, Nov. 1995.
11. T. Colin Campbell, keynote, conference, American Natural Hygiene Society, Hofstra U., Hempsead, NY, July 27, 1991.

REASON #20

1. Michael Pollan, "Power steer," *The New York Times Magazine*, Mar. 31, 2002.
2. Neill Smith, "Taking an integrated view of the biosphere: Grain production," Whole Systems Foundation, May 6, 2004.
3. Dale Allen Pfeiffer, *Eating Fossil Fuels*, Sherman Oaks, CA, Wilderness Publications, 2003.
4. M. Harris, *Cultural Anthropology*, 2nd ed. Harper & Row, 1987.
5. Walter Youngquist, "The post-petroleum paradigm," *Population and Environment*, Mar. 4, 1999.
6. David Pimentel, et al., "Impact of population growth on food supplies and environment," paper presented at the American Assoc. for the Advancement of Science annual meeting, Baltimore, Feb. 9, 1996.
7. Pfeiffer, *Eating Fossil Fuels*.
8. *The Rendering Industry: Economic Impact of Future Feeding Regulations*, Sparks Companies, McLean, VA, June 2001, p. 11.
9. "United States leads world meat stampede," news release, Worldwatch Institute, July 2, 1998.
10. "U.S. could feed 800 million people with grain that livestock eat, Cornell ecologist advises animal scientists," *Science Daily*, Aug. 12, 1997.
11. Richard Manning, "The oil we eat," *Harper's Magazine*, Feb. 2004.
12. Laurent Belsie, "How to feed the world," *The Christian Science Monitor*, Feb. 20, 2003.
13. Geoff McMaster, "How do we feed the world without destroying the environment," *Express News*, U. of Alberta, Oct. 14, 2003.
14. Manning, "The oil we eat."
15. Colin J. Campbell and Jean H. Laherrère, "The end of cheap oil," *Scientific American*, Mar. 1998.
16. David Pimentel and Marcia Pimentel, "The constraints governing ideal U.S. population size," Dept. of Entomology and Div. of Nutritional Sciences, Cornell U., Jan. 1995.
17. Lester R. Brown, "Food security deteriorating in the nineties: Grain prices more volatile," Worldwatch Institute, Mar. 6, 1997.
18. "World meat demand to rise animal disease fears, FAO," Reuters, Aug. 28, 2002.

REASON #21

1. Quoted in "Fewer fish in the sea," AP, May 14, 2003.
2. "The fishing industry: Heading for the final fillet," *The Economist*, Sept. 30, 2004.
3. William J. Broad and Andrew C. Revkin, "Overfishing imposes a heavy toll," *The New York Times*, July 29, 2003, p. F1.
4. Emma Duncan, "A whale of a tragedy," news release, WWF, June 13, 2003.
5. "Driftnet campaign," Greenpeace, fact sheet, www.greenpeacefoundation.com, no date (viewed Mar. 27, 2003).
6. Linda M.B. Paul, "High seas driftnetting: The plunder of the global commons," Earthtrust, May 1994.
7. "Earthtrust's 'DriftNetwork' program," fact sheet, Earthtrust, www.earthtrust.org /dnw.html, no date (viewed Feb. 2, 2004).
8. "Driftnet campaign."
9. Anouk Ride, "Dirty driftnet fishing continues in European waters," WWF, Oct. 16, 2002.

10. "Driftnets said decimating Mediterranean dolphins," Reuters, Nov. 21, 2002.
11. Ride, "Dirty driftnet fishing continues in European waters."
12. Otto Pohl, "Challenge to fishing: Keep the wrong species out of its huge nets," *The New York Times*, July 29, 2003, p. F3.
13. "Save the Albatross," campaign, www.birdlife.net, no date (viewed Apr. 18, 2004).
14. Kenneth R. Weiss, "Sea turtle is losing the race to poachers, fishing industry," *Los Angeles Times*, May 4, 2003.
15. "Trawlers, dredgers harm ocean floor, groups charge," AP, Dec. 16, 1998.
16. Emma Graham-Harrison, "Aggressive fishing threatens oceans—UN," Reuters, June 4, 2004.
17. Andrew C. Revken, "Deep peril for deep-sea corals," *The New York Times*, Sept. 19, 2000.
18. Quoted in Emma Graham-Harrison, "Aggressive fishing threatens oceans—UN," Reuters, June 4, 2004.
19. Michael Parfit, "Diminishing returns," *National Geographic*, Nov. 1995, pp. 15–17.

REASON #22

1. "McLibel verdict and the evidence: An analysis of the outcome and the judgment of the McLibel trial," www.McSpotlight.org, *circa* July 1997.
2. "Scientists question whether fast food is addictive," Reuters, Jan. 29, 2003.
3. David Barboza, "If you pitch it, they will eat," *The New York Times*, Aug. 3, 2003.
4. "McLibel verdict and the evidence."
5. Barboza, "If you pitch it."
6. Quoted in Annie Brown, "Operation burger kids," *Daily Record* (Scotland), Apr. 10, 2002.
7. Geraldine Sealey, "Whose fault is fat?" ABC News, Jan. 22, 2002.
8. *Broadcasting Bad Health: Why Food Marketing to Children Needs to be Controlled*, IACFO, (International Assoc. of Consumer Food Organizations, UK), 2003.
9. "Health groups warn: World's children at risk from junk food marketing," news release, The Food Commission (UK), July 29, 2003.
10. Erik Millstone and Tim Lang, *The Atlas of Food: Who Eats What, Where, and Why*, Earthscan, London, 2003.
11. Caroline E. Mayer, "KFC misled consumers on health benefits, FTC says," *Washington Post*, June 4, 2004.
12. "Court throws out 'Happy Cows' ad suit," *San Francisco Chronicle*, AP, Mar. 26, 2003.
13. Dominic Timms, "Food ads accused of endangering children's health," *The Guardian*, July 29, 2003.
14. J.M. Hirsch, "Obstacles in way of healthy school lunch," AP, Dec. 6, 2003.
15. Eric Schlosser, *Fast Food Nation*, Addison Houghton Mifflin, 2001 p. 128–29.
16. Ibid., p. 123.

REASON #23

1. John A. McDougall, *The McDougall Program: 12 Days to Dynamite Health*, Plume, New York, 1990, p. 7.
2. Norine Dworkin, "Heading off migraines, *Vegetarian Times*, Apr. 1998, p. 88.
3. Neal Barnard, *Foods That Fight Pain*, Three Rivers Press, New York, 1998, pp. 47–48.
4. "Ask the Mayo dietitian: Migraines and cheeses," Mayo Clinic/Health Oasis, Aug. 25, 1999.
5. Barnard, *Foods That Fight Pain*, p. 57.
6. John McKenzie, "Study links high cholesterol to memory loss," ABC News, Mar. 14, 2002.
7. "High-fat diets linked to poorer brain function," Reuters, Feb. 23, 2001.
8. "Studies say vegetables good against Alzheimer's," Reuters, Feb. 17, 2003.
9. "Can your diet affect Alzheimer's risk?" AP, Feb. 17, 2003.
10. "Soy, fish oil may protect against Alzheimer's, study," Reuters, Sept. 1, 2004.
11. Carol M. Coughlin, "A feast for the eyes," *Vegetarian Times*, Aug. 1997, p. 28.

REASON #24

1. Joel Fuhrman, *Fasting and Eating for Health*, St. Martin's Griffin, New York, 1998, p. 25.
2. "Diet and kidney stones," Food and Health Communications, Continuing Professional Education Courses, #2, www.foodandhealth.com, no date (viewed Feb. 18, 2003).
3. "Staying stone free," *Vegetarian Times*, Sept. 1996, p. 22.
4. Laura MacInnis, "Study links arthritis to women's heart attack risk," Reuters, Feb. 17, 2003.
5. John McDougall, et al., "Effects of a very low-fat vegan diet in subjects with rheumatoid arthritis," *Journal of Alternative and Complimentary Medicine*, Feb. 2002, pp. 71–75.
6. Neal Barnard, *Foods That Fight Pain*, Three Rivers Press, New York, 1998, p. 129.
7. Ibid., p. 127.
8. Ibid., pp. 82, 126–27, and 155.
9. Suzanne Rostler, "Low-fat vegetarian diet may reduce PMS symptoms," Reuters, Feb. 4, 2000.
10. Neal Barnard, *Food for Life: How the New Four Food Groups Can Save Your Life*, Three Rivers Press, New York, 1993, p. 96.

11. "Constipation tied to colon cancer," Reuters, June 16, 1998.
12. Susan Okie, "Colon susceptible to other woes besides cancer," *Washington Post*, Feb. 10, 1998, p. Z19.
13. Ibid.
14. Michael Greger, "Paratuberculosis and Crohn's disease: Got milk?" www.madcow.org, no date (viewed Jan. 2001).
15. Ibid.
16. Fuhrman, *Fasting and Eating for Health*, p. 164.
17. Patricia Reaney, "Study links animal bacteria to Crohn's disease," Reuters, Sept. 17, 2004.
Greger, "Paratuberculosis."
18. Quoted in Marian Jones, "The hard sell: Impotence rises from taboo to marketing tool," Fox News, June 10, 1999.
19. Neal D. Barnard, *The Power of Your Plate*, Book Publishing Company, Summertown, TN, 1995, p. 134.
20. "Impotence may be warning signal for heart disease," PRNewswire, news release, Loyola University Health System, May 31, 1998.

REASON #25

1. Quoted in Emily Green, "The bug that ate the burger: E. coli's twisted tale of science in the courtroom and politics in the lab," *Los Angeles Times*, June 6, 2001.
2. Green, "The bug that ate the burger."
3. Quoted in Green, "The bug that ate the burger."
4. Michael Pollan, "Power steer," *The New York Times Magazine*, Mar. 31, 2002.
5. "Meatpackers wage war on E. coli," AP, July 4, 2000.
6. "Escherichia coli O157:H7," fact sheet, CDC, Sept. 3, 2003.
7. "Half nation's feedlot cattle found to carry deadly E. coli," AP, Mar. 1, 2000.
8. Eric Schlosser, *Fast Food Nation*, Addison Houghton Mifflin, 2001, p. 203.
9. Ibid.
10. Green, "The bug that ate the burger."
11. Randy Fabi, "U.S. meat plants must do more against E. coli, says USDA," Reuters, Feb. 5, 2003.
12. "Meatpackers wage war on E. coli."
13. Julie Vorman, "USDA, meatpackers take aim at deadly bacteria," Reuters, Mar. 8, 1999.
14. Interview with Robert Tauxe, "Modern meat," draft transcript, PBS Online and WGBH/Frontline, Apr. 18, 2002.
15. Alex Pulaski, "Mad cow disease raises questions about hodgepodge that is hamburger," Newhouse News Service, Feb. 19, 2004.
16. "Pork Power," *60 Minutes*, CBS, Dec. 22, 1996.
17. Donovan Webster, "The stink about pork," *George* magazine, Apr. 1999, p. 110.
18. "Facts about pollution from livestock farms," fact sheet, NRDC, July 24, 2001.

REASON #26

1. Quoted in "CDC chief: Obesity top health threat," Reuters, Oct. 29, 2003.
2. "Fatter than other animals," survey, *The Economist*, Dec. 13, 2003, p. 5.
3. Danielle Knight, "World's overfed population rivals the number of hungry," Inter Press Service, Mar. 7, 2000.
4. Carolyn Lochhead, "It's fat city in America," *San Francisco Chronicle*, Apr. 8, 2002, p. B7.
5. Betsy McKay, "CDC concedes it overstated obesity-linked deaths," *The Wall Street Journal*, Jan. 18, 2005.
6. David Barboza, "If you pitch it, they will eat," *The New York Times*, Aug. 3, 2003.
7. "Report: Kids need obesity checkups," AP, Aug. 4, 2003.
8. "WHO: Some cancers due to fat, inactivity," AP, Apr. 6, 2001.
9. Susan Okie, "Study links excess weight to risk of heart failure," *Washington Post*, Aug. 1, 2002, p. A2.
10. "Weight linked to early heart attack," Reuters, Aug. 2, 2001.
11. Lindsey Tanner, "Study: Obesity ups risk of birth defects," AP, May 5, 2003.
12. "Diabetes, obesity on rise in United States," Reuters, Oct. 4, 2003.
13. "Can arginine save your toes?" *Time* magazine, Jan. 12, 2004, p. 78.
14. "Obesity may cancel health gains for older people," AP, May 26, 2002.
15. Fiona Symon, "Cost of obesity in the U.S. put at $75 billion a year," *Financial Times*, Jan. 22, 2004.
16. "CDC chief."
17. Michael Pollan, "When a crop becomes king," *The New York Times*, July 19, 2002.
18. Liz Else, "The true cost of meat," *The New Scientist*, Aug. 14, 2004.
19. Richard Manning, "The oil we eat," *Harper's Magazine*, Feb. 2004.
20. "The diet war: Low-fat vs. high protein with Dean Ornish," Live Events Transcript Archive, WebMD, July 16, 2002.
21. Jeanne Rattenbury, "All hail fiber!" *Vegetarian Times*, Apr. 1993, p. 50.
22. Michael Klaper, M.D., *A Diet for All Reasons*, video, Institute of Nutrition Education and Research, 1993.
23. Ridgely Ochs, "Obesity: Bad news, good news," *Los Angeles Times*, Aug. 6, 2001.

REASON #27

1. Transcript, M2 Communications, Ltd., Sept. 17, 2003.

2. "Forty percent of food land degraded, study finds," Reuters, May 22, 2000.
3. Anthony Boadle, "UN donors to fight loss of fertile soil," Reuters, Aug. 27, 2003.
4. "Food security and the environment," fact sheet, FAO/UN, Jan. 7, 2001.
5. "Meat production and consumption grow," *Vital Signs 2003*, Worldwatch Institute, pp. 30–31.
6. "Forty percent of food land degraded, study finds."
7. Ibid.
8. Bill McKibben, "A special moment in history," *The Atlantic Monthly*, May 1998.
9. Andrew C. Revkin, "UN predicts more harm to environment by 2032," *The New York Times*, May 23, 2002.
10. Jeremy Rifkin, *Beyond Beef: The Rise and Fall of the Cattle Culture*, Dutton, New York, 1992, p. 200.
11. Ed Ayres, "Will we still eat meat?" *Time* magazine, Nov. 8, 1999, p. 107.
12. "Food security and the environment," fact sheet, FAO/UN, Jan. 7, 2001.
13. Howard Lyman, *Mad Cowboy*, Scribner, New York, 1998, p. 145.
14. "U.S. soil erosion not as severe as thought," ENN, Aug. 23, 1999.
15. "U.S. could feed 800 million people with grain that livestock eat, Cornell ecologist advises animal scientists," news release, *Science News*, Cornell U., Aug. 7, 1997.
16. Alan Durning, "Eating green," *Nutrition Action Health Letter*, CSPI, Jan.–Feb. 1992, p. 6.
17. Lyman, *Mad Cowboy*, p. 145.
18. Jacques Leslie, "Running dry: Water scarcity," *Harper's Magazine*, Jul. 2000.
19. "Biting the silver bullet," *The Economist*, Mar. 25, 2000.
20. Anthony Boadle, "Poor nations agree on financing to stop deserts," Reuters, Sept. 3, 2003.

REASON #28

1. Emanuel Goldman, "Microbial risk assessment: Antibiotic abuse in animal agriculture, exacerbating drug resistance in human pathogens," *Human and Ecological Risk Assessment*, vol. 10, no. 1, 2004, p. 121.
2. "Of birds and bacteria," *Consumer Reports*, Dec. 11, 2002.
3. "Report raises concerns of human harm from antibiotics-fed chickens," AP, Dec. 9, 1999.
4. "Limit vital antibiotics in factory farm effluent," open letter to the EPA, Union of Concerned Scientists, Aug. 3, 2000.
5. Stuart B. Levy, "The challenge of antibiotic resistance," *Scientific American*, Mar. 1998, p. 47.
6. Rich Hayes, "Antibiotics overused in chickens," *Baltimore Sun*, July 23, 2001.
7. Levy, "The challenge of antibiotic resistance," p. 47.
8. "Of birds and bacteria."
9. Levy, "The challenge," p. 48.
10. Goldman, "Microbial risk assessment," pp. 129–130.
11. Levy, "The challenge of antibiotic resistance," p. 48.

REASON #29

1. Quoted in Anita Huslin, "Hope seen for poultry industry," *Washington Post*, July 25, 2003, p. B1.
2. "Farms are polluters of nation's waterways," AP, May 14, 1998.
3. "Managing nonpoint source pollution from agriculture," fact sheet (pointer no. 6): Polluted Runoff, EPA, Aug. 18, 2003.
4. "Nonpoint source pollution: The nation's largest water quality problem," fact sheet (pointer no. 1): Polluted Runoff, EPA, Aug. 18, 2003.
5. Tom Horton and Heather Dewar, "Feeding the world, poisoning the planet," *Baltimore Sun*, Sept. 24, 2000.
6. "Remarks by deputy secretary Rich Rominger," transcript, USDA, Nov. 15, 1999.
7. Ibid.
8. Tim Craig, "Bay cleanup criticized; oversight change urged," *Washington Post*, Aug. 22, 2003, p. B8.
9. "Suffocating the bay," editorial, *Washington Post*, Aug. 10, 2003.
10. David A. Fahrenthold, "Pennsylvania pollution muddies bay cleanup," *Washington Post*, May 16, 2004, p. A1.
11. Tom Horton, "Cleanup gets price tag," *Baltimore Sun*, Jan. 10, 2003.
12. Elizabeth Becker, "Big farms making a mess of U.S. waters, cities say," *The New York Times*, Feb. 10, 2002.
13. "Judge says EPA can set runoff limits for rivers," AP, Apr. 6, 2000.
14. Elliot Diringer, "In Central Valley, defiant dairies foul the water," *San Francisco Chronicle*, July 7, 1997, p. A1.

REASON #30

1. Karen Davis, *Prisoned Chickens, Poisoned Eggs*, Book Publishing Company, Summertown, TN, 1996, p. 99.
2. "What's bootiful about this?" *VivaLIFE*, (UK), Spring 2002, pp. 12–13.
3. Joy A. Mench and Paul B. Siegel, "Poultry," Animal Welfare Issues Compendium, South Dakota State U., http://ars.sdstate.edu/animaliss/poultry.html, Jul. 11, 2001.
4. Clare Druce and Bob Fromer, "Hidden suf-

fering," video, Farm Animal Welfare Network (UK), 1992.

5. "Leg problems in broilers: Disturbing new studies," *AgScene*, Spring 2000.
6. *Behind Closed Doors: The Truth About Chickens Bred for Meat*, Royal Society for the Prevention of Cruelty to Animals (RSPCA), UK, 2001, p. 13.
7. Jacky Turner, "The gene and the stable door," CIWF (UK), 2002, pp. 13–14.
8. Patrick Martins, "About a bird," *The New York Times*, Nov. 24, 2003.

REASON #31

1. Quoted in Rebecca James, "Terror on the farm: Agriculture experts fear farms will be the next targets of bioterrorism," *The Post Standard* (Syracuse), July 22, 2002.
2. Bryan Salvage, "Veterinarians are on the front lines in the global food-safety war," The Meating Place Web site, Aug. 8, 2002.
3. "The economic benefits of biosecurity in poultry farming," Antec International, www.antecint.co.uk, no date (viewed Oct. 26, 2003).
4. Web-posted video of Antec International, www.antecint.co.uk, viewed Oct. 26, 2003.
5. "Thompson fears terror attack on food," AP, Dec. 4, 2004.
6. William J. Broad, "Anthrax expert faces fine for burning infected carcasses," *The New York Times*, Mar. 1, 2002, p. A16.
7. Philip Brasher, "Congress seeking ways to safeguard food supply," AP, Oct. 26, 2001.
8. Ian Shapira, "Avian flu stops the show," *Washington Post*, Aug. 2, 2002, p. B1.
9. "U.S. food sector may be vulnerable to attack," Reuters, Feb. 25, 2004.
10. Daniel J. Wakin, "Report cites security flaws at Plum Island," *The New York Times*, Oct. 29, 2003.

REASON #32

1. Michael Greger, "USDA misleading American public about beef safety," Organic Consumers Assoc., Dec. 24, 2003.
2. "Bovine Spongiform Encephalopathy (BSE): Questions and answers," fact sheet, FDA, Feb. 27, 2004.
3. Geoffrey Cowley, "Cannibals to cows: The path of a deadly disease," *Newsweek*, Mar. 12, 2001, pp. 53, 56–57.
4. Sandra Blakeslee, "Stringent steps taken by U.S. on cow illness," *The New York Times*, Jan. 14, 2001.
5. Suzanne Daley, "Such a deal: A million tons of animal parts to go," *The New York Times*, Nov. 26, 2000, p. 10.
6. Christopher Drew, Elizabeth Becker, and Sandra Blakeslee, "Despite mad-cow warnings, industry resisted safeguards," *The New York Times*, Dec. 28, 2003.
7. Mary Pearl and Jonathan Epstein," Anatomy of an outbreak: Mad cow, mad elk, mad cat....Can we end the madness?" *San Francisco Chronicle*, Jan. 5, 2004.
8. E-mail correspondence with Michael Greger, Apr. 18, 2004.
9. Cowley, "Cannibals to cows," p. 54.
10. Lisa Belkin, "Why is Jonathan Simms still alive?" *The New York Times*, May 11, 2003.
11. Cowley, "Cannibals to cows."
12. Stuart Laidlaw, "Bizarre affliction first seen in cattle on British farm," *Toronto Star*, Apr. 19, 2003.
13. Donald G. McNeil, Jr., "Doubling tests for mad cow doesn't quiet program critics," *The New York Times*, Feb. 9, 2004.
14. Carey Gillam, "U.S. mad cow testing ignites criticism," Reuters, Aug. 3, 2004.
15. James Ridgeway, "Slaughterhouse politics," *The Village Voice*, Dec. 31, 2003.
16. Ira Dreyfuss, "Nationwide livestock IDs years away," AP, Feb. 7, 2004.
17. Lauran Neergaard, "Mad cow is one of many mystifying diseases," AP, Jan. 6, 2004.
18. Steve Mitchell, "No mad cow results for nearly 500 cows," UPI, Aug. 11, 2004.
19. "Bovine Spongiform Encephalopathy."
20. Ira Dreyfuss, "Panel: Undiscovered cases of mad cow likely to be in United States," AP, Feb. 4, 2004.
21. Thomas M. Burton and Martin Fackler, "U.S. can afford a wider BSE test to spot bad beef," *The Wall Street Journal*, Jan. 2, 2004.
22. Donald G. McNeil, Jr., "U.S. won't let company test all its cattle for mad cow," *The New York Times*, Apr. 10, 2004.

REASON #33

1. Quoted in "Vegetarian diet 'cuts heart risk'," BBC News, Dec. 15, 2002.
2. Lawrence Lindner, "Stone age soup," *Washington Post*, Feb. 13, 2001, p. HE9.
3. "National Cholesterol Education Program (NCEP) issues major new cholesterol guidelines," news release, NIH, May 15, 2001.
   Jane E. Brody, " 'Normal' blood pressure: Health watchdogs are resetting the risk," *The New York Times*, Aug. 12, 2003.
4. Jane E. Brody, "Statins: Miracles for some, menace for a few," *The New York Times*, Dec. 10, 2002, p. F7.
5. Denise Grady, "U.S. guidelines reassess blood pressure," *The New York Times*, May 15, 2003, p. A32.
6. Joe Graedon and Teresa Graedon, "Some users of cholesterol drug report memory impairment," *Los Angeles Times*, Mar. 12, 2001.
7. Paul Raeburn, "Drug safety needs a second opinion," *Business Week*, Sept. 20, 1999.

8. LuAnn Soliah, "A survey of nutrition in medical school curricula," *Today's Dietitian*, Feb. 2004.
9. "Veggie diet lowers cholesterol like drugs, study," CP (Canadian Press), July 22, 2003.
10. "Controlling cholesterol," fact sheet, PCRM, Nov. 17, 1998.
11. "Ask the Mayo dietitian: Cholesterol from plants?" Mayo Clinic, Mar. 22, 2000.
12. "High blood pressure," fact sheet, PCRM, Apr. 21, 1998.
13. Ibid.
14. Jane E. Brody, " 'Normal' blood pressure: Health watchdogs are resetting the risk," *The New York Times*, Aug. 12, 2003.
15. Ibid.
16. Ibid.
17. "What is high blood pressure?" fact sheet, NHLBI, www.nhlbi.nih.gov/health/dci/index.html, no date (viewed, Feb. 29, 2004).
18. Brenda Davis and Vesanto Melina, *Becoming Vegan,* Book Publishing Company, Summertown, TN, 2000, p. 22.

REASON #34

1. Michael Pollan, "When a crop becomes king," *The New York Times*, July 19, 2002.
2. Gale Norton and Ann Veneman, "There's more than one way to protect wetlands," *The New York Times*, Mar. 12, 2003.
3. Heather Dewar and Tom Horton, "Cycle of growth and devastation," *Baltimore Sun*, Sept. 25, 2000.
4. Verlyn Klinkenborg, "Keeping a lost world alive: A last remnant of Iowa's tall grass prairie," *The New York Times*, Aug. 7, 2003.
5. Ibid.
6. Richard Manning, "The oil we eat," *Harper's Magazine*, Feb. 2004.
7. Ibid.
8. Edythe Preet, "Thanks for the miracle of corn," *Los Angeles Times*, Sept. 8, 2000.
9. "Editorial: Corn and what's wrong with it," *Baltimore Sun*, Apr. 25, 2002.
10. *Feed Yearbook*, ERS/USDA, Apr. 25, 2002.
11. Terry Gross, producer, "Michael Pollan discusses the U.S. beef industry," *Fresh Air*, WHYY–NPR, Apr. 3, 2002.
12. Payal Sampat, "Deep trouble: The hidden threat of groundwater pollution," Worldwatch Paper 154, Worldwatch Institute, Dec. 2000, p. 9.
13. Dewar, "Cycle of growth and devastation."
14. Manning, "Oil we eat."
15. "Editorial: Corn and what's wrong with it."
16. John McChesney, "Profile: Growers of grass-fed beef hope to go beyond niche status," *Morning Edition*, NPR News, July 4, 2002.
17. Tom Appenzeller, "The end of cheap oil," *National Geographic*, June 2004, p. 98–99.
18. Jim Paul, "High grain prices mean higher costs for livestock producers," AP, Apr. 19, 2004.
19. Gross, "Michael Pollan discusses the U.S. beef industry."
20. Michael Pollan, "Power steer," *The New York Times Magazine*, Mar. 31, 2002.

REASON #35

1. Quoted in Lance Gay, "Clinton administration reduces standards for wholesome meats," *Seattle Post-Intelligencer*, July 17, 2000.
2. Charles E. Morris, "HACCP under the microscope," *Food Engineering*, Oct. 1, 2000.
3. Ibid.
4. Bud Hazelkorn, "Special report: Inspector abuse, how bad is it?" *Meat Processing*, July 2000.
5. Interview with Carol Tucker Foreman, "Modern meat," draft transcript, PBS Online and WGBH/Frontline, Apr. 18, 2002.
6. Mike Von Fremd, "Bad meat or bad policy? Judge knocks fed salmonella policy," ABC News, May 26, 2000.

REASON #36

1. Temple Grandin, "The way I see it: The dangers of trait over-selection," *Western Horseman*, Aug. 1998, pp. 120–124.
2. Tom Abate, "Origen far from chicken-hearted about bioengineering; Program may yield birds that grow faster, bigger," *San Francisco Chronicle*, July 10, 2000, p B1.
3. Anthony Browne, "Ten weeks to live…and they're the lucky organic ones," *The Guardian*, Mar. 10, 2002.
4. "Fact sheet 3: Pig farming," Animals Australia, www.animalsaustralia.org, no date (viewed July 6, 2002).
5. James E. Pettigrew, "Weaning age: A perspective," *American Protein*, Summer 1998.
6. Rod Smith, "Embryo transfer is 'next frontier' in reproductivity," *Feedstuffs*, May 25, 1998.
7. Harlan Ritchie, "Why is efficiency so important to the beef industry?" *Feedstuffs*, Feb. 21, 2000.
8. Terry Gross, producer, "Michael Pollan discusses the U.S. beef industry," *Fresh Air*, WHYY–NPR, Apr. 3, 2002.
9. Colin Tudge, "The freaks of the farmyard," *London Times*, Sept. 3, 1997.
10. Michael Laris, "DNA trail began in Virginia: Bull's genes could speed changes to feed millions around the world," *Washington Post*, June 30, 2002, p. A1.
11. Tudge, "The freaks of the farmyard."
12. Grandin, "The way I see it."
Anthony Browne, "Ten weeks to live…and

they're the lucky organic ones," *The Guardian*, Mar. 10, 2002.

13. Grandin, "The way I see it."
14. Megan Goldin, "Naked chicken plan may make feathers fly," Reuters, May 20, 2002.

REASON #37

1. Quoted in John Robbins, *May All Be Fed: Diet for a New World*, Morrow, New York, 1992, p. 75.
2. "Fruit," www.Healthwell.com, Aug. 2, 1999.
3. "Antioxidants and free radicals," www.Kroger.com, http://tinyurl.com/6qbku, Aug. 2, 1999.
4. Emily Esterson, "Phytonutrient warriors," www.Healthwell.com, Sept. 1999.
5. Jane E. Brody, "The color of nutrition: Fruits and vegetables," *The New York Times*, May 14, 2002, p. F8.
6. Charlene Laino, "Fruits, vegetables cut stroke risk," MSNBC, Oct. 5, 1999.
7. "Antioxidants in fruit, veg slow brain aging," Reuters, Oct. 2, 1998.
8. "Fighting heart disease with fruit," BBC News, Mar. 2, 2001.
9. Jane E. Brody, "Preserving a delicate balance of potassium," *The New York Times*, June 22, 2004.
10. "Black beans," The George Mateljan Foundation Web site (World's Healthiest Foods), www.whfoods.com, Jan. 2, 2004.
11. Doug Eborn, "The legumes," www.waltonfeed.com, Mar. 31, 2001.
12. "The fifty healthiest foods," *Ladies' Home Journal*, Nov. 1993, p. 266.
13. "Whole grains protect against cancer," Reuters, June 24, 1998.
14. "Whole grains: Reap the rewards," www.MayoClinic.com, Aug. 11, 2003.

REASON #38

1. Quoted in Elizabeth Becker, "Critics take aim at guidelines on standards for food safety," *The New York Times*, Nov. 2, 2002.
2. Elliot Jaspin and Mike Ward, "Chicken once tainted by feces salvaged, sold," *Austin American-Statesman*, June 18, 1998.
3. Richard Behar and Michael Kramer, "Regulation: Something smells fowl; The Espy scandal is minor compared with the way the USDA has favored the poultry industry," *Time* magazine, Oct. 17, 1994.
4. Richard Behar and Michael Kramer, "Something smells fowl: The Espy scandal is minor compared with the way the USDA has favored the poultry industry," *Time* magazine, Oct. 17, 1994.
5. Doris Stanley, "Steaming out the salmonella risk," *Agricultural Research* magazine, ARS/USDA, Oct. 1997.
6. "Study finds one in 100 poultry carcasses contaminated," AP, Mar. 21, 2000.
7. Mark Vosburgh, "Diseased chicken parts served up," *Plain Dealer Reporter*, Feb. 9, 2000.
8. "From cradle to gravy," *Consumer Reports*, Mar. 1998, pp. 14–15.
9. Beatrice Trum Hunter, "Overlooked threats of foodborne illness," *Consumers' Research* magazine, Oct. 1, 1995.
10. "From cradle to gravy," *Consumer Reports*, Mar. 1998, pp. 14–15.
11. "Is our food fit to eat?" *48 Hours*, CBS, Feb. 9, 1994.
12. Richard Behar and Michael Kramer, "Regulation: Something smells fowl; The Espy scandal is minor compared with the way the USDA has favored the poultry industry," *Time* magazine, Oct. 17, 1994.
13. "Cradle to gravy."
14. "Study finds one in 100 poultry carcasses contaminated," AP, Mar. 21, 2000.
15. John Larson, "Is the meat, poultry, and fish you buy as fresh as you think?" *Dateline NBC*, NBC, May 21, 2002.
16. Ibid.

REASON #39

1. "The promise of a blue revolution," *The Economist*, Aug. 9, 2003, p. 20.
2. "Farmed fish: Packing them in like sardines," *Business Week*, Nov. 11, 1996.
3. *America's Living Oceans: Charting a Course for a Sea Change*, Pew Oceans Commission, Arlington, VA, May 2003, p. 77.
4. Frank Langfitt and Heather Dewar, "China's prosperity turns seas toxic in a generation," *Baltimore Sun*, Sept. 27, 2000.
5. Kenneth R. Weiss, "Fish farms become feedlots of the sea," *Los Angeles Times*, Dec. 9, 2002.
6. Terry McCarthy and Campbell River, "Is fish farming safe?" *Time* magazine, Nov. 17, 2002.
7. *America's Living Oceans*.
8. Weiss, "Fish farms become feedlots of the sea."
9. Michael L. Weber, *What Price Farmed Fish: A Review of the Environmental and Social Costs of Farming Carnivorous Fish*, SeaWeb Aquaculture Clearinghouse, Providence, RI, 2003.
10. Walter Gibbs, "Fish-farm escapees threaten wild salmon," *The New York Times*, Oct. 1, 1996, p. C4.
11. Steve Cowan and Barry Schienberg, "Farming the seas," Habitat Media for PBS, Nov. 20, 2004.
12. Weiss, "Fish farms become feedlots of the sea."
13. Marc Kaufman, "Maine salmon face upstream battle as species returns dwindle

as aquaculture booms," *Washington Post*, Sept. 3, 2000.

14. "The promise of a blue revolution."
15. Weber, *What Price Farmed Fish.*
16. Nancy A. Melville, "The down side of fish farms," HealthScout, Sept. 23, 2000.
17. Carl Safina, "The world's imperiled fish," *Scientific American*, Nov. 1995. p. 49.
18. Ibid.

REASON #40

1. Verlyn Klinkenborg, "Cow parts," *Discover*, Aug. 2001.
2. *The Rendering Industry: Economic Impact of Future Feeding Regulations*, Sparks Companies, McLean, VA, June 2001, p. 12.
3. "Bovine Spongiform Encephalopathy (BSE): Questions and answers," fact sheet, FDA, Feb. 27, 2004.
4. Klinkenborg, "Cow parts."
5. J. Peder Zane, "It ain't just for meat: It's for lotion," *The New York Times*, May 5, 1996.
6. Klinkenborg, "Cow parts."
7. Steve Woodward, "Cattle byproducts are found in hundreds of products from soap to drugs," Knight-Ridder/Tribune, Jan. 4, 2004.
8. Klinkenborg, "Cow parts."
9. Emily Gersema, "FDA to limit what goes into animal feed," AP, Sept. 23, 2003.
10. Sandi Doughton, "Should U.S. follow UK on mad cow?" *The Seattle Times*, Feb. 5, 2004.
11. "Animal 'pharm': Making supplements and medicines from livestock plants," AP, Oct. 21, 2001.
12. Rukmini Callimachi, "Authorities recalling cow parts used in candles, poultry feed, and gardening soil," AP, Dec. 27, 2003.
13. Woodward, "Cattle byproducts are found in hundreds of products from soap to drugs."
14. Sandra Blakeslee, "Study finds broader reach for mad cow proteins," *The New York Times*, Jan. 21, 2005.

REASON #41

1. Quoted in Gail Eisnitz, *Slaughterhouse: The Shocking Story of Greed, Neglect, and Inhumane Treatment Inside the U.S. Meat Industry*, Prometheus Books, Amherst, New York, 1997, p. 24.
2. Jon Carroll, "Many amusing facts about the cow," *San Francisco Chronicle*, Aug. 23, 2001, p. E10.
3. Temple Grandin, re: "Modern meat: A brutal harvest," live online, *Washington Post*, Apr. 20, 2001.
4. Joby Warrick, "They die piece by piece," *Washington Post*, Apr. 10, 2001, p. A1.
5. Dena Jones, "Crimes unseen," *Orion Magazine*, July/Aug. 2004.
6. Quote from the transcript of a petition addressed to the Honorable Christine Gregoire, attorney general of the state of Washington, from the Humane Farming Assoc., May 31, 2000.
7. Ibid.
8. Warrick, "They die piece by piece."
9. Ibid.
10. Quoted in Joby Warrick, "A brutal harvest: Big Mac's voice in meat plants," *Washington Post*, Apr. 10, 2001.
11. Quoted in Wenonah Hauter, "Groups petition USDA to enforce Humane Slaughter Act," news release, Public Citizen, June 13, 2001.
12. Frederic J. Frommer, "Report finds spotty enforcement of humane slaughter law," AP, Feb. 28, 2004.

REASON #42

1. Quoted in Tara Burghart, "Tax break for hog farm neighbors may set precedent," AP, May 26, 1998.
2. Ken Midkiff, *The Meat You Eat*, St. Martin's Press, New York, 2004, p. 63.
3. Scott Mooneyham, "Study finds health problems around the hog farms," AP, Feb. 15, 2000.
4. Quoted in John H. Cushman, Jr., "Pollution by factory farms inspires industrial approach to regulation," *The New York Times*, Mar. 6, 1998, p. A12.
5. Bill Berkowitz, "Trouble on the farm," *The Nation*, June 25, 2002.
6. Quoted in Fern Shen, "Maryland hog farm causing quite a stink: Hog farming raises concern among neighbors, officials," *Washington Post*, May 23, 1999, p. A1.
7. Quoted in Frances X. Clines, "Perdue offers a plan to fight odor and pollution," *The New York Times*, Oct. 19, 1999, p. A16.
8. J. Kyle Foster, " 'Hog farming, tourism clash in Finger Lakes region,' *New York Times* says," Bloomberg, Aug. 12, 2001.
9. Michael Pollan, "Power steer," *The New York Times Magazine*, Mar. 31, 2002.
10. Chris Clayton, "Livestock groups, EPA agree on air-quality monitoring," *Omaha World-Herald*, Jan. 25, 2005.
11. Burghart, "Tax break for hog farm neighbors may set precedent."

REASON #43

1. Lisa Turner, "Strong bones without dairy," *Vegetarian Times*, Mar. 1998, p. 50.
2. "What is lactose intolerance?" fact sheet, *Your Health*, PCRM, Jan. 14, 2002.
3. Bob LeRoy, "Milk does not build strong bones," *Vegetarian Voice*, vol. 21, no. 4, North American Vegetarian Society, 1996.
4. T. Colin Campbell, "Dr. Campbell responds to *New York Times* reporter Jane E. Brody's milk 'editorials',"

www.VegSource.com, no date (viewed Nov. 14, 2000).

5. Anne Karpf, "Dairy monsters: Part I," *The Guardian*, Dec. 13, 2003.
6. Quoted in Ibid.
7. Michael Pollan, "Power steer," *The New York Times Magazine*, Mar. 31, 2002.
8. Jane E. Brody, "Debate over milk: Time to look at the facts," *The New York Times*, Sept. 26, 2000, p. F8.
9. "Consumer news: Facts and answers," USDA/ARS Children's Nutrition Research Center at Baylor College of Medicine, 1999.
10. Daphne Miller, "The juice on cows' milk for babies," WebMD, June 23, 1999.
11. "Constipation in children," editorial, *New England Journal of Medicine*, Oct. 15, 1998.
12. LeRoy, "Milk does not build strong bones."
13. Mary Jane Horton, "Skeleton crew," *Vegetarian Times*, July 1999, p. 84.
14. Anne Karpf, "Dairy monsters: Part I," *The Guardian*, Dec. 13, 2003.
15. Sandra G. Boodman, "The osteoporosis scare: Separating fact from fiction," *Los Angeles Times*, Oct. 16, 2000.
16. Marta D. Van Loan, "Boning up on osteoporosis," *Agricultural Research* magazine, ARS/USDA, Mar. 2003.

REASON #44

1. E-mail correspondence with William Harris, Feb. 4, 2000.
2. Joel Achenbach, "Soybeans & flapdoodles: Life on an Indiana farm," *Washington Post*, Sept. 7, 2001.
3. Elizabeth Becker, "Far from dead, subsidies fuel big farms," *The New York Times*, May 14, 2001, p. A1.
4. Quoted in Ibid.
5. "Senate OKs aid for hog farmers," AP, Mar. 19, 1999.
6. Elizabeth Becker, "Agriculture secretary vs. sacred cow," *The New York Times*, Dec. 14, 2001.
7. "What to do with a mountain of milk," AP, June 29, 2002.
8. Ellen Ruppel Shell, "New world syndrome," *The Atlantic Monthly*, June 2001.
9. "Grazing subsidy: $500 million or more a year," *Watersheds Messenger*, Fall 2002.
10. "Poultry feathers made into plastic mulch," ARS/USDA, Feb. 2005.
11. "Market Access Program (MAP)," fact sheet, Foreign Agricultural Service, USDA, June 2003.
12. Tamra Fitzpatrick, "U.S. fishing industry got $50 million for relief," Bloomberg, July 14, 2000.
13. "Bush wants $441 million for mad cow, food safety," Reuters, Feb. 2, 2004.
14. Lance Gay, "Dairy industry seeks $1.3 billion to kill diseased cows," Scripps Howard, May 11, 2000.
15. "Health crisis in America," Produce for Better Health Campaign, www.5aday.com, no date (viewed Feb. 22, 2002).
16. Reed Mangels, "Scientific updates: A review of recent scientific papers related to vegetarianism," *Vegetarian Journal*, Sept.–Oct. 1994.
17. Chris Edwards and Tad DeHaven, "Save the farms: End the subsidies," *Washington Post*, Mar. 3, 2002.
18. www.taxmeat.com.

REASON #45

1. Quoted in Andrew C. Revkin, "Commercial fleets reduced big fish by 90 percent, study says," *The New York Times*, May 15, 2003.
2. Emma Graham-Harrison, "Aggressive fishing threatens oceans—UN," Reuters, June 4, 2004.
3. "Fish 'massacre' in North Atlantic," BBC News, Feb. 16, 2002.
4. Ellen Barry, "Sea cukes? Cool," *The Boston Globe*, Oct. 24, 1999, p. A1.
5. Carl Safina, "The world's imperiled fish," special edition, the oceans, *Scientific American Presents*, Fall 1998, p. 60.
6. Ted Williams, "The exhausted sea," *Audubon*, Sept. 2003.
7. "EU is failing to halt overfishing in Africa, says WWF," Reuters, Oct. 24, 2003.
8. "Factoids: World fisheries in crisis," ENN, July 10, 1998.
9. "EU is failing to halt overfishing in Africa, says WWF."
10. "Going deep," survey, *The Economist*, May 23, 1998, p. 7.
11. William J. Broad, "Creatures of the deep find their way to the table," *The New York Times*, Dec. 26, 1995, p. C5.

REASON #46

1. *The Rendering Industry: Economic Impact of Future Feeding Regulations*, Sparks Companies, McLean, VA, June 2001, p. 12.
2. Sandra Blakeslee, "Fear of disease prompts new look at rendering," *The New York Times*, Mar. 11, 1997, p. C11.
3. *The Rendering Industry: Economic Impact of Future Feeding Regulations*, Sparks Companies, McLean, VA, June 2001, p. 12.
4. Suzanne Daley, "Such a deal: A million tons of animal parts to go," *The New York Times*, Nov. 26, 2000, p. 10.
5. "USA is concerned about meat and bone meal feed exports as EU plan to extend the ban on its use," *Meat News*, Feb. 12, 2002.
6. Daley, "Such a deal."
7. Denise Grady and Donald G. McNeil, Jr., "Rules issued on animal feed and use of

disabled cattle," *The New York Times*, Jan. 27, 2004.

8. Philip Brasher, "Many feed mills breaking FDA mad cow rules," AP, Mar. 24, 2001.
9. Marian Burros, "Warily searching for safer beef," *The New York Times*, Dec. 31, 2003.
10. Carol Ness and Kim Severson, "What shoppers need to know about mad cow: A guide to buying and eating beef," *San Francisco Chronicle*, Dec. 31, 2003.
11. Brad Knickerbocker, "Amending the U.S. beef business," *The Christian Science Monitor*, Jan. 7, 2004.
12. Steve Mitchell, "Mad cow: Follow the feed," UPI, Dec. 29, 2003.
13. Quoted in Ibid.
14. Knickerbocker, "Amending the U.S. beef business."
15. Beatrice Trum Hunter, "What is fed to our food animals?" *Consumers' Research* magazine, Dec. 1, 1996.
16. Michael Satchell and Stephen J. Hedges, "The next bad beef scandal?" *U.S. News and World Report*, Sept. 1, 1997.
17. Hunter, "What is fed to our food animals?"

REASON #47

1. David Perlman, "Early humans ate their way through species," *San Francisco Chronicle*, June 8, 2001.
2. Will Dunham, "Prehistoric humans blamed for mass extinctions," Reuters, June 14, 2001.
3. "What killed the megabeasts?" Discovery Channel, Aug. 2002.
4. "Study says early humans caused a quick extinction of flightless birds in New Zealand," AP, Mar. 23, 2000.
5. "Hunting gear," *Modern Marvels*, The History Channel, Mar. 4, 2004.
6. Quoted in Ibid.
7. Kenneth R. Weiss, "Overhunting has ravaged sea habitats, study finds," *Los Angeles Times*, July 27, 2001.
8. "The bushmeat trade: Killing off the ark," *The Economist*, May 15, 2003.
9. Kenneth R. Weiss, "Sportfishing blamed in depletion," *Los Angeles Times*, Aug. 27, 2004.
10. Richard B. Anderson and Gregory Helms, "Fish are the earth's canaries," *Los Angeles Times*, Feb. 28, 2002.
11. Jordan Kahn, "Fishing rules face historic changes," *Daytona Beach News-Journal*, Sept. 24, 2004.
    Maggie Fox, "Fishing just for fun damages stocks, study finds," Reuters, Aug. 30, 2004.
12. "Northeast warned on fish consumption," AP, May 28, 2004.
13. Lolly Merrell, "No magic bullet for wasting disease," *High Country News*, June 10, 2002.
14. Stephanie Simon, "Fear of disease triggers order to kill 25,000 deer," *Los Angeles Times*, Aug. 19, 2002.

REASON #48

1. Paul A. Lachance, "Apple-eaters breathe easy, study suggests," AP, Jan. 20, 2000.
2. Jennifer K. Nelson, "Apples, phytochemicals and cancer," Mayo Clinic, June 23, 2000.
3. Sheldon Margen and Dale A. Ogar, "With avocados, high-fat is good," *Los Angeles Times*, Dec. 28, 1998.
4. "Blueberries may restore some memory, coordination and balance lost with age," news release (0360.99), USDA, Sept. 10, 1999.
5. "A daily dose of blue: The tastiest way to get your antioxidants," Wild Blueberry Assoc. of North America, PRNewswire, Jul. 22, 1998.
6. Mary Duenwald, "Added beauty from blueberries," *The New York Times*, Aug. 31, 2004.
7. "Recently published study suggests cranberry may help fight ulcer-causing bacteria; benefits beyond urinary tract health," BW HealthWire, Mar. 7, 2001.
8. "Cranberry," www.deliciouslivingmag.com, http://tinyurl.com/5d2zn, Aug. 2001.
9. Amy Satterfield Gades, "Flax for what ails you," www.Healthwell.com, Aug. 2, 1999.
10. Jane E. Brody, "Study indicates that grapes and red wine may contain powerful inhibitor to cancer," *The New York Times*, Jan. 10, 1997, p. A17.
11. "All fruits are not created equal—kiwi is king," *Nutrition Science News*, Feb. 1998.
12. Jane E. Brody, "The fatty nut finds its place at the table," *The New York Times*, Feb. 8, 2000, p. F8.
13. Harvard University School of Health, "No matter how you crack them, nuts are a heart-healthy food," PRNewswire, Nov. 19, 1998.
14. "Nuts may help prevent diabetes, study of 83,000 women shows," *The New York Times*, Nov. 27, 2002, p. A19.
15. "New research puts the nut back in nutrition," Almond Board of the United States, PRNewswire, Apr. 20, 1998.
16. Maggie Fox, "Test could find healthiest foods, researcher says," Reuters, Feb. 8, 1999.

REASON #49

1. Peter Jaret, "Broccoli beats most other veggies in health benefits," WebMD, Apr. 13, 2000.
2. Ibid.

3. "Colon cancer curbed by high-selenium broccoli," *Agricultural Research* magazine, ARS/USDA June 2000.
4. "Vegetables," www.independent pharmacy.co.uk, Aug. 2, 1999.
5. Jean Carper, "Of cabbages and cancer," *USA Weekend*, Feb. 3–5, 1995.
6. "Don't give yourself an ulcer—eat broccoli," AP, May 28, 2002.
7. Tony Tantillo, "Reference shelf: Disease-fighting phytochemicals," The Fresh Grocer, Fresh Farms, LLC, www.tonytantillo.com, no date (viewed Nov. 4, 2003).
8. Jean Carper, "Six secret disease fighters," *USA Weekend*, Feb. 7, 1997.
9. "Study: Folic acid reduces birth defects," AP, Oct. 3, 2000.
10. Marian Burros, "One more reason to eat your greens," *The New York Times*, May 16, 2001, p. F1.
11. "Vitamin K: Another reason to eat your greens," *Agricultural Research* magazine, ARS/USDA, Jan. 2000.
12. "Eat spinach because it's good for your eyes," Business Wire, May 3, 1999.
13. Jean Carper, "Spinach vs. depression," *USA Weekend*, Feb. 6–8, 1998.
14. Winifred Yu, "Blue-chip foods," *Vegetarian Times*, June 1996, p. 76. (The others were avocados, broccoli, brown rice, cantaloupe, dried beans and peas, garlic, grapefruit, nutritional yeast, potatoes, tofu, and whole wheat bread.)
15. "Watermelon packs a powerful lycopene punch," *Agricultural Research* magazine, ARS/USDA, June 2002.

REASON #50

1. Virgil Butler, "Inside the mind of a killer," blog, The Cyberactivist, Aug. 31, 2003.
2. "What humans owe to animals," *The Economist*, Aug. 19, 1995, p. 11.
3. Karen Davis, *Prisoned Chickens, Poisoned Eggs*, Book Publishing Company, Summertown, TN, 1996, pp. 115–116.
4. Ibid., p. 118.
5. Ibid., p. 114.
6. Butler, "Inside the mind of a killer."
7. "Signed statement of Tyson employee, Virgil Butler," United Poultry Concerns, Jan. 30, 2003.
8. Ibid.
9. "KFC's house of horror," PETA TV, www.petatv.com/veg.html (viewed July 28, 2004).
10. Donald G. McNeil, Jr., "KFC supplier accused of animal cruelty," *The New York Times*, July 20, 2004.

REASON #51

1. "President Bush addresses National Cattlemen's Beef Assoc.," Denver, Colorado, www.cnn.com/transcripts, Feb. 8, 2002.
2. "Cardiovascular disease epidemic threatens developing countries, global economy," news release, American Heart Assoc., Feb. 16, 1998.
3. "Obesity problem goes global," *Meat and Poultry* magazine, May. 16, 2003.
4. Emma Ross, "WHO: Cancer may rise 50 percent by 2020," AP, Apr. 3, 2003.
5. "Report finds heart disease a global threat: No longer a disease of the aging rich," Reuters, Apr. 26, 2004.
6. Indira A.R. Lakshmanan, "Rise in obesity weighs on Asia," *The Boston Globe*, Feb. 27. 2001, p. A1.
7. Ellen Ruppel Shell, "New world syndrome," *The Atlantic Monthly*, June 2001.
8. Heather Dewar and Tom Horton, "Seeds of solution to nitrogen glut," *Baltimore Sun*, Sept. 28, 2000.
9. "Overview," no. 58, *The Strategic Global Investors Newsletter*, Siena Financial Services, Dec. 23, 2002.
10. Richard Manning, "The oil we eat," *Harper's Magazine*, Feb. 2004.
11. *Food and Agriculture Policy: Taking Stock for the New Century*, USDA, Washington DC, Sept. 2001, p. 39.
12. Elizabeth Becker, "Western farmers fear Third-World challenge to subsidies," *The New York Times*, Sept. 9, 2003.
13. Elizabeth Becker, "U.S. corn subsidies said to damage Mexico," *The New York Times*, Aug. 27, 2003.
14. Howard Lyman, *Mad Cowboy*, Scribner, New York, 1998, p. 42.
15. *Summary Annual Report*, McDonald's Corporation, Oak Brook, IL, 2002.
16. "Farm Animal Genetic Resources," *SD Dimensions*, FAO/UN, Sustainable Development Dept., FAO/UN, Feb. 1998.
17. *The Detrimental Impacts of Industrial Animal Agriculture: A Case for Humane and Sustainable Agriculture*, CIWF (UK), 2002, p. 6.
18. "Food security and the environment," FAO/UN, Jan. 17, 2001.

REASON #52

1. Quoted in Tim Lengerich, "Dispelling the cowboy myth," *EarthSave News*, Summer 2003, p. 1.
2. Marc Robichaux, "Scientists fight fires by trying to outwit a very persistent weed," *The Wall Street Journal*, Sept. 1, 2000, p. A1.
3. George Wuerthner and Mollie Matteson, eds., *Welfare Ranching: The Subsidized Destruction of the American West*, Island Press, Foundation for Deep Ecology, Sausalito, CA, 2002, p. 7.
4. Todd Oppenheimer, "The rancher sub-

sidy," *The Atlantic Monthly*, Jan. 1996, p. 28.

5. Mike Hudak, "Public lands ranchers: Heading for the last roundup," *Veg-News*, Oct. 2002, p. 12.
6. "Something fishy about those cattlemen's ads," NRDC, Mar. 12, 1997.
7. Oppenheimer, "The rancher subsidy."
8. Paul Rogers, et al., "Cash cows," reprint ed., *San Jose Mercury News*, Nov. 7, 1999, p. 3S.
9. "U.S. could feed 800 million people with grain that livestock eat, Cornell ecologist advises animal scientists," news release, *Science News*, Cornell U., Aug. 7, 1997.
10. Rogers, "Cash cows."
11. Robichaux, "Scientists fight fires by trying to outwit a very persistent weed," p. A6.
12. Martin Taylor, "Grazing policy is the cause of our wildfires," *Tucson Citizen*, Aug. 25, 2000.
13. Ibid.
14. "USGS studies wildfire ecology in the Western United States," *Science Daily*, Sept. 22, 1999.
15. Robichaux, "Scientists fight fires by trying to outwit a very persistent weed," p. A1.
16. Jack Rosenberger, "Wasting the West: How welfare ranchers and their livestock are damaging public land, "*E/The Environmental Magazine*, Oct. 8, 2004.
17. Paul Rogers, "Taxes support a Wild West holdover that enriches ranchers, degrades land," *San Jose Mercury News*, Mar. 12, 2002.
18. "Is there an alternative to expensive grazing subsidies?" *The Economist*, Mar. 7, 2002.
19. Rogers, "Taxes support a Wild West holdover that enriches ranchers, degrades land."

REASON #53

1. Quoted in P.C. Pethick, "Seven days in a chicken coop," *Centertown News* (Canada), Nov. 7, 1997.
2. Mark Lewis, "The natural history of the chicken," WETA–TV, July 11, 2001.
3. Clare Druce and Bob Fromer, "Hidden suffering," video, Farm Animal Welfare Network (UK), 1992.
4. Karen Davis, "The battery hen: Her life is not for the birds," *Poultry Press*, vol. 3, no. 1, 1993.
5. "Egg-Ribusiness," video, Farm Sanctuary, Watkins Glen, NY, date not noted.
6. Lance Gay, "Hen starvation to boost egg production draws fire," Scripps Howard, Aug. 2, 2001.
7. Anthony Browne, "Ten weeks to live," *The Guardian*, Mar. 10, 2002.
8. Davis, "The battery hen."
9. Peter Singer and Karen Dawn, "Back at the ranch, a horror story," *Los Angeles Times*, Dec. 1, 2003.

REASON #54

1. Quoted in "USDA researchers create new product that reduces salmonella in chickens," news release, USDA, Mar. 19, 1998.
2. "Watch the water," *The Economist*, Sept. 23, 1999.
3. "Economics of foodborne disease," ERS/USDA, May 12, 2003.
4. Peter Perl, "Poisoned package," *Washington Post*, Jan. 16, 2000, p. W8.
5. "Gut warfare," *Journal of the American Veterinary Medical Association*, Mar. 1, 2003.
6. "FDA concerned anti-salmonella products could create new health problems," AP, Nov. 20, 2000.
7. Ibid.
8. Jill Lee, "Zapping airborne salmonella and dust," *Agricultural Research* magazine, ARS/USDA, Mar. 2000.
9. Beverly Cheng, "Producer claims cherries may shut down E. coli O157:H7 in cattle," The Meating Place Web site, Jan. 22, 2001.
10. "Hay cuts E. coli in slaughter cattle," *Hay & Forage Grower*, Jan. 1, 1999.
11. John Gregerson, "Technology update: Bacteria busters," *Food Engineering*, Sept. 1, 2001.
12. "Minnesota company markets electronically pasteurized beef," AP, May 17, 2000.
13. Steve Raabe, "Packer: Process makes beef cleaner, juicier," *Denver Post*, May 10, 2002.
14. "USDA to allow use of liquid nitrogen to freeze beef, pork," Dow Jones, May 22, 1997.
15. "PristineOyster.com clears the NASD," news release, www.PristineOyster.com, Feb. 11, 1999.
16. Melinda Fulmer, "Putting the squeeze on germs," *Los Angeles Times*, Aug. 2, 2001.
17. Bryan Salvage, "New instrument under development detects carcass fecal matter," The Meating Place Web site, June 27, 2000.
18. Samuel Epstein and Wenonah Hauter, "Preventing food poisoning: Sanitation not irradiation," PR Newswire, June 6, 2000.
19. Michael Colby and Samuel Epstein, "Risks of radiation: Too many questions about food safety," *USA Today*, Jan. 22, 1992.
20. Janelle Carter, "Food safety regulators back new strips to test for spoiling," AP, Feb. 14, 1999.
21. Ann Bagel, "New pathogen detection devices could have industry application," The Meating Place Web site, July 19, 2000.
22. Stacey Higginbotham, "A silver bullet for bacteria," *Business Week*, July 5, 1999, p. 8.
23. Naomi Freudlich, "Playing catch-up with

'hamburger disease'," *Business Week*, Dec. 2, 1996.

REASON #55

1. Quoted in "UPC attends First International Symposium on the Artificial Insemination of Poultry," *Poultry Press*, United Poultry Concerns, Fall–Winter 1994, p. 3.
2. "Cattle ranches," *Modern Marvels*, The History Channel, May 8, 2002.
3. Peter Lovenheim, *Portrait of a Burger as a Young Calf*, Harmony Books, New York, 2002, p. 38.
4. "Cattle ranches."
5. Lovenheim, *Portrait of a Burger as a Young Calf*, p. 39.
6. "Advantages to using artificial insemination in swine breeding programs," *Livestock Updates*, Virginia Cooperative Extension, Sept. 1999.
7. "Cattle ranches."
8. Lovenheim, *Portrait of a Burger*, p. 45.
9. Richard A. Battaglia, *Handbook of Livestock Management Techniques*, 2nd ed., Prentice Hall, Upper Saddle River, NJ, 1998, p. 121.
10. Lovenheim, *Portrait of a Burger*, p. 49.
11. "Swine production management: Artificial insemination (collection)," College of Veterinary Medicine, Iowa State U., www.vetmed.iastate.edu, no date (viewed Mar. 20, 2004).
12. Ibid.
13. "In the turkey breeding factory," *Poultry Press*, United Poultry Concerns, Fall–Winter 1994, pp. 1–2, 7.

REASON #56

1. Quoted in Rebecca Renner, "Do cattle growth hormones pose an environmental risk?" *Environmental Science & Technology*, May 1, 2002.
2. J.J. Miller, "Impact of feedlots on water quality," presentation, 34th Annual Western Canada Trace Organic Workshop, Calgary, Alberta, Apr. 28, 1999.
3. "Animal waste pollution in America: An emerging national problem," report, Minority Staff of the U.S. Senate Committee on Agriculture, Nutrition and Forestry, Dec. 1997.
4. Marla Cone, "Feedlot effluent damaging fish, report claims," *Los Angeles Times*, Dec. 11, 2003.
5. Renner, "Hormones pose an environmental risk?"
6. Janet Raloff, "Hormones: Here's the beef," *Science News*, Jan. 5, 2002, p. 10.
7. Kim McGuire, "Animal drugs may taint water: CSU study finds antibiotics for livestock in Cache la Poudre," *The Denver Post*, Oct. 20, 2004.
8. Miller, "Impact of feedlots on water quality."
9. Mark Bourrie, "Chemical gender bender," *National Post* (Canada), Feb. 9, 1999.
10. "Drugs used in the salmon farming industry," fact sheet, David Suzuki Foundation, www.davidsuzuki.org, no date (viewed Apr. 23, 2003).

REASON #57

1. Quoted in "Specialization shifting production into efficient but fewer operations," *Feedstuffs*, Mar. 6, 2000.
2. Ibid.
3. Ibid.
4. Ben Sutherly, "Industry giants leave little room for competition," *Dayton Daily News*, Dec. 3, 2002.
5. William Claiborne, "Fighting the 'new feudal rulers'," *Washington Post*, Jan. 3, 1999, p. A3.
6. Keith Collins, chief economist, USDA, "The outlook for the farm economy," address to the USDA American Agricultural Bank Assoc. annual meeting, Nov. 3, 1999.
7. Michael Pearson, "Hog farming profitable again," AP, Apr. 21, 2000.
8. Jim Phillips and Gregg Hillyer, "Hanging tough with hogs," *Progressive Farmer*, Mar. 1999.
9. Harold Brubaker, "Meatpacker adapts through buyout," *Philadelphia Inquirer*, May 13, 2001, p. C1.

REASON #58

1. Quoted in James Sterngold, "Urban sprawl benefits dairies in California," *The New York Times*, Oct. 22, 1999.
2. Jack Norris, "But it doesn't hurt the cow," essay, Vegan Outreach, Mar. 1, 2000.
3. Dan Looker, "The milk meisters," *Successful Farming*, Nov. 1998.
4. Verlyn Klinkenborg, "Holstein dairy cows and the inefficient efficiencies of modern farming," *The New York Times*, Jan. 5, 2004.
5. "Waterbeds tested to keep cows comfy, productive," AP, Nov. 8, 1999.
6. Jon Carroll, "Many amusing facts about the cow," *San Francisco Chronicle*, Aug. 23, 2001, p. E10.
7. C. David Coats, *Old MacDonald's Factory Farm*, Continuum, New York, 1989, p. 55.
8. Elizabeth Weise, "PETA: 'Happy cows' ad is a lie," *USA Today*, Dec. 11, 2002.
9. Richard A. Battaglia, *Handbook of Livestock Management Techniques*, 2nd ed., Prentice Hall, Upper Saddle River, NJ, 1998, p. 196.
10. Bernard E. Rollin, *Farm Animal Welfare: Social Bioethical, and Research Issues*, Iowa State University Press, 1995, p. 103.

REASON #59

1. Quoted in Tim King, "What's the beef?"

The Christian Science Monitor, Jan. 22, 2004.

2. Elizabeth Weise, "The farmer in the lab," *USA Today*, Sept. 22, 2002.
3. Andrea Graves, "Cloned chickens on the menu," *New Scientist*, Aug. 15, 2001.
4. James Meek, "Britain urged to ban GM salmon," *The Guardian*, Sept. 4, 2002.
5. Kenneth R. Weiss, "It came from the gene lab," *Los Angeles Times*, May 14, 2003.
6. "Experts confirm that bioengineered animals are an environmental threat," Reuters, Sept. 23, 2002.
7. Weiss, "It came from the gene lab."
8. Andrew Pollack, "Concerns raised over altered fish," *The New York Times*, Jan. 15, 2003.
9. Carol Lewis, "A new kind of fish story: The coming of biotech animals," *FDA Consumer*, Jan./Feb. 2001.
10. Justin Gillis, "Old laws, new fish," *Washington Post*, Jan. 15, 2003, p. E1.
11. Pollack, "Concerns raised over altered fish."
12. Justin Gillis, "Cloned livestock expected to add to food supply soon: U.S. farmers breeding many cows, pigs," *Washington Post*, Sept. 17, 2002.
13. Ulysses Torassa, "Dolly euthanized for lung disease: Six-year-old sheep the center of ethical, scientific maelstrom," *San Francisco Chronicle*, Feb. 15, 2003.
14. Maggie Fox, "U.S. says all clones genetically abnormal," Reuters, Sept. 11, 2002.
15. Justin Gillis, "Ready for a big side of clone? Some say 'yuck' to FDA's thumbs-up," *Washington Post*, Oct. 31, 2003.
16. James Gerstenzan, "Cloned products could blend into food supply," *Los Angeles Times*, Nov. 1, 2003.

REASON #60

1. Quoted in Joby Warrick, "Death in the Gulf of Mexico," *National Wildlife*, June 1, 1999.
2. "UN warns about ocean 'dead zones'," AP, Mar. 29, 2004.
3. Tom Horton and Heather Dewar, "Sea grasses vanish, marine life in peril," *Baltimore Sun*, Sept. 26, 2000.
4. "UN warns about ocean 'dead zones.' "
5. Ibid.
6. Janet McConnaughey, "Scientists seek ways to bring marine life back to world's 'dead zones'," AP, Aug. 8, 1999.
7. Michael McCarthy, " 'Dead zones' in world's oceans are growing, say alarmed UN scientists," *The Independent*, Mar. 30, 2004.
8. Sarah Simpson, "Political uncertainty could stall a plan to rein in deadly waters in the Gulf of Mexico," *Scientific American*, July 2001.
9. Warrick, "Death in the Gulf of Mexico."
10. McConnaughey, "Scientists seek ways to bring marine life back to world's 'dead zones.' "
11. Many U.S. coastal areas damaged by polluting runoff, report says," AP, Apr. 5, 2000.
12. Simpson, "Political uncertainty could stall a plan to rein in deadly waters in the Gulf of Mexico."
13. Horton, "Sea grasses vanish, marine life in peril."
14. Timothy B. Wheeler, "Bay loses 5,740 acres of grasses," *Baltimore Sun*, May 29, 1999.
15. Tom Horton and Heather Dewar, "Feeding the world, poisoning the planet," *Baltimore Sun*, Sept. 24, 2000.
16. Horton, "Sea grasses vanish, marine life in peril."

REASON #61

1. Payal Sampat, "Deep trouble: The hidden threat of groundwater pollution," Worldwatch Paper 154, Worldwatch Institute, Dec. 2000, p. 9.
2. Danielle Nierenberg, "Factory farming in the developing world," *Worldwatch*, May/June 2003, p. 13.
3. Ed Ayres, "Will we still eat meat?" *Time* magazine, Nov. 8, 1999, p. 106.
4. Fred Pearce, "Asian farmers sucking the continent dry," *New Scientist*, Aug. 28, 2004.
5. Jacques Leslie, "Running dry: Water scarcity," *Harper's Magazine*, Jul. 2000.
6. Ibid.
7. Sampat, "Deep trouble," p. 5.
8. Ibid., pp. 13–14.
9. Leslie, "Running dry."
10. Mark Johnson, "Study urges water conservation on farms," AP, Jan. 10, 2005.
11. Richard Cowen, "Chapter 18: Mining Ground Water," lecture notes, Geology 115, Earth Science, History, and People, Dept. of Geology, UC Davis, California, Mar. 2003.
12. Carey Gillam, "Fight on to save Plains water source," Reuters, Dec. 1, 2003.
13. Fen Montaigne, "Water pressure," *National Geographic*, Sept. 2002, p. 50.
14. Ginger Otis, "A world without water," *The Village Voice*, Aug. 21–27, 2002, p. 63.
15. "Memorial Day weekend signals start of peak meat grilling season," news release, American Meat Institute, May 23, 2003.

REASON #62

1. Lynn Jacobs, *Waste of the West: Public Lands Ranching*, published by the author, 1991, p. 303.
2. Paul Rogers, "Taxes support a Wild West holdover that enriches ranchers, degrades

land," *San Jose Mercury News*, Mar. 12, 2002.

3. Jacobs, *Waste of the West,* p. 253.
4. George Wuerthner and Mollie Matteson, eds., *Welfare Ranching: The Subsidized Destruction of the American West*, Island Press, Foundation for Deep Ecology, Sausalito, CA, 2002, p. 247.
5. Steve Lustgarden, "War on wildlife," *Vegetarian Times*, Mar. 1994, pp. 70, 72.
6. Wuerthner, *Welfare Ranching,* p. 248.
7. Lustgarden, "War on wildlife," p. 73.
8. Jacobs, *Waste of the West,* p. 252.
9. Nicole Rosmarino, "The ultimate underdog: The battle over prairie dogs on the Great Plains," *Animals' Agenda*, July–Aug. 1999, p. 25.
10. Les Line, "A taste for catfish lands a bird in trouble as farmers seek to arm," *The New York Times*, Oct. 7, 1997, p. F9.

REASON #63

1. Kenneth B. Kephart, "Handling hogs," PENPages: College of Agricultural Sciences, Penn State U., Oct. 15, 1997.
2. Matthew Wilde, "Something to squawk about," *Waterloo, Cedar Falls Courier* (Canada), Aug. 16, 2004.
3. Gene Bauston, *Battered Birds, Crated Herds: How We Treat the Animals We Eat*, Farm Sanctuary, Watkins Glen, NY, 1996, p. 46.
4. Gail Eisnitz, *Slaughterhouse: The Shocking Story of Greed, Neglect, and Inhumane Treatment Inside the U.S. Meat Industry*, Prometheus Books, Amherst, New York, 1997, p. 100.
5. Bauston, *Battered Birds, Crated Herds,* p. 44.
6. Ibid, p. 46.
7. "Cows go wireless," *The Economist*, Mar. 13, 2004, p. 10.
8. C. David Coats, "The transport of livestock in the United States," *The Animals' Voice* magazine, July–Aug.–Sept. 1993, p. 21.
9. "Briefing room/hogs: Trade," ERS/USDA, Apr. 30, 2003.
10. "Ship carrying controversial shipment of Australian sheep docks in Kuwait," AP, Oct. 3, 2003.
11. Kephart, "Handling hogs."
12. Karen Davis, *Prisoned Chickens, Poisoned Eggs*, Book Publishing Company, Summertown, TN, 1996, p. 109.

REASON #64

1. Peter Benchley, "What will be the catch of the day?" *Time* magazine, Nov. 8, 1999, p. 105.
2. "The tragedy of the oceans," *The Economist*, Mar. 19, 1994, p. 22.
3. "Five countries set up team to tackle illegal fishing," AP, Dec. 3, 2003.
4. "California eateries to pull Chilean bass," AP, May 19, 2002.
5. Beth Daley, "With fish piracy on rise, agents cast worldwide net," *The Boston Globe*, May 18, 2003.
6. Kenneth R. Weiss, "Panel presses new ocean safeguards," *Los Angeles Times*, Apr. 21, 2004.
7. William J. Broad and Andrew C. Revkin, "Overfishing imposes a heavy toll," *The New York Times*, p. F2.
8. Jeffrey Tayler, "The caviar thugs," *The Atlantic Monthly*, June 2001, p. 28.
9. Megan Lindow, "South Africa's abalone plundered: Appetite for valued mollusk fueling social, environmental crisis," *San Francisco Chronicle*, Nov. 28, 2003.
10. Dick Russell, "Smugglers are using tuna boats to transport cocaine," *Defenders* magazine, Defenders of Wildlife, Summer 2002.
11. Lolita C. Baldor, "More sanctions demanded for fishing quota violations," AP, Oct. 30, 2003.
12. *Pirate fishing: Plundering West Africa*, Greenpeace International, Netherlands, Sept. 2001, p. 4.
13. Judith Achieng, "Local fishermen battle foreign trawlers," Inter Press Service, Mar. 26, 1999.
14. "Illegal fishing threatens Cambodia's fish stocks," Kyodo World News Service (Japan), June 17, 2000.
15. "Cambodia vows to stop 'anarchic' fish poaching," Reuters, Apr. 9, 1999.
16. Larry Rohter, "Big fish, little fish battle over the Amazon's bounty,' *The New York Times*, Oct. 26, 2004.
17. "Battle over ecosystem in Ecuador's Galapagos Islands," AP, Dec. 28, 2000.
18. Tim Weiner, "In Mexico, greed kills fish by the seaful," *The New York Times*, Apr. 10, 2002, p. A1.
19. Frank Clifford, "U.S. to slash limits on 83 species of Pacific fish," *Los Angeles Times*, Dec. 28, 1997.
20. Daley, "With fish piracy on rise, agents cast worldwide net."
21. "The EU action plan to eradicate IUU fishing: A Greenpeace critique," news release, Greenpeace, Oct. 2001.
22. Alexander Marjin, "Black caviar may be rarer as Russia stops sturgeon fishing," Deutsche Presse-Agentur, July 25, 2001.

REASON #65

1. "Cattle hormones: Hot flushes," *The Economist*, May 15, 1999.
2. Judy Foreman, "Q: Should I be worried about bovine growth hormones in milk?" *The Boston Globe*, May 11, 2004.
3. Roger Runningen, "Monsanto milk hormone needs added review, group says," Bloomberg, Dec. 15, 1998.
4. "Raising valid beefs about meat testing,"

The Globe and Mail (Canada), Nov. 12, 2000.

5. Andrew Pollack, "Maker warns of scarcity of hormones for dairy cows," *The New York Times*, Jan. 27, 2004.
6. Susan Gilbert, "Fears over milk, long dismissed, still simmer," *The New York Times*, Jan. 19, 1999, p. F7.
7. Runningen, "Monsanto milk hormone needs added review, group says."
8. Jeff Kamen, "Formula for disaster: An investigative report on genetically engineered bovine growth hormone in milk and consequences for your health," *Penthouse* magazine, Mar. 1999.
9. "Udder confusion," *The Economist*, July 3, 1999.
10. E-mail correspondence with Robert Cohen, www.notmilk.com, Dec. 11, 2003.
11. "Udder confusion."
12. "Chemicals in food: Uncowed," *The Economist*, Mar. 26, 1994, p. 32.
13. Michael K. Hansen and Jean Halloran (both of the Consumer Policy Institute, a division of Consumers Union), "Yes, ask why we need this stuff in our milk: Make them label it," letters, *The New York Times*, Feb. 21, 1994.
14. Fact sheet, Humane Farming Assoc., 1991.
15. "EU affirms ban on some beef imports," Bloomberg, Oct. 16, 2003.
16. "The use of steroid hormones for growth promotion in food-producing animals," FDA/CVM, July 2002.

REASON #66

1. Kerry Bowman, "Please don't eat the animals," Bell Globemedia Interactive, July 7, 2003.
2. "Bushmeat trade could spell disaster for the chimps," People and the Planet (UK), www.peopleandplanet.net, Feb. 18, 2003.
3. "MEPs take on bushmeat trade," www.EUpolitix.com, Jan. 13, 2004.
4. Denis D. Gray, "Quest for health, sex, exotic food in China wiping out wildlife in Southeast Asia," AP, Mar. 27, 2004.
5. Gary Strieker, "Elephant meat for sale," CNN, Mar. 13, 2002.
6. Doug Struck, "Japanese whaling culture endangered, not extinct," *Washington Post*, Aug. 22, 2000, p. A1.
7. "Japan 'buys' pro-whaling votes," CNN, July 18, 2001.
8. "Avian influenza: Wings across the world?" *The Economist*, Jan. 29, 2004.
9. Jeremy Laurance, "New diseases pose threat to world health," *The Independent*, Jan. 14, 2004.
10. "A year on from first SARS case and much still unknown," Agence France Presse, Nov. 11, 2003.
11. Denise Grady, "On an altered planet, new diseases emerge as old ones re-emerge," *The New York Times*, Aug. 20, 2002.
12. "Ebola caused by wild boar meat," News24 (South Africa), Nov. 10, 2003.
13. Bowman, "Please don't eat the animals."

REASON #67

1. Quoted in Pam Smith O'Hara, "A little protein is all it takes: Many Americans get much more than they really need," *Washington Post*, Mar. 24, 1998, p. Z20.
2. Brenda Davis and Vesanto Melina, *Becoming Vegan,* Book Publishing Company, Summertown, TN, 2000, p. 39.
3. Mark Bittman, "Need more protein? Probably not," *The New York Times*, Oct. 27, 1993.
4. "Red meat and health," *Vegetarian Nutrition & Health Letter*, Loma Linda University, Apr. 1, 2001.
5. Jane E. Brody, "Huge study of diet indicts fat and meat," *The New York Times*, May 8, 1990, p. A1.
6. Anne Karpf, "Dairy monsters: Part I," *The Guardian*, Dec. 13, 2003.
7. "Too much protein may cause reduced kidney function," *Harvard University Gazette*, Mar. 13, 2003.
8. "Position of the American Dietetic Assoc. and Dietitians of Canada: Vegetarian diets," *Journal of the American Dietetic Association*, June 2003, p. 749.
9. Davis, *Becoming Vegan,* p. 43.
10. Sally Squires, "Heart Association skewers Atkins diet: High-protein plans called unproven, risky," *Washington Post*, Oct. 9, 2001, p. HE1.
11. Jane E. Brody, "High-fat diet: Count calories and think twice," *The New York Times*, Sept. 10, 2002, p. F6.
12. "Vegetarianism, Atkins diet to be addressed at local talks," *Dunn County News* (Wisconsin), Oct. 4, 2004.
13. E.J. Mundell, "High-protein diets dehydrate even the very fit," Reuters, Apr. 22, 2002.
14. Sally Squires, "Low-carb diets take a punch," *Washington Post*, July 6, 2004, p. HE1.
15. Ibid.
16. Ibid.
17. Ridgely Ochs, "Obesity: Bad news, good news," *Los Angeles Times*, Aug. 6, 2001.
18. "Four popular diets get thumbs up," Reuters, Nov. 9, 2003.
19. Lawrence Lindner, "Stone age soup," *Washington Post*, Feb. 13, 2001, p. HE9.
20. "Position of the American Dietetic Assoc. and Dietitians of Canada: Vegetarian diets," *Journal of the American Dietetic Association*, June 2003, p. 750.
21. Karin Horgan Sullivan, "The iron file," *Vegetarian Times*, July 1996, p. 62.

22. Karin Horgan, "A possible cancer link," *Vegetarian Times*, June 1994, p. 19.
23. "Iron content of meat linked to heart attack," Reuters, Mar. 1, 1999.
24. "Too much iron, not anemia, problem in U.S.—study," Reuters, Feb. 23, 2001.
25. Ed Edelson, "Too much zinc ups prostate cancer risk," HealthDay, July 2, 2003.

REASON #68

1. Quoted in John Duce, "Scientists demand 'fish parks'," BBC News, Feb. 17, 2001.
2. Andrew C. Revkin, "Commercial fleets reduced big fish by 90 percent, study says," *The New York Times*, May 15, 2003.
3. Dan Vergano, "Study: Ninety percent decline of big oceangoing fish," *USA Today*, May 14, 2003.
4. Severin Carrell, "Ban fishing in third of all seas, scientists say," *The Independent*, Aug. 31, 2003.
5. Jane Kay, "U.S. urged to better regulate its fisheries: Panel calls for reserves, coordination of conservation efforts," *San Francisco Chronicle*, June 5, 2003, p. A8.
6. William Broad, "Researchers find fish thriving in protected waters," *The New York Times*, Mar. 21, 2000, p. F4.
7. Kenneth R. Weiss, "Big fish near marine reserves called weighty evidence that bans work," *Los Angeles Times*, July 22, 2002.
8. "Marine conservation: Net benefits," *The Economist*, Feb. 24, 2001, p. 83.
9. Tom Uhlenbrock, "Farmland ruined in 1993 flood teems with wildlife, plants," *St. Louis Post-Dispatch*, June 1, 1999.
10. Bijal P. Trivedi, "Marine reserves found to boost nearby fishing grounds," *National Geographic Today*, Dec. 4, 2001.

REASON #69

1. Quoted in Gary Polakovic, "Getting the cows to cool it," *Los Angeles Times*, June 7, 2003.
2. "No doubts global warming is real, U.S. experts say," Reuters, Dec. 3, 2003.
3. "Study: Warming to doom many species," AP, Jan. 7, 2004.
4. Kenneth Chang, "As earth warms, the hottest issue is energy," *The New York Times*, Nov. 4, 2003.
5. "Study: Warming to doom many species."
6. "Great Barrier Reef faces major coral destruction," Reuters, Feb. 24, 2004.
7. Christopher C. Williams, "Toting up the potential toll of global warming," *Barrons*, Apr. 19, 2004, p. 13.
8. Mark Townsend and Paul Harris, "Now the Pentagon tells Bush: Climate change will destroy us," *The Observer* (London), Feb. 22, 2004.
9. "No doubts global warming is real, U.S. experts say."
10. Polakovic, "Getting the cows to cool it."
11. "Cow power," Riverdeep Interactive Learning, Ltd., Mar. 25, 2002.
12. "Methane and other gases: Sources of methane," EPA, Nov. 4, 2003.
13. Ibid.
14. Gerard Seenan, "Cowabunga! Cutting cattle flatulence to save the planet," *The Guardian*, Mar. 1, 2003.
15. "Cow burps make for a bad air down under," ENN, July 21, 2000.
16. Polakovic, "Getting the cows to cool it."
17. "Methane and other gases: Scientific background and current research," EPA, Nov. 4, 2003.
18. E-mail correspondence with Ralph Cicerone, Sept. 8, 2004.
19. "Methane and other gases."
20. "The Amazon: The price of success," *The Economist*, Apr. 17, 2004, p. 35.
21. Michael Astor, "Soybeans: The new threat to Brazilian rainforest," AP, Dec. 18, 2003.
22. Larry Rohter, "Relentless foe of the Amazon Jungle: Soybeans," *The New York Times*, Sept. 17, 2003.
23. Jim Lobe, "Hamburger consumption spurs Amazon deforestation," OneWorld.net, Apr. 9, 2004.
24. Keay Davidson, "Huge Amazonian fires may spawn fierce tempests in South America," *San Francisco Chronicle* Feb. 27, 2004.
25. Axel Bugge, "Amazon fires change weather, speed deforestation," Reuters, July 28, 2004.
26. Lobe, "Hamburger consumption spurs Amazon deforestation."
27. "Brazil's government announces measures to slow Amazon deforestation," AP, July 4, 2003.

REASON #70

1. Quoted in Anita Manning, "If you eat a lot of fish, you may run health risk," *USA Today*, Nov. 4, 2002.
2. Nita Bhalla, "Whales reveal man's damaging impact on oceans," Reuters, Dec. 8, 2003.
3. DeNeen L. Brown, "Poisons from afar threaten Arctic mothers, traditions," *Washington Post*, Apr. 11, 2004.
4. Jane Kay, "Alarming find on mercury levels in canned tuna," *San Francisco Chronicle*, June 19, 2003.
"High levels of chemicals in beef, pork: Montreal report," CBC (Canada), Sept. 16, 2002.
Marian Burros, "Farmed salmon is said to contain high PCB levels," *The New York Times*, July 30, 2003.
5. "Fishing warnings up due to mercury pollution—EPA," Reuters, Aug. 24, 2004.
6. "Questions and answers about dioxins," EPA, Jan. 2003.

7. Ibid.
8. Marlene Cimons, "EPA report declares dioxin a cancer-causing agent," *Los Angeles Times*, June 13, 2000.
9. Cindy Skrzycki and Joby Warrick, "EPA links dioxin to cancer; risk estimate raised tenfold," *Washington Post*, May 17, 2000.
10. Laura Hamburg, "Tainted catch in San Francisco Bay: Oakland, San Francisco officials resolving to end dioxin pollution in waters," *San Francisco Chronicle*, Feb. 2, 1999, p. A13.
11. Elizabeth Olson, "U.S. is urged by panel to tell women about dioxins," *The New York Times*, July 2, 2003.
12. Kay Lazar, "Tests show babies get doses of toxins in mom's breast milk," *Boston Herald*, May 20, 2003.
13. Quoted in Skrzycki, "EPA links dioxin to cancer."
14. "Questions and answers about dioxins."
15. Skrzycki, "EPA links dioxin to cancer."
16. "Questions and answers about dioxins."
17. Maggie Fox, "Mercury damage seen in children of fish eaters," Reuters, Feb. 6, 2004.
18. Elizabeth Shogren, "Estimate of fetuses exposed to high mercury doubles," *Los Angeles Times*, Feb. 6, 2004.
19. Devlin Barret, "IQ loss linked to mercury costs $8.7 billion," AP, Feb. 28, 2005.
20. Manning, "If you eat a lot of fish, you may run health risk."
21. Jane Kay, "Eating lots of fish tied to high mercury levels," *San Francisco Chronicle*, Oct. 21, 2004, p. A7.
22. Quoted in Lauran Neergaard, "FDA under fire for planned advice about mercury in fish," AP, Dec. 10, 2003.
23. "Polychlorinated biphenyls (PCBs) update: Impact on fish advisories," fact sheet, EPA, Sept. 1999.
24. Rob Edwards, "Farmed salmon more contaminated than wild," *New Scientist*, Jan. 8, 2004.
25. Gina Kolata, "Farmed salmon have more contaminants than wild ones, study finds," *The New York Times*, Jan. 9, 2004.
26. Michael Grunwald, "Monsanto held liable for PCB dumping," *Washington Post*, Feb. 23, 2002, p. A1.

REASON #71

1. Yvette la Pierre, "Taking stock: Environmental effects of recreational fishing," *National Parks*, May 1, 1993.
2. David S. Pilliod and Charles R. Peterson, "Evaluating effects of fish stocking on amphibian populations in wilderness lakes," USDA Forest Service Proceedings, RMRS-P-15-Vol. 5, 2000.
3. "Travel east, travel west: Same fish put to test," ENN, May 5, 2000.
4. La Pierre, "Taking stock."
5. "Amphibian population decline in the interior West," *RMRScience*, USDA Forest Service, Rocky Mountain Research Station, Feb. 2002.
6. David Perlman, "California biologist solves mystery of disappearing Sierra frogs," *San Francisco Chronicle*, May 13, 2004.
7. Gene Johnson, "Scientists criticize government over salmon rules," AP, Mar. 25, 2004.
8. Jeff Barnard, "ESA salmon listings grow one more with consideration of hatchery fish," AP, May 27, 2004.
9. David Shook, "No time to let anglers off the hook," *Business Week*, Aug. 9, 2001.
10. La Pierre, "Taking stock."
11. Pete Thomas, "Fair game: It's raining trout. Should it?" *Los Angeles Times*, Oct. 14, 2003.
12. Quoted in Marla Cone, "Ecosystem decline tied to whaling," *Los Angeles Times*, Sept. 23, 2003.
13. Cone, "Ecosystem decline tied to whaling."
14. "Collapse of seals, sea lions and sea otters in North Pacific triggered by overfishing of great whales," *Science Daily*, Sept. 24, 2003.
15. Amy Mathews-Amos, report to the Science Advisory Board, NOAA, Jan. 1999.
16. "Aleutian otters take a nosedive," ENN, July 6, 2000.
17. William K. Stevens, "Search for missing otters turns up a few surprises," *The New York Times*, Jan. 5, 1999, p. F1.
18. Cone, "Ecosystem decline."
19. "Alaska sea otters' disappearance a mystery," Reuters, Feb. 4, 2004.

REASON #72

1. Quoted in Steve Mitchell, "Mad cow: Follow the feed," UPI, Dec. 29, 2003.
2. Upton Sinclair, *The Jungle*, New American Library, Signet Classics, New York, 1905, p. 100.
3. Elliot Jaspin, "Meat with scab, pus, and tumors is OK, USDA says," Cox, June 30, 2000.
4. Joshua Lipsky, "Details from British poultry scam show inexperienced vets, massive corruption," The Meating Place Web site, Sept. 9, 2003.
5. "Emerging pathogens and grinding and cooking of comminuted beef," retail meat and poultry processing training material, FSIS/USDA, Mar. 19, 1998.
6. "Crackdown on water in chicken scam," Food Standards Agency (UK), June 19, 2003.
7. "Canada investigating whether human remains in meat from farm of accused serial killer," AP, Mar. 10, 2004.

8. Beatrice Trum Hunter, "Overlooked threats of foodborne illness," *Consumers' Research* magazine, Oct. 1, 1995.
9. "USDA tells poultry industry to disclose water content," Bloomberg, Jan. 5, 2001.
10. "Meat derived by Advanced Meat Recovery (AMR)," fact sheet, American Meat Institute, Feb. 2004.
11. "USDA begins sampling program for Advanced Meat Recovery (AMR) systems," news release, FSIS/USDA, Mar. 3, 2003.
12. Lance Gay, "Potomac watch: Agency to reduce standards for wholesome meat," Scripps Howard, July 17, 2000.
13. James Ridgeway, "Slaughterhouse politics," *The Village Voice*, Dec. 31, 2003.

REASON #73

1. Quoted in Kieran Mulvaney, "Boss hog and the killer algae," ENN, 1996.
2. Tony Bartelme, "The scientists track the 'phantom'," *The Post and Courier* (Charleston, NC), Sept. 1, 1996.
3. E-mail correspondence with JoAnn M. Burkholder, July 12, 2002.
4. William J. Broad, "A spate of red tides menacing coastal seas," *The New York Times*, Aug. 27, 1996, p. C1.
5. Michael Satchell, "The cell from hell," *U.S. News and World Report*, July 28, 1997.
6. " 'The Blob' sighted on East Coast: Toxic alga, a fish killer, may also affect divers," *UnderWater* magazine, Fall 1994.
7. Satchell, "The cell from hell."
8. Ira Flatow, "North Carolina coastal issues: Health of fish populations and the dynamics of the state's sandy shores," *Talk of the Nation Science Friday*, NPR, May 4, 2001.
9. " 'The Blob' sighted on East Coast."
10. Ginny Carroll, "Are our coastal waters turning deadly?" *National Wildlife*, Apr. 14, 1998.
11. "Harmful algal blooms," fact sheet, National Centers for Coastal Ocean Science, Feb. 4, 2003.
12. Heather Dewar and Tom Horton, "Across globe, algae blooms spread disease and death," *Baltimore Sun*, Sept. 27, 2000.

REASON #74

1. Quoted in "Chinese diet heart-healthy, study finds," Reuters, Nov. 10, 1999.
2. Marian Burros, "The pyramid that calls for more olive oil," *The New York Times*, Mar. 29, 1995, p. C4.
3. "Albanian longevity linked to diet," Reuters, Dec. 22, 1997.
4. Rudy Ruitenberg, "A drink a day, fish once a week can cut heart risk, doctors say," Bloomberg, Aug. 30, 1999.
5. Richard Saltus, "The secret of life: Okinawans, the world's longest-lived people, have a lot to teach Americans on the art of reaching age 100," *The Boston Globe*, May 22, 2001, p. A14.
6. Connie Lauerman, "The Okinawa factor," *Chicago Tribune*, June 24, 2001.
7. Norimitsu Onishi, "On U.S. fast food, more Okinawans grow super-sized," *The New York Times*, Mar. 30, 2004.
8. James Conaway, "Soy and green tea for you and me?" www.Onhealth.com, Dec. 9, 1998.
9. "Chinese diet heart-healthy, study finds."
10. "Diet credited for fall in Polish heart deaths," Reuters, Apr. 6, 1998.
11. John Robbins, *Diet for a New America*, Stillpoint Publishing, 1987, p. 152.

REASON #75

1. Quoted in Janelle Carter, "Lift beef ban or face retaliation, says U.S.," AP, May 6, 1999.
2. "Russians hit U.S. poultry standards," AP, Apr. 12, 2002.
3. Dan Chapman, "Georgia poultry farmers wary of free trade," *Atlanta Journal-Constitution*, Dec. 31, 2002.
4. DeNeen L. Brown, "On Saskatchewan farm, a mad cow mystery," *Washington Post*, Aug. 25, 2003, p. A11.
5. Ira Dreyfuss, "Consumers will pay less for meat this year because of mad cow case," AP, Feb. 19, 2004.
6. Raf Casert, "Belgian stores yank steak, eggs," AP, June 4, 1999.
7. Dan Morgan, "Catfish farmers under siege from Vietnam," *Washington Post*, Sept. 16, 2001.
8. Jonathan Friedland, "Eco-threats: Redefining national security," *The Wall Street Journal*, Nov. 25, 1997.
9. Soo-Jeong Lee, "As crab season peaks, so do confrontations between north and south," AP, June 4, 2003.

REASON #76

1. Greg Stohr, "Smithfield loses bid to topple $12 million fine for bay pollution," Bloomberg, Oct. 2, 2000.
2. Peter S. Goodman, "Waste trucked to Maryland thanks to loophole," *Washington Post*, Aug. 2, 1999, p. A11.
3. Ibid.
4. Peter S. Goodman, "An unsavory byproduct: Runoff and pollution," *Washington Post*, Aug. 1, 1999, p. A1.
5. Ibid.
6. Peter S. Goodman, "Permitting a pattern of pollution," *Washington Post*, Aug. 2, 1999, p. A1.
7. "Central Industries pleads guilty to 26 felony violations in Mississippi water pollution case," news release, U.S. Department of Justice, Nov. 2, 2000.

8. Tom Meersman, "Company fined $4 million for polluting; Texas renderer dumped animal waste into river," *Minneapolis Star Tribune*, Dec. 17, 1996, p. 1B.
9. Joe Mozingo, "Rendering aid," *Los Angeles Times*, May 28, 1998.
10. Stohr, "Smithfield loses bid to topple $12 million fine for bay pollution."
11. "The rapsheet on animal factories," Sierra Club, Aug. 2002.
12. Ibid.

REASON #77

1. Brenda Davis and Vesanto Melina, *Becoming Vegan,* Book Publishing Company, Summertown, TN, 2000, p. 54.
2. Melissa Diane Smith, "The fats you need," www.Healthwell.com, Aug. 2, 1999.
3. Michael Greger, "Optimum vegetarian nutrition: Surprising new research on omega-3's and vitamin B12," lecture, www.veganmd.org/talks (viewed June 15, 2004).
4. Neal D. Barnard and Cindy S. Spitzer, "Don't mistake seafood for health food," *Journal-Bulletin* (Providence, RI), May 23, 1998.
5. Davis, *Becoming Vegan,* p. 68.
6. Barnard, "Don't mistake seafood."
7. "Fish oils," PDRhealth/Thomson Healthcare, www.gettingwell.com, no date (viewed June 6, 2004).
8. "FDA says jury still out on benefits of fish oil," Reuters, Nov. 2, 2000.
9. "Now fish too can suffer version of mad cow disease," Asian News International, Feb. 2, 2003.
10. "FDA says jury still out on benefits of fish oil," Reuters, Nov. 2, 2000.
11. Davis, *Becoming Vegan,* p. 67.
12. Karen Pallarito, "Walnuts may protect the heart: They lower cholesterol and improve artery function, study suggests," HealthDay, May 6, 2004.
13. Greger, "Optimum vegetarian nutrition."

REASON #78

1. Matt Claeys, "Castration: Not cutting will cut profits," *Animal Husbandry Newsletter*, Jan.–Feb. 1996.
2. Bernard E. Rollin, *Farm Animal Welfare: Social Bioethical, and Research Issues*, Iowa State University Press, 1995, p. 62.
3. Claeys, "Castration."
4. Joy A. Mench and Paul B. Siegel, "Poultry," Animal Welfare Issues Compendium, South Dakota State U., http://ars.sdstate .edu/animaliss/poultry.html, Jul. 11, 2001.
5. Rollin, *Farm Animal Welfare*, p. 64.
6. Ibid., p. 58.
7. Ibid., p. 94.
8. Ibid., p. 105.
9. Karen Davis, *Prisoned Chickens, Poisoned Eggs*, Book Publishing Company, Summertown, TN, 1996, p. 48.
10. Mench, "Poultry."
11. "Ducks liberated from factory farm reveal bill mutilation," news release, Viva! USA, June 3, 2002.

REASON #79

1. Quoted in Melinda Fulmer, "Tainted meat prompts outcry," *Los Angeles Times*, July 27, 2002.
2. Melody Petersen and Christopher Drew, "New safety rules fail to stop tainted meat," *The New York Times*, Oct. 10, 2003.
3. Jane E. Allen, "Tainted meat not always recovered," *Los Angeles Times*, May 3, 2004.
4. Eric Schlosser, "Bad meat: The scandal of our food safety system," *The Nation*, Sept. 16, 2002, p. 7.
5. "From cradle to gravy," *Consumer Reports*, Mar. 1998, p. 14.
6. Julie Vorman, "USDA calls ConAgra meat recall ineffective," Reuters, Oct. 3, 2003.
7. Ibid.
8. Sankar Vedantam, "Illness prompts recall of beef," *Washington Post*, July 20, 2002, p. A1.
9. Fulmer, "Tainted meat prompts outcry."
10. Daniel Enoch, "U.S. meat testing is deficient, Congressional investigators say," Bloomberg, Sept. 19, 2002.
11. Petersen, "New safety rules fail to stop tainted meat."
12. "Government's ground beef testing program leaves consumers vulnerable to dangerous bacteria: USDA records show systemic breakdown in salmonella testing regimen," news release, Public Citizen, May 23, 2002.
13. "Revolutionizing turkey production: Functional genomics is the driving force," ARS/USDA, Sept. 2004.
14. "Government: Salmonella declining in raw meat," AP, Nov. 24, 2003.
15. Vedantam, "Illness prompts recall of beef."
16. David Migoya, "E. coli-tainted meat mixed with fresh, sold," *Denver Post*, Sept. 3, 2002, p. A1.

REASON #80

1. Quoted in Rochelle Detweiler, "The Buckeye of the storm," *The Animals' Agenda*, Nov.–Dec. 2000, p. 10.
2. Barbara Hagenbaugh, "Heat blamed for seven million chicken deaths," Reuters, July 19, 1998.
3. James D. Martin, "Storm damages poultry houses across the South," *Feedstuffs*, Feb. 7, 2000.

4. "Cowboys rope flood-swept cattle," AP, Oct. 22, 1998.
5. David Whitman, "Hell in high water," *U.S. News and World Report*, Oct. 4, 1999, p. 22.
6. "Rolling blackouts pose threat to California chickens," *Washington Post*, May 13, 2001, p. A9.
7. "Nearly three million young salmon suffocate when fire destroys oxygen-pumping system," AP, May 16, 2003.
8. Kevin Cantera, "Farm plans burial for thousands of swine killed in fire," *Salt Lake Tribune*, Aug. 3, 2001.
9. Kelly Pedro, "Pigs found dead, dying: Seven men have been charged over the grim discovery involving 10,000 animals," *The London Free Press* (Canada), Oct. 15, 2003.

REASON #81

1. Quoted in "New scientific thinking implicates body fat as cancer promoter: Excess fat may act as continuous 'hormone pump' raising risk," news release, AICR, July 11, 2002.
2. "New scientific thinking implicates body fat as cancer promoter."
3. Jacqueline Stenson, "Study suggests Western diet tied to prostate cancer," Reuters, Apr. 28, 2003.
4. Maggie Fox, "Animal fat linked with breast cancer in U.S. study," Reuters, July 16, 2003.
5. "Lifelong vegetarians may have lower risk of breast cancer," Reuters, May 8, 2002.
6. Neal Barnard, *Foods That Fight Pain*, Three Rivers Press, New York, 1998, p. 129.
7. Neal D. Barnard, "Women and cancer: Opportunities for prevention," *PCRM Update*, Sept.–Oct. 1991.
8. "New scientific thinking implicates body fat as cancer promoter."
9. Jane E. Brody, "Huge study of diet indicts fat and meat," *The New York Times*, May 8, 1990, p. A1.
10. Neal D. Barnard and A.R. Hogan, "Cancer commentaries: Got prostate cancer? Maybe milk's to blame," The Cancer Project, www.cancerproject.org/comms/comm06.html, no date (viewed Feb. 13, 2003).
11. "Several sobering facts," *Los Angeles Times*, June 15, 1998.
12. John Carey, "Money floods in to fight a killer," *Business Week*, May 10, 1999, p. 104.
13. "Animal fat may raise prostate cancer risk," Reuters, Mar. 5, 1999.
14. Stenson, "Study suggests Western diet tied to prostate cancer."
15. "Prostate cancer," National Library of Medicine, NIH, Nov. 1, 2002.
16. "Nutrition and prostate cancer: The complete report (The case for nutrition)," fact sheet, Prostate Cancer Foundation, www.prostatecancerfoundation.org, no date (viewed May 31, 2004).
17. Jane E. Brody, ed., *The New York Times Book of Health*, The New York Times Company, 1997, p. 322.
18. Christopher Snowbeck, "Low-fat diet, exercise help fight prostate cancer," Scripps Howard, Apr. 14, 2002.

REASON #82

1. Quoted in "Trout trauma puts anglers on the hook?" news release, The Royal Society (UK), Apr. 30, 2003.
2. Colin Adams, et al., "Briefing paper 2: Fish welfare," Fisheries Society of the British Isles, Granta Information Systems, Oct. 29, 2002.
3. "Trout trauma puts anglers on the hook?"
4. Lynne U. Sneddon, et al., "Do fish have nociceptors: Evidence for the evolution of a vertebrate sensory system," Roslin Institute, Apr. 30, 2003.
5. James Meek, "Fish don't scream," *The Guardian*, July 31, 2001.
6. Quoted in Richard Schwartz, "Do you eat fish?" *Tikkun*, Nov. 1999.
7. Quoted in Barry Kent MacKay, "Fish don't cry," *Animal Issues*, Spring 2002.
8. "Cold as a fish?" *PETA's Animal Times*, May–June 1995, p. 9.
9. Peter Singer, *Animal Liberation*, 2nd ed., New York Review/Random House, 1990, pp. 171–174.
10. Jennifer Smith, "Scientific can of worms: Dueling reports disagree on whether fish are capable of feeling pain on the hook," *Newsday*, July 13, 2003.
11. Maggie Fox, "Fishing just for fun damages stocks, study finds," Reuters, Aug. 30, 2004.
12. James D. Martin, "Cage culture increases fish stress," *Feedstuffs*, Jan. 29, 2001.
13. Patrick Bateson, "The pain league for animals: Decision cube for animal suffering," *New Scientist*, Apr. 25, 1992, p. 30.
14. Singer, *Animal Liberation*.
15. Adams, "Briefing paper 2: Fish welfare."
16. Ibid.
17. "Fish feelings focus of fight," Sentinel Wire Services (Holland), May 17, 2001.

REASON #83

1. Verlyn Klinkenborg, "Pox populi," *The New York Times*, May 6, 2001.
2. Beverly Cheng, "Texas animal health officials fear spread of foot and mouth disease," The Meating Place Web site, Mar. 2, 2001.
3. John J. Goldman, "Bigger risk seen of U.S. foot and mouth outbreak," *Los Angeles Times*, Apr. 18, 2001.
4. "World meat demand to rise along with

animal disease fears," *Render* magazine, Oct. 2002.

5. "Foot and mouth may halt UK agriculture for year," Reuters, Mar. 18, 2001.
6. Anthony Deutsch, "Disease threatens rare breeds of farm animals," AP, Apr. 6, 2001.
7. Fiona Houston, "For British farmers, a disease destroys without touching," *Washington Post*, Mar. 21, 2001, p. C1.
8. "The carcasses pile up," *The Economist*, Mar. 17, 2001, p. 57.
9. "World meat demand to rise along with animal disease fears."
10. Stephen Pincock, "Britain investigates health risk of animal pyres," Reuters Health, Apr. 23, 2001.
11. Juliet Gellatley, "Foot the bill and shut your mouth," *Viva!LIFE*, Viva!, (UK), Summer 2001, p. 25.
12. Joshua Lipsky, "The birth of a crisis: The foot and mouth disease timeline," The Meating Place Web site, Mar. 1, 2001.

REASON #84

1. Quoted in Robin McKie, "New market for old farts? Free trade or protection?" *The Observer* (London), July 25, 1999.
2. Robbin Marks, "Cesspools of shame: How factory farm lagoons and sprayfields threaten environmental and public health," NRDC and the Clean Water Network, July 2002, p. 18.
3. "Action plan: Component I: Atmospheric Emissions," national programs, manure and byproduct utilization, ARS/USDA, www.ars.usda.gov/research/programs.htm, no date (viewed June 15, 2004).
4. Scott A. Sheeder, et al., "Modeling atmospheric nitrogen deposition and transport in the Chesapeake Bay watershed," *Journal of Environmental Quality*, June 29, 2001.
5. *Airsheds and Watersheds III: A Shared Resources Workshop*, Chesapeake Bay Program, EPA Great Waters Program, et al., Nov. 15–16, 2000.
6. Heather Dewar and Tom Horton, "Cycle of growth and devastation," *Baltimore Sun*, Sept. 25, 2000.
7. Heather Dewar and Tom Horton, "Seeds of solution to nitrogen glut," *Baltimore Sun*, Sept. 28, 2000.
8. "Options for managing odor: A report from the Swine Odor Task Force," North Carolina State U., Mar. 1, 1995.
9. Joby Warrick and Pat Stith, "New studies show lagoons are leaking: State's groundwater and rivers affected by waste," *The News & Observer* (Raleigh, NC), Feb. 19, 1995.
10. McKie, "New market for old farts?"
11. "Industrial livestock systems and the environment," chapter 4, Livestock and Environment Toolbox, FAO/UN.
12. Lowry A. Harper and Ron R. Sharpe, "Soil-plant-animal-atmosphere research," USDA, ARS, www.spcru.ars.usda.gov/SPAA.html, no date (viewed May 7, 2002).
13. Dina Cappiello, "Barbecue's fatty fumes add to haze," *Houston Chronicle*, Mar. 17, 2003.
14. Marla Cone, "Smog agency seeks to put lid on restaurant broilers," *Los Angeles Times*, Sept. 2, 1994, p. A1.
15. "AQMD adopts quick-service restaurant control measure," news release, South Coast Air Quality Management District (CA), Nov. 14, 1997.

REASON #85

1. Katie Couric, testimony before the Senate Select Committee on Aging, Mar. 9, 2000.
2. "New tests predict prostate, colon cancer better," Reuters, Apr. 7, 2004.
3. Kate Murphy, "New weapons against a killer," *Business Week*, July 26, 1999, p. 120.
4. "Conditions A–Z: Colorectal cancer," OnHealth Network Company, www.onhealth.com, no date (viewed on Aug. 11, 1998).
5. Alison McCook, "More evidence vegetarian diet may cut cancer risk," Reuters, Feb. 16, 2004.
6. Ibid.
7. Anastasia Toufexis, "Red alert on meat: The link between high-fat diets and colon cancer gets stronger," *Time* magazine, Dec. 24, 1990, p. 70.
8. Gina Kolata, "Animal fat is tied to colon cancer," *The New York Times*, Dec. 13, 1990, p. A1.
9. "White meat linked to colon cancer risk," Reuters, Oct. 16, 1998.
10. Emma Ross, "Study focuses on red meat, cancer," AP, June 23, 2001.
11. Ibid.
12. James J. Kenney, "Fiber, fruits, vegetables, and risk of colon cancer," Food and Health Communications, Continuing Professional Education Courses, Oct. 2003.

REASON #86

1. "Grassley: Independent producers need amendment to limit packer ownership," press release, Charles Grassley, U.S. Senator, Jan. 29, 2002.
2. Brian Halweil, "The bioterror in your burger," Worldwatch Institute, Nov. 6, 2001.
3. "Glickman statement on meat concentration report," FWN Financial News, June 6, 1996.
4. Bruce Ingersoll, "Meatpacking industry target of U.S. probe into competition," *The Wall Street Journal*, June 4, 1997.

5. "USDA panel urges more disclosure of livestock prices," Bloomberg, June 6, 1996.
6. Philip Brasher, "Senate OKs meat-regulation bill," AP, Oct. 24, 2000.
7. Philip Brasher, "USDA lacks staff to investigate meat industry, GAO says," AP, Sept. 22, 2000.
8. "Senators blast packers' livestock ownership," *Omaha World-Herald*, July 19, 2002.

REASON #87

1. Temple Grandin, "Farm animal welfare during handling, transport, and slaughter," *Journal of the American Veterinary Medical Association*, Feb. 1, 1994.
2. "Downed animals," *Farm Sanctuary News*, Farm Sanctuary, Spring 1999, p. 3.
3. Grandin, "Farm animal welfare during handling, transport, and slaughter."
4. Clifford Rothman, "Last frontier of animal rights?" *Los Angeles Times*, July 6, 1995.
5. Donald G. McNeil, Jr., "Doubling tests for mad cow doesn't quiet program critics," *The New York Times*, Feb. 9, 2004.
6. Kevin Diaz, " 'Downer' cattle ban is targeted," *The Sacramento Bee*, Apr. 13, 2004.

REASON #88

1. Denise Grady, "As heart attacks wane, heart failure is on the rise," *The New York Times*, May 4, 1999, p. F1.
2. Gina Kolata, "New studies question value of opening arteries," *The New York Times*, Mar. 21, 2004.
3. Grady, "As heart attacks wane."
4. Ibid.
5. *Heart Disease and Stroke Statistics—2004 Updates*, American Heart Assoc., Dallas, TX, 2003, p. 23.
6. Grady, "As heart attacks wane."
7. " 'Western' diet raises stroke risk—U.S. study," Reuters, July 2, 2004.
8. *Heart Disease and Stroke Statistics*, p. 13.
9. William Bulman, "Life after stroke: A primer for stroke survivors and their families," www.strokecenter.org, Mar. 12, 2001.
10. Ibid.
11. *Heart Disease and Stroke Statistics*, p. 11.
12. "Arterial grafts carried blood equally well, study finds," Reuters, Apr. 21, 2004.
13. Joseph Epstein, "Taking the bypass," *The New Yorker*, Apr. 12, 1999, p. 63.
14. "Improving the heart's blood supply," Mayo Clinic, Nov. 6, 2000.
15. Sandeep Jauhar, "Saving the heart can sometimes mean losing the memory," *The New York Times*, Sept. 19, 2000, pp. F1, F4.
16. Rani Hutter Epstein, "Facing up to depression after a bypass," *The New York Times*, Nov. 27, 2001, p. F8.
17. "Improving the heart's blood supply."

REASON #89

1. Quoted in Elliot Blair Smith, "Stench chokes Nebraska meatpacking towns," *USA Today*, Feb. 14, 2000, p. 1B.
2. "Options for managing odor: A report from the Swine Odor Task Force," North Carolina State U., Mar. 1, 1995.
3. "Health and safety issues in sludge handling," Solids Technology International Limited, Wexford, Ireland, www.solidstechnology.com.
4. "Options for managing odor."
5. "Health and safety issues in sludge handling."
6. Jennifer 8. Lee, "Neighbors of vast hog farms say foul air endangers their health," *The New York Times*, May 11, 2003.
7. Ibid.
8. Perry Beeman, "Livestock air law has no penalties," *The Des Moines Register*, Sept. 15, 2004.
9. Blair Smith, "Stench chokes Nebraska meatpacking towns."
10. "Meatpacker must cut hydrogen sulfide emissions at Nebraska plant; U.S. and IBP sign agreement aimed at public health threat," news release, EPA, May 25, 2000.
11. "Options for managing odor."
12. Tom Spears, "Huge pig farms are health menace, federal report: Manure and urine pollute soil and water, fumes defile the air," *Ottawa Citizen*, Mar. 27, 2002.
13. Gary Polakavic, "Fumes force dairies out to pasture," *Los Angeles Times*, May 6, 2003.
14. Tim Molloy, "Pollution rules targeting manure could force dairies to relocate," AP, June 28, 2004.
15. Erin McCormick, "Too young to die, part II: Toxic Legacy," *San Francisco Chronicle*, Oct. 4, 2004, p. A1.
16. Carol Pogash, "Faced with new air standards, California's earthbound farmers are wary," *The New York Times*, July 1, 2004.
17. "Emissions from cow manure targeted," AP, Sept. 28, 2001.

REASON #90

1. Mindy S. Kursban, "Taking on the 'sacred cow': PCRM challenges the Food Pyramid," *Satya*, May 2000.
2. "Vegetarian diets," position paper, American Dietetic Assoc., 2003.
3. "Proper diets best defense against cancer," *Fresno Bee*, Jul. 10, 1997.
4. "Dietary guidelines," fact sheet, American Heart Assoc., www.americanheart.org, no date (viewed Feb. 22, 2004).
5. "Nutrition and cancer risk," *ACS News Today*, American Cancer Society, Nov. 15, 1999.
6. "Resolve to reduce your risk of cancer,"

ACS News Today, American Cancer Society, Dec. 30, 2003.

7. Conversation with Mindy S. Kursban, PCRM, Feb. 24, 2004.
8. Kursban, "Taking on the 'sacred cow.' "
9. Sally Squires, "USDA loses a battle in war on diet guides," *Washington Post*, Oct. 4, 2000.
10. Neal D. Barnard and A.R. Hogan, "Wanted: Honest dietary guidelines," commentary, PCRM Web site, *circa*, 2000.
11. Marian Burros, "Diet panel mixes politics and chicken fat," *The New York Times*, Jan. 25, 2000, p. F7.
12. Ibid.
13. *Dietary Guidelines for Americans*, USDA, 2000, p. 14.
14. Marian Burros, "U.S. diet guide puts emphasis on weight loss," *The New York Times*, Jan. 13, 2005.

REASON #91

1. "Listeriosis," fact sheet, CDC, Mar. 6, 2001.
2. Dan Murphy, "Special report: The NAMP [North American Meat Processors] expert targets top ten food-safety challenges," The Meating Place Web site, Oct. 9, 2002.
3. Jan Suszkiw, "New tool on tap for fighting listeria," ARS/USDA, May 27, 2003.
4. Jennifer Dixon, "Workers: Sara Lee plant managers knew meat was bad," Knight-Ridder/Tribune, Aug. 29, 2001.
5. Murphy, "Special report."
6. Julie Vorman, "Hot dog plants to fight bacteria with high-tech," Reuters, June 18, 1999.
7. "Listeria monocytogenes: An emerging foodborne pathogen," Animal Health Forum, Government of Alberta, Canada, June 28, 2000.
8. Vorman, "Hot dog plants to fight bacteria with high-tech."
9. Quoted in Ibid.
10. Catherine Strong, "Government tries to contain listeriosis," AP, Feb. 11, 1999.
11. "USDA: Companies must share listeria plans," AP, June 5, 2003.
12. Bud Hazelkorn, "Poultry plant slow to report sharp increase in bacteria," *The New York Times*, Dec. 21, 2002.
13. Barbara Dunaway, "Listeriosis and pregnancy," *Moberly Monitor* (Missouri), Apr. 9, 2003.
14. Emily Gersema, "Meat companies must share tests, plans for preventing listeria, USDA says," AP, June 4, 2003.
15. Melody Petersen and Christopher Drew, "New safety rules fail to stop tainted meat," *The New York Times*, Oct. 10, 2003.

REASON #92

1. Quoted in Fred Pearce, "Southeast Asia's coral reefs at risk from cyanide fishing," *The Boston Globe*, Apr. 29, 2003, p. C1.
2. Dirk Bryant, et al., *Reefs at Risk*, World Resources Institute and the UN Environment Program, et al., 1998, p. 7.
3. Andrew Bridges, "Survey: Coral reefs in bad shape," AP, Aug. 26, 2002.
4. Patricia Reaney, "Study: Traditional fishing damages coral reefs," Reuters, May 4, 2004.
5. Alex Kirby, "Ten richest coral areas pinpointed," BBC News, Feb. 14, 2002.
6. Michael McCarthy, " 'Rainforests of the sea' ravaged: Overfishing and pollution kill 80 percent of coral on Caribbean reefs," *The Independent*, July 18, 2003.
7. "Scientists call for better management of Indonesia's coral reefs," news release, World Resources Institute, May 21, 2002.
8. Bryant, *Reefs at Risk*, p. 9.
9. Ibid., p. 13.
10. Pearce, "Southeast Asia's coral reefs at risk from cyanide fishing."
11. Bridges, "Survey: Coral reefs in bad shape."
12. Bryant, *Reefs at Risk*, p. 8.
13. Ibid., p. 7.

REASON #93

1. Quoted in "Serious holes in seafood safety net," AP, Feb. 13, 2001.
2. Leon Jaroff and Janice M. Horowitz, "Is your fish really foul?" *Time* magazine, June 29, 1992, p. 70.
3. "Worm dangers in sushi," Reuters, July 21, 1998.
4. "Millions in Vietnam at risk of worms from raw fish," Reuters, Nov. 26, 2002.
5. Subhash Chandra Parija, et al., "Trematode infections," www.Emedicine.com, Apr. 10, 2003.
6. Melinda Fulmer, "GAO seeks better shellfish safety rules: Report finds the FDA's lack of staff and regulations is leaving consumers at risk," *Los Angeles Times*, July 20, 2001.
7. H.H. Huss, *Assessment and Management of Seafood Safety and Quality*, FAO Fisheries Technical Paper, #444, FAO/UN, 2003.
8. Hoi Ho, "Vibrio infections," www.Emedicine.com, May 22, 2002.
9. "Vibrio vulnificus," fact sheet, CDC, Mar. 29, 2000.
10. Steve Hymon, "State oyster ban sticks in Gulf Coast craw," *Los Angeles Times*, Aug. 2003.
11. "Paralytic shellfish poisoning: The Alaska problem," *Marine Resources*, Oct. 1996.
12. Bill Egbert and Henri E. Cauvin, "Tuna sinks 29 at lunch," *Daily News* (New York), June 24, 1998, p. 5.
13. W. Steven Otwell, "Scombroid poisoning: An advisory note," flyer, FDA, Center for Food Safety and Applied Nutrition, 1989.

14. Melinda Fulmer, "Study: System for seafood safety inspections flawed," *Los Angeles Times*, Feb. 14, 2001.
15. Caroline Smith DeWaal and Michael F. Jacobson, "Weak links in the food chain: Guess what's coming for dinner?" *San Francisco Chronicle*, Feb. 21, 2003.
16. "Serious holes in seafood safety net."
17. R.W. Apple, Jr., "In the quest for safer seafood, one company follows its nose," *The New York Times*, Nov. 29, 2000, p. F1.
18. Fulmer, "Study: System for seafood safety inspections flawed."
19. Kenneth R. Weiss, "Panel presses new ocean safeguards," *Los Angeles Times*, Apr. 21, 2004.
20. *Federal Oversight of Seafood Does Not Sufficiently Protect Consumers*, Report to the Committee on Agriculture, Nutrition, and Forestry, U.S. Senate, GAO, Jan. 2001, p. 6.

REASON #94

1. "Dairy cows," fact sheet, Farm Sanctuary, www.factoryfarming.com, no date (viewed Feb. 6, 2004).
2. "Development of the special-fed veal industry," www.veal.org, no date (viewed Feb. 6, 2004).
3. "Slaughter report positive," The Meating Place Web site, Aug. 2, 2002.
4. "The welfare of calves in veal production: A summary of the scientific evidence," *Farm Sanctuary News*, Fall 2000.
5. "Veal fact sheet," Humane Society of the United States, www.hsus.org/ace/13973, no date (viewed, Feb. 6, 2004).
6. "Campaigns: HFA's national veal boycott," fact sheet, Humane Farming Assoc., www.hfa.org, no date (viewed, Feb. 5, 2004).
7. "Veal: A cruel meal," fact sheet, PETA, www.goveg.com/active/res-facts4.html, no date (viewed Feb. 6, 2004).
8. "Family veal farming: A portrait from the heart of America," promotional booklet, American Veal Assoc., no date, obtained at the Pennsylvania State Farm Show in Harrisburg in January 1998.
9. "Factory milk and veal production," fact sheet, Farm Sanctuary, www.factory farming.com, no date (viewed Feb. 6, 2004).

REASON #95

1. Quoted in Julie Vorman, "USDA unveils 'Bac' to fight foodborne illness," Reuters, Oct. 24, 1997.
2. Peter Van Sant, "Touchy Subject," *48 Hours*, CBS, Sept. 28, 2000.
3. E-mail correspondence with Charles Gerber, June 4, 2003.
4. Joe Palca, "NPR special report: How safe is the food supply? Foodborne illnesses often start at home," Weekend Edition, NPR, Aug. 18, 2001.
5. Lauran Neergaard, "Videotapes show pigs in the kitchen," AP, June 20, 2000.
6. Greg Hamilton, "For many, food safety put on the back burner," *St. Petersburg Times*, July 9, 2000.
7. Neergaard, "Videotapes show pigs in the kitchen."
8. Hamilton, "For many, food safety put on the back burner."
9. Jane E. Brody, "A recipe for disaster on your kitchen counter," *The New York Times*, Apr. 13, 2004.
10. "Americans' food-handling habits improving," *The Atlanta Journal-Constitution*, Sept. 27, 2002.

REASON #96

1. Keith Beaty, "Soy long, meat: Mock meats are tastier than they used to be and lower in that frightful duo, calories and fat," *Toronto Star*, July 30, 2003.
2. Sora Song, "Going soy crazy: A longtime staple of the Asian diet goes mainstream," *Time* magazine, Aug. 25, 2003.
3. Maggie Fox, "Heart Association recommends soy as a daily food," Reuters, Nov. 14, 2000.
4. Laura Lane, "How good is soy?" CNN, June 26, 2000.
5. "Soy soothes cellular circuits," *Agricultural Research* magazine, ARS/USDA, Feb. 2000.
6. Virginia Messina and Mark Messina, "Soybeans and cancer prevention," *Vegetarian Journal*, May–June 1993. p. 19.
7. Debra Goldschmidt, "The nutty health benefits of soy," CNN, Nov. 20, 2002.
8. Barbara Isaacs, "Soy diet could help lower cholesterol as well as popular drugs," Knight-Ridder/Tribune, July 22, 2003.
9. Marian Burros, "For soy, the time may finally have come," *The New York Times*, Aug. 4, 1999.
10. "Soy may help keep postmenopausal arteries healthy," Reuters, Aug. 21, 2002.
11. Sally Squires, "Eat your soy, boy," *Washington Post*, May 4, 2004, p. HE1.
12. John Robbins, "What about soy?" The Food Revolution Web site, www.foodrevolution.org, no date (viewed Mar. 11, 2004).
13. Rosie Mestel, "In light of troubling study on soy, moderation seen as key," *Los Angeles Times*, Mar. 27, 2000.
14. Kate Murphy, "The dark side of soy," *Business Week*, Dec. 18, 2000, p. 236.

REASON #97

1. "Specialization shifting production into efficient but fewer operations," *Feedstuffs*, Mar. 6, 2000.
2. Dan Fesperman and Kate Shatzkin, "The

plucking of the American chicken farmer," *Baltimore Sun*, Feb. 28, 1999.
3. Ibid.
4. Kate Shatzkin and Dan Fesperman, "Unprotected and alone," *Baltimore Sun*, Mar. 2, 1999.
5. Dan Fesperman and Kate Shatzkin, "Taking a stand, losing the farm," *Baltimore Sun*, Mar. 1, 1999.

REASON #98

1. Ted Williams, "The exhausted sea," *Audubon*, Sept. 2003.
2. William J. Broad and Andrew C. Revkin, "Overfishing imposes a heavy toll," *The New York Times*, p. F2.
3. Beth Daley, "With fish piracy on rise, agents cast worldwide net," *The Boston Globe*, May 18, 2003.
4. Jim Doyle, "Rough waters," *San Francisco Chronicle*, Apr. 19, 2002.
5. Mitchell Anderson, "The cod's gone, yet the deadly dragger boats remain," *The Globe and Mail* (Canada), Apr. 30, 2003, p. A17.
6. Williams, "The exhausted sea."
7. Anderson, "The cod's gone, yet the deadly dragger boats remain."
8. Raf Casert, "EU fisheries ministers call reform package a breakthrough for stock protection," AP, Dec. 19, 2003.
9. Jonathan Amos, "Fish 'massacre' in North Atlantic," BBC News, Feb. 16, 2002.
10. "Mixed reaction to cod plan," BBC News, Nov. 11, 2002.
11. "Global cod stocks may be gone by 2020," *The Boston Globe*, May 13, 2004.
12. Doyle, "Rough waters."
13. Hal Bernton, "Northwest rockfish face chancy future," *Seattle Times*, July 31, 2000.
14. Glen Martin, "U.S. likely to impose bottom-fishing ban on West Coast rockfish stocks," *San Francisco Chronicle*, June 3, 2002.
15. Bernton, "Northwest rockfish face chancy future."
16. Doyle, "Rough waters."
17. Bernton, "Northwest rockfish face chancy future."
18. Tomas Alex Tizon, "Buy the fleet to save fishery," *Los Angeles Times*, Nov. 14, 2003.
19. Pietro Parravano and Lee Crockett, "Who should own the oceans?" *San Francisco Chronicle*, Sept. 25, 2000.
20. Felicity Barringer, "Federal oceans commission finds decline along coasts," *The New York Times*, Apr. 21, 2004.
21. Ibid.

REASON #99

1. Quoted in Patricia Leigh Brown, "Foie gras fracas: Haute cuisine meets the duck liberators," *The New York Times*, Sept. 24, 2003.
2. "Get informed," fact sheet, AnimalWatch, 2002.
3. Michelle Locke, "Activists want to shut gourmet food company," AP, Dec. 17, 2003.
4. Brown, "Foie gras fracas."
5. "Foie gras: Liver disease as 'gourmet' treat," *Farm Sanctuary News*, Spring 2000.
6. Brown, "Foie gras fracas."
7. Peter Finn, "To Hungarian professor, what's good for the goose is good for the goose liver industry," *Washington Post*, Jan. 31, 2000, p. A13.
8. "Forced feeding: The facts behind foie gras production," fact sheet, World Society for the Protection of Animals, http://ww2.wspa-international.org, no date (viewed Feb. 5, 2004).
9. "Get informed."
10. Brown, "Foie gras fracas."
11. Clay Chandler, "A golden goose in Red China? Entrepreneur bets millions that foie gras will fatten export figures," *Washington Post*, Aug. 1, 2000, p. E1.
12. Nick Ravo, "A cornucopia of native foie gras," *The New York Times*, Sept. 24, 1998.
13. Brown, "Foie gras fracas."
14. "John Gielgud reveals the grief behind foie gras," online movie, PETA TV, www.petatv.com/veg.html, no date (viewed Feb. 5, 2004).
15. Brown, "Foie gras fracas."
16. "The grief behind foie gras," fact sheet, PETA, www.goveg.com, no date (viewed Feb. 3, 2004).
17. Ibid.

REASON #100

1. Michael Greger, "Optimum vegetarian nutrition: Surprising new research on omega-3's and vitamin B12," lecture, www.veganmd.org/talks (viewed June 15, 2004).
2. C. Claiborne Ray, "Vegetarians' life span," *The New York Times*, Aug. 3, 2004. "Eating less meat boosts longevity, says German report," Reuters, Mar. 10, 2003.
3. E-mail correspondence with Michael Greger, Sept. 13, 2004.

REASON #101

1. Henry Spira, "Let's start eating right," letters, *The New York Times*, Feb. 21, 1995.
2. Jeff Barnard, "Scientists: Saving salmon must address population, human nature," AP, June 12, 2003.
3. Glen Martin, "Group's surprising beef with meat industry," *San Francisco Chronicle*, Apr. 27, 1999.
4. "DNS helps develop out-of-this-world

food," *Nutrition Newsletter*, Cornell U., Spring 1998.

5. "Reap what you sow," *New Scientist*, Apr. 21, 2001, p. 11.
6. David Tilman, et al., "Forecasting agriculturally driven global environmental change, *Science*, p. 283.
7. David Tilman, "Global environmental impacts of agricultural expansion: The need for sustainable and efficient practices," paper presented at the National Academy of Sciences colloquium: "Plants and Population: Is There Time?" Irvine, CA, Dec. 5, 1998.
8. "A forecast for 2050: Scarcities will force a leaner U.S. diet," *The New York Times*, Feb. 18, 1995.
9. Ibid.

Index

Of Related Interest from Lantern Books

The Vegan Diet as Chronic Disease Prevention
Evidence Supporting the New Four Food Groups
Kerrie K. Saunders, PhD, MS, LLP

"*The Vegan Diet as Chronic Disease Prevention* is a compelling and concise argument for the overwhelming benefits to the human being of a pure vegetarian diet. Doctors and scientists should know these facts, and every person should live by these principles."—**John McDougall, MD**, Director, McDougall Residential Program; Author, *McDougall Program books*

The Lantern Vegan Family Cookbook
Brian P. McCarthy

Chef McCarthy has created over 400 simple vegan recipes with easy-to-find ingredients for traditional favorites like biscuits, corn bread, stews, pastas, pizzas, cakes, pies, and even eggnog. All the recipes come from the McCarthy home kitchen and have passed the test of many family meals. For individuals or families who are concerned about animals, the environment, or their health, mealtimes just got a whole lot easier.

Senior Fitness
The Diet and Exercise Program for Maximum Health and Longevity
Ruth E. Heidrich, PhD

"Ruth Heidrich has compiled a comprehensive, easy-to-read guide to maintaining and even improving your health and fitness levels using simple, logical principles that your doctor might have neglected to tell you about."—**Neal Barnard, MD**, author, *Eat Right, Live Longer* and *Foods That Fight Pain*

A Primer on Animal Rights
Leading Experts Write about Animal Cruelty and Exploitation
Edited by Kim W. Stallwood, Foreword by Jeremy Rifkin

This book is a collection of articles that document how animals are cruelly mistreated and commercially exploited for profit. Contributors include: Jim Mason, Marc Bekoff, Mike Markarian, Betsy Swart, Norm Phelps, Wayne Pacelle, Pat Derby, Gene Bauston, Karen Davis, Richard Schwartz, and many others.

Move the Message
Your Guide to Making a Difference and Changing the World
Josephine Bellaccomo

Consultant and activist Josephine Bellaccomo delivers a step-by-step process, complete with tips, tactics, strategies, examples and exercises, to ensure that your message is focused, powerful and unstoppable. Whether the difference you want is local or global, this guide is essential for activists and concerned individuals working to create lasting change.